Living Beyond Breast Cancer

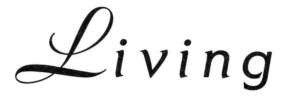

Living

Beyond Breast Cancer

*A Survivor's Guide for When
Treatment Ends and the Rest of
Your Life Begins*

MARISA C. WEISS, M.D.,

AND

ELLEN WEISS

TIMES 𝕋 BOOKS

RANDOM HOUSE

This book cannot and must not replace hands-on medical care or the specific advice of your doctor. Use it instead to help you ask the right questions, make the right choices, and work more closely with your doctor and other members of your health-care team.

LIVING BEYOND BREAST CANCER is a service mark of Living Beyond Breast Cancer (LBBC), a Pennsylvania nonprofit corporation located at 111 Forrest Avenue, Narberth, Pennsylvania 19072, which provides educational and support services for women affected by breast cancer. Telephone: 610-668-1320. Fax: 610-667-4789.
Internet: dvbiznet.com/lbbc
Limited use of the service mark has been granted to Dr. Weiss, president and founder of LBBC, in connection with the publication of this book. All responsibility for the contents of the book *Living Beyond Breast Cancer* belongs to Marisa Weiss and Ellen Weiss—not any other individual or organization.

Library of Congress Cataloging-in-Publication Data
Weiss, Marisa C.
Living beyond breast cancer / Marisa C. Weiss and Ellen Weiss.
p. cm.
Includes index.
ISBN 0-8129-2689-7 (alk. paper)
1. Breast—Cancer—Popular works. 2. Breast—Cancer—
Psychological aspects. 3. Adjustment (Psychology) I. Title.
RC280.B8W396   1997
616.99'449—dc21   97-1165

Printed in the United States of America on acid-free paper
98765432
First Edition
Book design by Susan Hood

To Edith, Rosie, Kitty, and Ellen

Acknowledgments

So many voices are heard in this book: the women who shared their stories with us, the patients and their families Marisa has had the privilege of taking care of, and those we met at the many Living Beyond Breast Cancer$_{SM}$ conferences. Each one contributed in her own personal style—eagerly or reluctantly, expansively or cautiously—but each one with honesty and courage and verve. The book would have fallen flat without the voices of these many friends, moved by their desire to help others. Privacy and discretion were essential, so all names were changed, but the quotes are true and speak from the heart. We are so grateful to each person who became part of this book.

We want to acknowledge the extraordinary volunteers, staff, and board members of the Living Beyond Breast Cancer$_{SM}$ organization who have labored with diligence, dedication, and unflagging spirit. It's impossible to thank them enough. And many thanks to the Cancer Center Staff at Paoli Memorial Hospital—a great team.

We also had help from a generous and willing group of professionals, and we want to thank them: Jayne Antonowsky, Michelle Battistini, Keith Block, Dan Brookoff, Irene Card, Constance Carino, Mary Daly, Milly Fink, Barbara Fowble, Adele Friedman, William Grizos, Barbara Hoffman, Cynthia Kling, Anton Kris, Julie Miller, Linda Miller, Martha Morse, Lois Eisner Murphy, Sue Murray, Greg Ochsner, Marlana Ottinger, Bill Reiss, Lewis Rowland, Abby Ruder, David Sachs, Jean Sachs, Romayne Sachs, Alan Saltiel, Marie Savard, Leslie Schover, Gloria Shattil, Walter Troll, Alice Weiss, Eve Weiss, Leon Weiss, Philip Weiss, Sara Manny Weiss, Stephen Weiss, Lisa

Weissmann, Wendy Wolf, Anna K. Wolff, Maureen Yelovich, and Richard Yelovich.

Kris Dahl helped us get started and made the connection to our editor, Betsy Rapoport, who is the best. Betsy watched the book grow, and grow, and grow—in shock but never in dismay, and always upbeat, encouraging, and insightful. Special thanks to "class mother" Nancy Inglis, for always being there with warm words of support and advice at the other end of a line. We are grateful to Marjorie Wexler for her thoughtful, intelligent reading, and to the people at dix! for their sharp-eyed patience. We are in John Rambow's debt for his care and attention to so many details.

Always there for support, advice, comfort, care, and feeding, our families patiently endured our neglect and absence as we worked away at this book. Thank you, Elias, Henry, Isabel, David, and Leon—you who waited with such good grace till all this book business was finished and still remembered who we were.

And we want to thank each other: for patience and good humor, for holding back and holding on, for drive, energy, and the right word. Close as we are, as mother and daughter, we have a new appreciation for each other's depths and gifts.

Marisa Weiss and Ellen Weiss

Contents

Introduction

Living Beyond Breast Cancer

Over 2 million women in the United States are living with breast cancer. One in eight women is at risk. Each year, over 200,000 cases are diagnosed.* If you've had breast cancer, you probably know these numbers by heart. With the progress we are seeing in early detection and the increasingly effective treatment of breast cancer, more women are surviving longer. More and more women are now living beyond breast cancer.

I am a physician specializing in breast cancer treatment, and I have the privilege of taking care of some of the women who make up these numbers. It wasn't long after I started treating women with breast cancer, over ten years ago, that I realized patients who had finished treatment continued to feel distressed. Instead of feeling thrilled to have the breast cancer experience behind them, they were uneasy, sometimes anxious. What do I do now? Am I really cured? Is it safe for me to get pregnant? Can I take hormones? Will my daughter get breast cancer? What should I tell the man I've just met? Will my cancer diagnosis affect my ability to get health insurance? My patients desperately wanted an intelligent, in-depth response to their questions as they moved from "I have breast cancer" back to "I am leading a normal life."

I found myself saying over and over, "We don't have good answers to your questions." I'm a hands-on, can-do person, and it was enormously frustrating to me to leave my patients dissatisfied and fum-

---

* Including 185,000 cases of invasive breast cancer, and 30,000 cases of noninvasive (intraductal) breast cancer.

bling about for answers to these vital questions. I felt I had to do something to tackle this astonishing void of information.

The whole point of early detection and effective treatment of breast cancer is to provide long life, and good quality of life, after treatment is over. Support and education are crucial parts of your care; you need them to nurture and sustain your physical, emotional, and financial health. I decided the most effective way to help my patients was to create educational conferences designed for their needs—not unlike the kinds of conferences physicians organize to keep up to date and informed—with seminars featuring expert speakers, panel discussions, and small group workshops where women could ask the experts the questions on their minds, and where we could hope for answers from those at the cutting edge of new work. So, in 1992, the organization Living Beyond Breast Cancer_{SM} was born in the spare room on the third floor of my busy and overcrowded home.

To date, we've had over a dozen conferences in the Philadelphia area, with attendance close to 1500 women for a single program. We've recruited internationally recognized experts (including Drs. Leslie Schover, Wendy Schain, Keith Block, David Spiegel, and David Eisenberg) as speakers. Twenty-seven medical institutions in the Philadelphia–Delaware Valley have been full participants. Twenty-five thousand survivors are individually invited to each of our programs and our educational newsletters reach over 9,000 members four times a year. We recently started a survivors' telephone helpline to provide information, support, and referrals. And we're on the Internet (http://www.dvbiznet.com/lbbc). No other single organization in the world has enlisted such full support of these diverse medical institutions nor reached out to as many women and families with education on living beyond breast cancer. With our two large-scale yearly conferences, multiple community-based workshops, and educational newsletters, we are in contact with our members perhaps more often than they are in contact with their own physicians. "I arrange my life around these conferences. I am always informed and never patronized."

Today we have a full staff, a proper office in a small commercial building just a few blocks from my home, major individual grant and corporate support, and many small regional conferences as well as our big ones. The Living Beyond Breast Cancer_{SM} organization has become an extension of my family.

My immediate family includes my three children: Elias, who is nine years old, and seven-year-old twins, Henry and Isabel. They love cooking with me, putting together the wacky birthday parties we have in our home, and fooling around with each other and their pets (we have three dogs: small, medium, and large). I've promised them we'll write a book together now that Grandma—my coauthor—and I have finished ours. My husband is a pediatrician in research, and while I zip around doing my thing, he quietly goes his way, stepping in to make dinner or scooping the kids off to ice-skating or fishing. (I am not great at organized—or unorganized—sports, and I grit my teeth when I'm forced to exercise.) The best of times, though, are the family get-togethers, where the kids match up with their treasured cousins and there's a regular free-for-all of activity and talk—we are all big-time talkers.

I think it's this love of family and the people in it that carries over to the work I do. Our family has been seriously affected by breast cancer, although my mother and I have not had breast cancer ourselves. I think and care a great deal about my patients and the thousands of women who are members of Living Beyond Breast Cancer$_{SM}$, and I try to provide as much support, up-to-date and timely information, and advice as I can, so they feel informed and empowered to make the best decisions for themselves.

Doctors and patients today work as partners. No book, including this one, can ever replace the services of your physicians and support staff, but I hope that reading this book will help to strengthen that partnership. My patients know what they want and I must listen to what my patients are telling me before I start telling them what their options are.

Listening to my patients and thinking about the profound effect breast cancer has had on their lives, and wanting to make a positive difference in their lives, has led to this book. The topics we've covered at the Living Beyond Breast Cancer$_{SM}$ conferences inspired the subject matter.

Although the book occasionally speaks to women who are at the point of initial diagnosis, the purpose of this book is not to deal with your initial treatment decisions. It is designed to help you *after* you have established your treatment, to help you focus on the issues that you may face as you go through treatment and beyond. When treatment is over, you may no longer be doing anything active to fight the cancer, and everyone thinks you're back to normal, you may be unprepared for, and overwhelmed by, a sense of bewilderment, loss, and separation anxiety. This book will help you manage your ongoing relationships with your doctors, nurses, and other health care professionals, empowering you to work to your best interest with your health care team. And it will show you how to find support beyond your immediate physical needs.

What kinds of tests do you need to monitor your health and the risk of recurrence? What information will help you make treatment decisions for reconstruction, tamoxifen, pain, or complementary medicine? I have included a description of the tests and breast self-examination technique that help you and your doctors evaluate the presence or absence of cancer—how you examine yourself after getting breast cancer is very different from how you conducted breast self-examination before.

I'll also offer an explanation for the lingering side effects of treatment, such as hair loss, breast and arm edema, and fatigue. For those who want to know how the body fights breast cancer, and why some women are more vulnerable to breast cancer than others, there are chapters on the immune system and the breast cancer genes. You may also need advice to get back to living a normal life, managing your love life, and having a child.

I've included a chapter on how to grow older and navigate through troubling menopausal symptoms, particularly when they come on abruptly and prematurely with chemotherapy, and how to cope with sudden termination of hormone replacement therapy upon diagnosis. A normal life includes dealing with job and health care issues, and wills, so there are chapters to help you plow through those parts of your life.

Most of you want to know what *you* can do to become as healthy as possible for as long as possible; how you improve your nutrition, control your weight, and add exercise to your agenda. I've tried to address all of these issues.

The big fear for all women who have had breast cancer is recurrence, and there are five chapters devoted to this: whether you can live cancer free; when cancer recurs, how to manage local and regional recurrence, metastatic disease, and pain management.

Some women do not outlive cancer. Chapters on endings and hospice are meant to help with quality of life, quality of death, and the overwhelming physical, emotional, spiritual, and financial issues that attend the close of life.

Last, and into the future, are hopes for cure and prevention, and what each of you can do to reach out to others and to help put an end to breast cancer altogether.

You can pick this book up and put it down many times over the years after your diagnosis and treatment as issues evolve for you— from surmounting infertility to battling hot flashes to cooking a healthful meal to figuring where the next "cure" may come from. I hope that the information and suggestions I provide in this book are respectful of your concerns and address the issues in your life with honest and reasonable answers, although in some cases, the "right" answer may not yet be available.

As a breast cancer survivor, you want so much to live well and long; you've been given what many call a "second chance." This book is geared to that second chance, to making every day of the rest of your life *better*—whether by helping you manage your general medical concerns, by encouraging you to adopt life-enhancing eating and exercising habits, or by getting you and yours to appreciate your special virtues and celebrate the life you share together.

This book has been a joint effort with my mother, Ellen Weiss. It represents the combined energy of two generations of women working together toward a mutual productive goal, in a loving (if sometimes embattled) effort to find the right word or the right direction for what we're laboring to present to you.

Living Beyond Breast Cancer$_{SM}$ is a nonprofit organization, and now it is a book, too, for women of many generations to come together for support, warmth, camaraderie, and clear information that will enrich and direct you to what we all hope will be a long, happy, healthy, and fulfilling life.

ONE

Treatment Over, On with Your Life

1

Over, Not Over

Normal is never what it used to be. You've got to face it, accept it, and work it through. You can't go back. The only thing is to go forward, one step at a time. It's time to move on, time to get on with the rest of your life. What choice do you have?

It's over. Treatment, that is. You've survived the initial ordeal. Now what? Maybe it's been two weeks, maybe two years, maybe twenty. Breast cancer is never completely over. "I never forget. Cancer has become part of my consciousness, part of my society. With every cancer death, my heart turns over. I'm always amazed at how other people take their lives for granted, as if they'll live forever."

Breast cancer represents a fear common to all women. Clearly, the women in my practice who have a personal or family history of breast cancer worry a lot more about its dangers, and have more to fear than women who have not. But whomever breast cancer haunts needs empathy and support.

Treatment may have been a full-time occupation for you—bills, taxes, job, vacation, housework, even children, were put on hold. All the chores and work and pleasures that waited till you had strength, interest, and enough time to get back to them combine now with the fears, stress, and accumulated fatigue that so frequently build up during treatment. You may actually be feeling worse than ever, worn down and worn out, and full to bursting. "I took my husband to an auction, my first post-treatment outing, and he went—something he wouldn't normally do, but he was still treating me extra nice. I bought a few things, and he asked me, 'What are you going to do with this junk?' I exploded: 'You should be down on your knees thanking God that I'm interested in *something* again!' " Thirteen years after this episode Dina still spoke of it with heat and intensity.

Limbo: Life Beyond Treatment

Many women find themselves escorted through treatment with love and support from sources and in ways they could hardly have imagined. Newfound neighbors, friends, children's friends' parents, co-workers, church members, family, and partners offer themselves. "My neighbors got together and delivered dinner every weekday for months!" "My twelve-year-old would run in from school each day and ask, 'What can I get you?' Then half an hour later she'd be back: 'Can I get you anything else?' " "I hadn't seen my sister for years, but she showed up at the hospital with a bunch of dirty magazines to make me laugh, and then she went back to my house and filled up my freezer with home-cooked meals." "My husband took off every morning to bring me in for radiation, waited with me, and got me settled back at home before he went off to work. He was with me each step of the way; he stayed with me while I cried, screamed, took my anger and frustration out on him. He showed me what a true soul mate is."

The support you get from family and friends can vary tremendously. Some of you may have very little in the way of support or comfort. (See the next chapter on support groups.)

After months or more of concentrated attention on you, your illness, and your therapy, you come to that moment when the days mapped out for you by hour and procedure come to an end. You are dismissed. " 'Come back in three months,' the doctor said. I felt like I was *dumped,* and I was so frightened," Janet recalled. Your health care team provided support you may not have fully appreciated when so many things were happening to you at once. It may not be till the whirlwind of your treatment experience subsides that the reality of the breast cancer diagnosis really sinks in. "I felt more scared after treatment was over than I did before it started," said Gena. "During treatment I had peace." The scheduled routine and plan of attack were very comforting, and now they're gone.

Your family and friends generally conclude the disease is beaten and done with, congratulate you, and celebrate with appropriate enthusiasm. "I dreaded going to my own end-of-treatment party." You're expected to feel great and back to normal and ready to get on with your life, but instead you feel lost, kind of nowhere, with the veiled fear that the cancer might grow back because you are not doing anything active to keep it away. Then you may worry whether the treatment really worked, whether you're fit to be discharged. Separation anxiety takes on new meaning.

A string of troubling questions dog you: What do I do now?

Shouldn't I be doing *something?* Where's my support? Where's my lifeline? Can I really get along without my doctors and nurses? When do I get to see my doctor again? Now that I don't see my doctors every day or every week, how do I get all my questions answered? *Can I walk the walk on my own again?*

Coping with the New "Normal"

You can, you must, cope with this new, "normal" life. Countless women have done it, are doing it. But you may feel as wobbly inside as a new toddler, especially because few seem to appreciate this vulnerable, exhausted you that may be hidden by a cheerful front.

"I didn't know what to do with myself," Christy recalled of this limbo period. Annamarie's coping mechanism was ceaseless activity: "I got depressed not doing anything more. Cancer was still on my mind, twenty-four hours a day. I started looking for things I could do, things I still had to decide about, like diet, exercise, tamoxifen, anything I could possibly do to avoid recurrence. I kept very busy."

"Right after treatment I felt very *old,* and lost, like I was looking into my grave. I got help, and it took a while, but I came around to feeling reborn, reinvented," said Clara, bringing an almost religious fervor to her recollections. Other survivors speak of that newness, of a transformation of attitude and self. "I became assertive, someone I'd never been. I had a new voice. I said whatever I felt, like a cranky old lady. I knew nobody would stop me."

Cancer Worry

Even if you've been discharged by your doctors, you still keep a corner of your head reserved for Cancer Worry. "Every time something hurts or I get sick, I think it's come back. Automobile accidents are better: you *almost* lose your life, and then it's over and in the past."

As years pass, Cancer Worry will ebb, but it will always stand ready to expand again with any new unidentifiable pain or symptom, and to shrink back again when that sign turns out to be benign. It's something you learn to live with. "Like a whale that moves into your living room" is how one wry patient described her lingering fears of breast cancer. "Over time, the whale gets smaller, but it never quite goes away. A tenant you can't get rid of. Maybe it's down to the size of a magazine rack and once in a while you bump into it, and sometimes it swells up into your face again, like when you have a mammogram and they call you back for extra views."

Most of the women I take care of who have had a breast cancer diagnosis bear Cancer Worry as a conscious burden. They carry it with them indefinitely, like a badge that marks them and separates them somehow, even as year after year after year proves them disease free. The burden gradually gets processed.

A few women, however, close the door and say it's over and done with. That may be the only way for them to deal with what's happened. Five, ten, or more years may pass without processing that cancer experience: pushed off and away, important issues remain unresolved, fear and anxiety remain buried deep. Some women go on to other things without any difficulty, living their lives free of trying resolution, succumbing at last to some other ailment or simple old age. Denial is not an issue. Others go their way till they get brought up short by a suspicious mammogram, a bout of arm edema, the onset of natural menopause, a daughter who has reached her mother's age at diagnosis, or worst of all, recurrence or a new cancer—issues that drag back the cancer history. Buried emotions erupt, and what wasn't resolved before now clamors for closure.

Of one thing you're sure: You don't want friends unburdening sad tales to you. Annamarie would stop people mid-breath: "I only listen to stories with happy endings." It's hard to understand how reasonable people can be so thoughtless with misplaced reassurance. Maybe they think they must say something, but they don't quite know what or how. Or maybe they're expressing their own fears. Whatever the reason, these stories about sickness and death that others may want to unload can wound. Stop them the moment you sense what's coming. Use Annamarie's "happy endings" line. There are plenty of stories with good outcomes for you to hear.

The uncertainty that has entered your life, of what has happened and is happening to you, can be overwhelming and exhausting. "Not knowing what will be is worse than knowing the worst. It was a living hell." I'm convinced that the hardest thing to deal with is this uncertainty—it can consume all your energy. You are busy doing little or nothing other than finishing up treatment and getting better. Even high-energy women are laid low. "I gave up on my superwoman image. It was costing too much and it was beyond my available resources." Lily was satisfied to lead an uneventful life for a while. Some of these formerly high-powered women feel discouraged, useless, and unable to accomplish anything important. "It takes all day to do one thing!"

So there you are, projects waiting, not knowing where to start, still exhausted, but now finished. And there's your family, waiting for you to take over again, looking for the attention they've been wanting and missing for some time. They, too, may be exhausted by all you and they have been through, relieved that you're done, unable (unwilling, even) to give any more, and looking to you for reassurance, draining your meager strength. Christy recalled, "I had to act like I could just flip a switch and not be a cancer patient—as if it were possible!"

Is it any wonder that many women become depressed at this point? You are most vulnerable to depression at the time of diagnosis and again when your treatment is completed, and you can see why. "I thought I was dealing with everything just fine, but I wasn't. I couldn't. Everything fell in on me. I became clinically depressed shortly after the end of my chemotherapy."

It's a normal phenomenon to find yourself angry, sad, and depressed in this period of transition. Usually your mood improves in a month or two, but if it doesn't, you should seek help. Time by itself may not solve things; don't neglect troubling symptoms. *Take care of yourself.*

Finding Your New Support Network

You can't expect family members to meet all of your needs at this point, especially those problems that require specialized attention. For Donna's husband, the issue was simple. "I don't want to hear about your illness anymore. Put it away. It's done." "If there are no support receptors in your family, you may not be able to put them there," commented Molly. Support can be as much a part of your medicine as anything else; unfortunately, you may need it most when you find it dwindling.

This may be the time for you to connect with a support group. Here are people who know what you have been through and how you are feeling at this moment. You don't need to explain—they understand. If nothing else, it's a safe haven, with people who have a strong shared concern. Florrie explained: "I decided to go someplace where others knew it wasn't over, where I could tell this complete stranger about my history and feelings, knowing what we share." This can be another level of friendship for you.

Word of mouth will lead you to some groups, but your most likely resource for a reference is your treatment center or a local breast cancer organization. Some women organize support groups on their own, when nothing else seems available. It's especially difficult for women in small towns, where other women in a similar situation are few and far between. (See Chapter 2.)

Support groups don't work for everyone. "I couldn't sit there and listen to all those painful histories. I had enough to do just taking care of myself; I can't deal with other women's complaints, as justified as they may be. I felt I was doing better than they were, and they were dragging me down."

There are women, on the other hand, who are having an especially hard time and who may appreciate, and need, the company of other women fighting similar battles.

For many women, the Living Beyond Breast Cancer_{SM} conferences, where over a thousand survivors gather in one place for information and support, are a powerful source of strength. "It's incredible, that combined power," Vivian declared. "I've been to every one. I'll go anywhere to be part of that experience."

One-on-one support with a mental health professional, a member of the clergy, or another supportive person, may be the right choice for you. Please regard your emotional and psychological needs as deserving treatment and attention as much as your physical needs. Take care of the whole you.

Telling

Another problem you may be struggling with is the question of whom to tell about your cancer. Years ago people did not talk about cancer, period—as though it were a shameful disease. Another reason it was kept private was that often the patient herself was not told she had cancer, especially if it appeared to be fatal and the family thought the information would alarm or overwhelm her. Now, most doctors tell their patients the whole story, leaving it to the patient to tell everybody else. For an occasional patient, this may be too burdensome.

Judging how much to tell, when to tell, and how much to tell at one time, needs to be carefully assessed for each individual you tell: partner, child, mother, boss, or neighbor. You must take into account human weakness and vulnerability. The news might be more than some can bear; others will respond to the information with strength, comfort, and support. There are people you want to tell, and there are others you feel don't need any explanation whatever.

"Telling my mother was the hardest thing I had to do: 'Oh, and by the way, I'm going in for a mastectomy next Thursday.' After I got past telling my mom, breast cancer was just another 'ordinary' detail of my life I'd mention whenever it fit into a conversation."

Paula described how her daughter revealed the news of her double mastectomy: "I had no idea she was in any kind of difficulty. She was trying to protect me because I was still mourning the death of her sister from colon cancer. We talked as usual on the phone, and then I went to join her and all the family on our annual holiday. She picked me up at the train, brought me home to the gang, and there in the bosom of the family casually remarked, 'By the way, I had a double mastectomy six weeks ago.' I looked around, everyone was relaxed and unworried, as was my daughter, so I figured if they could absorb it that well, so could I. That was fifteen years ago. I'm now ninety-one, and she's sixty-seven. I won't be around, but I think she'll make it for another twenty."

Any woman who has had to tell a young daughter old enough to understand, about her breast cancer diagnosis, knows telling *her* was the hardest of all. "I felt I was passing on a death sentence to my daughter, but I knew I had to tell her about it, that whatever she would imagine about what was happening to me would be worse than the truth."

Telling others about your breast cancer can be hard, or easy. Sometimes it just happens. "I didn't want to talk about it, and then this woman I'd just met at a party mentioned her work with breast cancer survivors, and I found myself telling her things I'd never told anyone, years and years after I'd been through with it. Maybe I was just waiting for the right moment, or the right person." Molly was a well-balanced, self-assured woman who surprised herself with the release of this flood of suppressed feelings.

Some of the women I've worked with are so self-conscious about their illness, they feel almost as though they're wearing a sign and they need to explain: "I stood there in the supermarket, telling this sympathetic checkout clerk my entire history!" Others, however, mull over whether or not to share this painful experience with their closest friends. And how do you tell a new boyfriend or lover? (See Chapter 12.)

Sylvie told everyone she had breast cancer. "I felt it was part of my responsibility to others, to tell. I don't think it's good for anybody to be quiet about this disease. Not if we want to find a cure, find the money for research, get women active in the cause." Lily came from a prominent business family in a major city, and telling her story brought her into the public eye on TV and in the newspapers. "I was deluged. All kinds of organizations asked me to speak to their members, and I did. I believe a lot of women went and got mammograms because of my story, as they did with Betty Ford, Happy Rockefeller, and Nancy Reagan. Look, today is a gift—that's why they call it 'the present'—and I need to share mine."

Gena wasn't altruistic or open. "I decided not to tell my friends—and my doctor told me not to. This was years ago. I was young. I didn't want people clucking over me, feeling sorry for me, being nice to me just because I'd had breast cancer. I kept my mouth shut for twenty years. It was a different time." Betsy would have agreed with Gena. "People ask me, 'How *are* you?' with this woeful eye. Like I'm so brave but really dying. Or they say, 'How good you look!' with real surprise, as though I should look half-dead. Or I *do* look half-dead and they lie through their teeth and say, 'How great you look!' Who needs all that?"

Telling may help others deal with your situation but may do little to help you. You're the one who can end up giving support, often getting the energy sucked out of you to help someone else. You soon find out which friends have the capacity to understand what's happening to you, and can give you important attention, love, and support.

Most women do tell their friends and co-workers. "I don't like to be with people who don't know," said Florrie. "It makes it so much easier at work. And everyone is so supportive and kind, in many loving ways. Maybe I talk about it too much." Ginnie told her friends but she felt she had to hide it at work because she was worried about keeping her job and her health insurance.

What never ceases to amaze me is how intense and vivid the retelling can be. In one interview after another, women ten, twenty, even thirty years later speak of their experiences with an energy that suggests it all happened only a few days before.

Getting Back to Normal: Setting Priorities

Many breast cancer patients come away from this experience with a clearer view of what matters most in life, and tell how cancer has changed their lives. And maybe not surprising to you, but surely surprising to people without cancer, is the repeated comment, "My life is so much better now," or, "We're a much closer family now than we ever were before." That does not include, however, the small but important number of individuals and families that come apart, unable to manage this crisis. Between these extremes are the women who chug along like everybody else, dealing with everyday issues and keeping their past health problems on a short leash.

"I've chucked so much garbage." "I don't waste time." "I don't suffer fools." "I take risks I never did before." "I take better care of myself." "I'm more assertive." "I don't worry about unimportant details." "I won't let people take advantage of me." "I'm able to make changes I always needed to make." "I stop and look around at new things." "I'm much kinder to myself." "I take nothing for granted." "I don't waste time."

So many women who have been diagnosed with breast cancer have said to me, "I want to find meaning in and derive fulfillment from each day. I want to build memories." Workaholics take time off. Trivial matters are seen for what they are. "I used to get all worked up in traffic; now I'm happy just sitting there." Laughter and merriment are prized; hugging takes on major importance.

Many women say they no longer put off what they really want to do. "Eat dessert first." "I'm doing things I'd talked about doing for years: I'm going to graduate school, for starters," Vivian told me with pride. But it can backfire. Jenny was irritable and tired: "I've been trying so hard to do all the things I enjoy. I find it's too stressful—it's wearing me out!"

Take Care of Yourself

Indulge yourself. Give yourself a reward. Treat yourself better. Go on a vacation. "Each year on my anniversary I am in a beautiful place, celebrating life." Jo told me: "If you feel like crying, do it. If you need help, get it. Give yourself time—the biggest gift—for recovery. Don't let anyone make you feel guilty, and don't take on things you're not ready for. It isn't as easy as one might think to put yourself first. Grab what you want and need. I was too brave, always protecting others. Now it's my time."

Don't let your family's expectations get out of hand. Expectations should be totally realistic for *you,* and no one else. You may know someone who sailed through treatment, back to work full time the week after surgery, house, husband, and kids all cared for—but so what! If that's not you (or most women I know), it's not relevant. Your experience and feelings are what are at issue here. Keep your head, and make your family see you as you are and treat you as you need to be treated.

You Do Have a Future

No normal human being has the time or emotional wherewithal to process this whole experience until the major thrust of treatment is completed. It gets stored away, waiting for when fatigue has receded and your life is on the way back to normal. Maybe that's another reason that the end of treatment is such an unexpectedly hard time. "My stress and anxiety became more apparent to me after I finished therapy than when I was going through it," Donna reflected. "Enough time has finally gone by so that now I have confidence. I was given this really big test—and I passed. I can wake up and not think first thing about cancer. I can go to work and feel good all day. There is life after cancer! I am who I am; I am not defined by that disease. Breast cancer is behind me."

Gena, too, was in charge of her life. "I didn't choose this disease and I wasn't going to let it control me. I had a good life before, and this bad thing wasn't going to change my life for me. I was going to make life good again. You don't want to disappoint yourself; you don't want to let yourself down. So you make yourself come through. That was twenty years ago—and it has been good!"

Form your own conclusions about what your life beyond breast cancer should be, because no one can quite supply the answers you need. "I live one day at a time. I value each and every day." Many of you want to think of and plan for your future but are afraid to presume that you *have* a future. Don't let fear stop you. *You do have a future,* and you're not daring fate to think about it and plan what you want to do for yourself, your family, your children, vacations, or retirement. You're no different from anyone else on this score, although you may bring a sharper appreciation for the idea of "future." It's reasonable to hope that your "future" will be years and years of a good life.

2

Support Groups

I needed to go someplace where others knew it wasn't over, like going through an invisible wall, cancer people on one side, everyone else on the other. I didn't need to explain—they understood. That was my support group. They helped me learn to trust my instincts, *to take care of myself*—nobody else can or will. That's what a support group does.

Why a Support Group?

It takes a while to sort through and process the emotional turmoil that comes with the diagnosis of breast cancer. You may consider joining a support group to be with other women like yourself, to talk about what's on your mind, what you don't understand, what worries you, what scares you, and to express all this, out loud, to someone else. You need to hear that you are not alone, that other women with the same condition have similar feelings. The strain starts with the diagnosis of cancer; isolation may follow because people still have a hard time getting the word *cancer* out of their mouths—it's "the Big C." But each woman in the support group knows what it is and can learn to say the words, talk about it, and get back the energy no one can spare.

The goal of a support group is to restore your confidence in the future that the diagnosis of cancer has shattered, to reclaim the control of your life that cancer has stolen from you, and to draw you into a community of understanding people who allow you to connect to others, to share good and bad news, and to simply recover.

What Is a Breast Cancer Support Group?

A breast cancer support group is a number of women who gather together on a scheduled basis, for a period of time, in the presence of a facilitator who is usually a trained therapist. The nature of the group can vary. The women may all be newly diagnosed breast cancer patients, or women experiencing a recurrence, or women with metastatic disease, or women at mixed stages of breast cancer. The women may have nothing in common with each other but this one thing, cancer.

The group may be organized around one theme, perhaps "Life after Treatment," or it may be a group of women with very mixed concerns that finds its focus as it goes along, influenced by the dynamics of individual participants. The emphasis can be on personal issues and resolution, education, or a hybrid of both. It can plumb these issues in depth; it can be topical and pragmatic, or wide-ranging, reflective, and spiritual.

The women may meet once a week or once or twice a month for a one- or two-hour session, usually on a weekday evening. Participants may come and go or a fixed number may stay through a prescribed session. A minimum of six women in a session is desirable. "After all, it's not a group experience unless you have a group." Some consider ten an ideal number that cannot be exceeded without sacrificing a sense of trust and intimacy, but I've seen groups of twenty-five women that work.

Some groups bring in an occasional speaker to address a particular issue; other groups provide guest speakers on a regular schedule. The guest presents an educational topic, a point of view, or advice, and the group may use the talk as a springboard—a combination of information and support.

Support groups are usually sponsored by a hospital or allied medical organization like the American Cancer Society or the Wellness Community and are located preferably in a neutral, comfortable, safe, and readily accessible setting. A hospital location may be off-putting—the sights and smells may have too many unpleasant associations—but a hospital may be the only reasonable, convenient place for this kind of program.

Who's in Charge?

The person who guides the group is called a facilitator: someone who takes a neutral role in assisting the progress of the group toward recovery. The group needs delicate guidance, which is different from being led or directed. It's important to have an experienced facilitator who knows how to keep the focus on what the group is there for: a tolerant atmosphere, a hopeful attitude, newfound control in the lives of each individual, and the reversal of isolation.

The facilitator should be nonjudgmental, sincere, knowing, and caring, creating a safe environment so people can open up and share and trust that their feelings won't be trivialized and that their disclosures won't leave the room. The facilitator is there for support, to empower each participant, and to provide security.

There are women who would prefer that their support group facilitator be a breast cancer survivor like themselves, but most facilitators are not breast cancer survivors. Most, but not all, facilitators are women. What is most important for the facilitator of a cancer support group is a background in dealing with illness, treatment, health, and loss, and a sense of compassion, dedication, and open-mindedness.

An effective facilitator starts out in a fairly active role, then lets the group evolve and become the main actor in the support group process. The facilitator draws out the group participants in quiet, subtle ways. There is no pressure for anyone to participate; no one is put on the spot. If one member takes over and monopolizes the discussion, the facilitator usually steps in gently, deftly, thanks the speaker for her contribution, for sharing her feelings with the others, and moves on to someone else.

Often when buried feelings finally start to come forward, there is no knowing how disturbing the feelings may be to the woman expressing them, and to the women listening. The group talks about pain, about coming apart, and about loss, as well as about ordinary, mundane subjects and the good things that make life worth living. The facilitator must be familiar with this process and know how to deal with varied reactions. What if someone goes off the deep end? It can happen. Participation in a support group can be a powerful experience, and only a trained professional can contain that power and deflect and channel it for the benefit of all present.

It's not unusual to have two facilitators run a support group, which may afford greater availability and flexibility of scheduling, and a capacity to handle a larger spectrum of ideas and issues.

Jayne Antonowsky, a psychotherapist who works with support groups, occasionally brings in a panel of long-term breast cancer survivors to her support group for women with newly diagnosed breast cancer, to introduce them to women in a different place in their lives. These survivors are comfortable talking about the struggles they have handled and the challenges they have overcome. The success these women have had in handling their difficulties gives the support group participants a boost, and also stimulates further communication.

Facilitators may be objective, but they can get emotionally involved with the people in their group. And they can't avoid feeling stress—and loss. In a well-run program, facilitators should have access to supervision and support for themselves.

Some support groups are run by a person without the credentials of a trained facilitator. While it may not be an ideal situation, it can work very well.

How a Support Group Works

The group tends to work as an ensemble, helping individual members to express what's on their minds. Each member of the group introduces herself, and tells something about herself and her breast cancer experience, why she has come to the group, and what her expectations may be. The facilitator needs to be consistently attentive, no matter how inconspicuous she may appear to be at times. Her first priorities are to establish the safe environment a support group must have and to ease the participants into open, meaningful communication.

A few ground rules: One person speaks at a time, no interruptions; everybody else sits quietly and attentively. No one is obliged to talk. Each person is expected to respect the privacy and confidences of the others in the group. One stipulation—the only one—of the Wellness Community, a national organization providing psychological and social support to cancer survivors, is to let the group know if you will be absent. "Otherwise, we worry: Is she sick? in the hospital, still alive? It makes everyone anxious when anyone is absent without explanation. We develop a real emotional investment in one another."

Limited-time support groups, who meet, say, for ten weeks, often insist on mandatory attendance. It's a privilege to get into a group; there are women, after all, who don't make the cutoff, so most group organizers don't want a casual attitude about showing up. A lot must be accomplished in a short space, and each individual plays an important role. Other groups have a looser approach to attendance, especially if the group has not been working too well, or where interest and commitment to the group may be lacking.

The Power of a Group

Even if you have people within your family or support network to talk to, it may be hard to tell them what scares you. "My family needs *my* support! I just can't burden them." You may be anxious to protect your family from your own worst fears, to avoid adding to their stress, worried that they can't handle all that's been happening to you. So you pretend to each other and to yourself. "I/You look great! I'm/You're doing so well. I'm/You're going to be fine." The hidden message is: I won't tell you how I feel if you don't tell me how you feel about how I feel.

women lack experience reaching out and asking for help. It's a Big hing. It's not okay in their eyes to be needy. They're care*givers,* not *kers.* Joining a support group calls for an overhaul of their whole alue system and "method of operation."

Those women who do come to a support group tend to be take-harge people. They enjoy talking and learning how to cope, and they vant all the information they can get their hands on about all the echniques available to help them fight cancer and stay alive. Support ecomes one more opportunity. They use the socialization of a breast ancer support group to help overcome their fear of cancer, to reestab-sh control of their lives, and to connect to a community they under-tand. Professionals say a take-charge woman tends to recover faster han the woman who feels she is a victim and is stuck in a disaster, un-ble to move on to any constructive action.

Some women simply can't bring themselves to join a group; they ind they must work out their problems on their own. Bernice couldn't get past what she considered complaining. "I couldn't sit around listening to that stuff. That's not me. They needed something I didn't." For some women, it may be a function of denial; they push heir anguish out of mind: "I got it. I had it cut out. I don't want to alk about it again." And they don't. Not even those who are terrified inside. And it may not *do* to try to break through this protective bar-rier; it's working. "If it ain't broke, don't fix it."

Not everybody should join a support group; not everybody is ready for a support group; not everybody *needs* a support group. There are always a few women who probably should not be in a group at all but who could benefit from one-on-one therapy. Remember, very little gets censored in a group; a newcomer can be startled, or disturbed. At times, a group can simply be too stressful: You listen to talk of recur-rence, metastases, and dying. The good things talked about, the ordi-nary problems that occupy most time in a group, may not register by comparison. Sylvia went to one support meeting. "Breast cancer am-plifies everything. The women there were so scary. There were too many of other people's issues and feelings I wasn't prepared to deal with." These may be women who have difficulty dealing directly with their feelings, or they feel too exposed. Or they've been overwhelmed by their diagnosis and they aren't yet ready to listen or share.

The lure of a support group is that the stress and isolatio
become such a burden to you can be alleviated. Sadness an
have been buried, repressed, denied. "I'm afraid that my sa
pecially if I talk about it—will make my cancer come bacl
considerable emotional energy to keep all that trouble buri
better spent someplace else in your life. Stress that isn't r
some way or other can be destructive. Being with other wo
have had breast cancer, empathizing with each other, or ma
nally acknowledging your fear and telling it to somebody el
minish the fear and make things better. Slowly, you reclaim
You restore equilibrium and meaning to your day-by-day ex
making some sense out of what has happened to you and v
come.

That's the strength of a support group. You talk about y
cerns, and you take what you've learned home to your fan
may also find there are a lot of issues you hadn't considered
Here in the group, you are talking about ideas that surprise y
ulate you, and move you to understand yourself as you ne
before.

A landmark study demonstrated the power and effects of
groups on the lives of women with metastatic breast cancer
randomized study at Stanford University, Dr. David Spiegel
the progress of women with metastatic disease who particip
support groups, and an equal number of women who did not.
as surprised as anyone that the women in the support groups l
most twice as long, after the study began, as those who were r
of a support group. In addition, the women in the support
were more satisfied with their lives. Although no other inves
has yet been able to duplicate the survival benefit, all therapists
nize the importance of support groups for improved quality of l

Who Joins a Support Group, and Who Doesn't

Women throughout history tend to be talkers, sharers, and s
tellers. They problem-solve with words. A support group is a na
mode for them, but in fact only 10 percent of cancer survivors tak
vantage of support groups. Some can handle it; others can't even s
Reaching out for support is as great a challenge for some women
coping with the concept of cancer. They know there are issues to
with that go beyond the issue of breast cancer. And, as I've said, a

The Right Group for You:
When and What Kind of Group?

You can go into a group too soon; perhaps you need to wait. Some-time later, six months or a year after your diagnosis, or more, your feelings will have settled down and focused, and you may find your-self ready to look for personal exploration and renewal. Mary: "It was a year till I had the energy for a support group." Normally, you'll know when you're ready and when you're in the right group.

If choice is available, the facilitator will help place you in the most suitable group for your needs. Nancy left her support session in tears: "Everyone there had someone at home for them. I had no one, no hus-band, no lover—and my mother had just passed away. There should be a group for someone who has nobody." Without choices, you may find yourself in an inappropriate group, and you'll have to decide if it's worth it to continue. If you are a woman with noninvasive breast can-cer (which doesn't go to lymph nodes or other parts of the body) and you share a group with women undergoing bone marrow transplanta-tion for advanced breast cancer, you may leave the group's session worried and convinced that it's only a matter of time before you need to have your own transplant. Unless you can ventilate anxiety of this sort, you might want to look for a more suitable group.

It sometimes becomes evident that one woman needs more help than her support group can provide. The facilitator may have to tell her, "I think you would benefit from individual counseling. You have a lot more to work out than we can manage in the group. I'll be happy to arrange a referral." The suggestion may be accepted, or not.

Problems within a Support Group

Occasionally, one person takes over a group, talking much more than others. The facilitator must then step in to restore balance, both to the group and to this particular individual. Or perhaps another woman is convinced that the stress of her divorce caused her breast cancer. Without making judgments, the facilitator may try to generalize the situation for the group: "If this is how you're feeling, no one can be the expert about yourself but you. If what you're telling us makes sense to you, that's fine. But what you've been talking about is what is past. How do you plan to go on from here? How are you going to cope with your life now? That's what we want to help you with."

Another woman may be quiet, too quiet. When someone asks her something, she's stunned that she's been noticed and valued. She's accustomed to feeling insignificant; her self-esteem is in the basement. She doesn't know how to express what she wants or needs; she has no practice in asking. She's embarrassed at the thought of people taking care of *her*. She needs permission to acknowledge her needs and accept help, to escape the high expectations she's established for herself, such as trying to carry on as usual, doing all of Thanksgiving or Christmas for the family, as she has in the past. "I'm a coper, I'm there to help others who need me." With the help of the facilitator, a few women may begin to pick up these signs, to catch on, to draw her out and encourage her to practice self-help skills. Instead of offering advice, women in the group learn to say, "This has worked for me. . . ." And they learn to accept different ways of coping. They learn to be respectful of one another; they may even acquire the nonjudgmental habits of the facilitator.

Sometimes it seems a struggle: A woman expresses only a measure of her fears; the group wants her to explore her feelings further. "People who care about you won't let you off the hook. They urge courage, honesty—but they do it with great kindness and affection. It can be magic, what goes on in a group." The support group really wants you to think about yourself, to devote more to what's happening in your life. "It's time you came first."

Burnout is not an uncommon feature of support groups, particularly groups that have been in existence for a long time, as some have. Energy may flag; women may lose interest, especially if there have been a number of deaths within the group, or if an admired facilitator gets sick or leaves. If you feel burned out, or your support group is not helping you because it keeps rehashing the same issues as new people join the group, or if a few people are really irritating or upsetting you, or an individual is polarizing the group with her anger, or the group is poorly organized, then talk about it with the group's facilitator. The facilitator may need to reassess the group's purpose and goals, and talk with other members to see if their needs are being met. Maybe you can work something out. A new group may emerge with another focus, the same group may be revitalized, individual members may shape up or ship out, the members may reaffirm their commitment to start and end the sessions on time, or you may decide to look for something different.

Self-Help Groups and Others

If you find yourself in a group unsuited to your needs, there are other options. You might be better served by a coffee klatch, a book club, or a self-help group. Self-help groups are peer-led groups, formed by women with similar interests and needs, sometimes quite spontaneously, and without the overseeing auspices of a professional or service organization. They tend to be informal, organized perhaps to serve an educational, informational purpose. They often have more participants than a typical support group, plus an easy come-and-go arrangement. "It's another level of friendship. We deal with loneliness, isolation, fear—many of the issues I explored in the hospital-sponsored support group I was part of for a year; it's emotional support, but nobody 'spills her guts' here. We tend to keep a little distance. We bring in speakers and focus more on education than unloading."

Help for Partners and Families

There are also support groups for partners or spouses who are dealing with the stress of breast cancer. Partners often are in real need of ventilating the concerns and tension that they are loath to express at home to the woman who is actually suffering from breast cancer. Hospitals or wellness centers are generally the organizers of these groups, having a large pool to draw upon. Lesbian partners may have a harder time adjusting to this type of support group, because most participants are men. Some centers offer support groups specifically for children.

Limited Access to Support Groups

You may live too far from any existing support groups, or support may be inaccessible for other reasons: you don't have reliable transportation, you can't get a sitter, or the available groups all meet at night and you're too tired by then. What can you do?

First, don't drop the idea of support. Support groups can really improve your sense of well-being. Seventy percent of women diagnosed with breast cancer believe that stress in their lives contributed to the cause of their cancer. How stress affects cancer is not known, but clearly the quality of your life is profoundly affected by stress. Breast cancer increases stress; support groups help relieve it. You need to address more than your physical needs as you return to a normal pattern of life. Also, support groups are free to you—a compelling factor after the cumulative expense of this illness. It does, however, require a commitment of time, energy, and social skills.

If your hospital does not offer a support group, approach your doctor, nurse, and your hospital and urge them to come up with suggestions and ideas for establishing a support group or help network. They know other breast cancer survivors with needs similar to yours. They must know resource people who can search out alternatives. Don't be reluctant to start out modestly. If you can create a beginning, perhaps the hospital can come through with a facilitator. And don't overlook your church or synagogue as a source of support: Your priest, minister, or rabbi may be able to organize a support group along your needs, as well as offering you immediate spiritual support.

We do need to find new ways to serve women in far-off places, who are isolated physically and emotionally. Can electronic systems help? Telephones? Telemedicine? Support groups on-line? Women have found each other on the Internet: Chat groups hook up, share personal experience, and offer comfort to each other. Maybe it's not the conventional mode of support, but it seems to work for the women who call and connect. Let's use whatever we can find that works.

TWO

Additional Care Beyond Treatment

3

You and Your Doctors: Continuing Care

I had a very good, calming doctor; she listened thoughtfully to whatever I asked her. I trusted her to tell me everything. She explained it all in detail, and gave me the statistics with a positive spin. She *cared* about me. She's still a great source of support. I need to trust my doctor completely. If you don't have that, you don't have the full value of medical care you're entitled to.

From Now On

You and your doctors have come through an exhausting, demanding, emotional, intimate, and frightening experience. You probably feel older and wiser, and, I hope, still confident in your doctors.

When you were given that diagnosis of breast cancer, you became dependent overnight on a team of health care professionals responsible for your life. You had to choose doctors you could trust, or your choices may have been limited by your health care plan. You had to become an expert on a subject you may have known little about, and to make critical choices you may have felt unprepared to make.

Now that treatment is nearing completion, or is over, you may want to reassess, reaffirm, reshape, or reconsider your relationship with your medical team. Have you been satisfied? Have you been happy with this team? Are they the people you want to take care of you in the future, or do you feel like making a change?

Continuing Care

As treatment ends, you have a multitude of mixed feelings to sort out and compose. You're thrilled treatment is over—enough of doctors and tests! A big part of you yearns to close the door on your illness and the people associated with it, but deep down you might find such isolation frightening, without the attention of the team you've learned to depend on and trust. You may be anxious and worried about the termination of your treatment and close supervision by your medical team. The information and support, the frequency of your meetings with that team, have carried you past diagnosis through treatment. What now?

You're not about to be abandoned, if that's one of your fears. After your cancer treatment has concluded, you will be scheduled for regular visits with the physicians who have participated in your cancer care. While reassuring, all this scheduling may once again be overwhelming—so many appointments, and you so tired. And with all that has been waiting for your return to health, you may find yourself hard-pressed to fit in so many doctors' visits. But it is important. Your doctors want to monitor any unresolved side effects, evaluate your response to treatment, ease your adjustment back to a full life, assess your overall health status, watch for signs and symptoms of possible recurrence, and focus on cancer prevention and the promotion of your health and sense of wellness.

Now is a good time to review your relationship with your cancer care team and see if those relationships are meeting your needs. Perhaps you weren't too happy with your doctor, but you didn't have the energy to do the work required to find a new one. Perhaps you just didn't want to change horses in midstream. Perhaps your experience with your doctor was adequate, but at this point, you want a relationship that gives you more. Now that the crisis is past and you're looking into your future, take the time and effort to be sure you're getting what you need from your doctor. Maybe you can make changes to improve an existing relationship, or maybe you should start fresh.

What Makes a Good Doctor?

There are certain qualities I feel are essential in my own doctors. Trust and respect are key elements to a good doctor-patient relationship. "The best thing about my doctor? He *listens*." Over and over that's what women truly appreciate. "He takes the time to listen." "She listens." Listening is essential in a good doctor-patient relationship. A doctor who listens, respects you.

"She's always available for questions—I wanted a doctor who didn't have one foot out the door." "She is never too busy to answer my questions. I felt I could really talk to her." "He answered all my questions, directly and honestly, didn't pull any punches." "He always returned my phone calls—explained everything."

And reassurance: " 'You didn't cause this disease; no one knows what caused it.' I finally didn't feel guilty." Concern for you as an individual: "He asks about my husband, about my farm animals, things like that." An optimistic outlook: "I loved his positive attitude. He transmitted the belief that I would live a long life. His attitude and his body language said: *You will prevail*." "My doctor communicated his optimism to me. He was always cheerful." "My surgeon was always upbeat. 'We can handle this.' That 'we' is so important. The better the sense of teamwork, the greater my sense of well-being."

Most important, I suspect, to how you feel about your doctor, is the matter of trust: whether you can trust your doctor to tell you the truth, the whole truth—even the awful truth. "Could you trust a doctor who never brought up the ultimate subject, who never mentioned the possibility of dying?" Patients worry that their doctor may be withholding information, that there may be collusion to keep a bad diagnosis hidden.

I make a definite point of telling my patients I will be direct and straightforward about all information, but I do respect those few women who don't want to know everything. I had a patient with a particularly aggressive type of cancer, inflammatory breast cancer. At the start of our first meeting, she explicitly told me she did not want to talk about her prognosis in any way. She knew her chances were not very good, because her cancer was progressing despite chemotherapy and wasn't responding well to radiotherapy, but she was still hopeful and certain she would beat the disease. It was hard to take care of her, because I was constantly having to avoid topics like how the treatment was going—and when she was beset by pain and refused hospice, I knew she could be receiving much better pain control if only she would let me tell her about it. But some lines can't be crossed, and truth does not suit everyone. Nonetheless, I believe truth and honesty, handled gently and with sensitivity, are the preferred course.

Complaints

What upsets people most about their doctors? Being given a misdiagnosis. Being told they're going to be fine, and then the tests come back: cancer. It happens. "I told him my symptoms, more than once. He missed the diagnosis. I know my body, I knew something was wrong, even when he said there wasn't. When they finally did a biopsy, he told me the frozen section looked good, go to work. Three nights later

I'm eating dinner, the phone rings: my doctor. 'It's malignant.' And I'm in total shock. You mustn't let anyone tell you it's nothing till they absolutely know it's nothing."

The shock of bad news after good expectations (for example, from a premature upbeat prognosis) can be devastating. "I can't take any more of these optimistic predictions. They were all wrong. First they said the lump was perfectly round and so small there was only a very remote possibility of cancer. When it turned out to be cancer, they said it was so small there was virtually no significant risk of node involvement—and then there were eight out of fifteen nodes with disease. Why bother with optimism for a few days of supposed peace of mind when they don't know what's really there? I failed each of their predictions and, on top of everything else, I had the peculiar feeling I'd disappointed both my doctors and myself. I was ready to come apart."

Doctors want the best for you, but they are human. The preliminary view looks okay, and they really think they "got it all," and they want to pass on good news. You desperately need reassurance. But then, over the next few days, the pathologist who does the staining and checking of all the slides may find malignant cells. Given the statistics—80 percent of breast biopsy results show no cancer—doctors are generally not far off in their optimism. But if you are part of that other 20 percent, that optimism is misleading. It's a delicate balancing act, figuring how to be reassuring without giving unrealistic expectations.

How do you separate the message from the messenger? The message "You have breast cancer" is devastating; the messenger, usually a physician, tries to present the information with all the sensitivity and support possible, which can sometimes be too reassuring.

Besides mistakes in diagnosis, women resent arrogance and condescension. "My doctor thought I just wanted attention—and there I was so sick I ended up in the hospital again." Catherine was bitter about her doctor's indifference to her reported symptoms. June still bristles over the reception she got from a new doctor: "I went to this specialist—he didn't even look at me. 'Whom do you know that got you this appointment with me?' What an egotistical jackass!"

"I had this list of questions I'd been writing down about what was bothering me. 'You don't need to know all that stuff,' my doctor told me. He didn't welcome any questions. I was left with all my worries and he made me feel like a dunce." "He never told me what to expect." "He took it for granted I didn't want or need to know anything. I was never included in making decisions regarding my care. Being a patient became synonymous with losing all control of my life."

Another major complaint: insensitivity. "I'd be sitting there with my husband, and my doctor would be talking to *him,* like I was invisible. 'Do I exist?' I wondered. And later, I'm lying there almost naked while he unwraps the bandages five days after the mastectomy—in a roomful of students, all of them in their clothes, me more than naked. I call that cruel and unusual punishment. I was so young. I got so old after that. I have rights. Now I speak up—that's what my voice is for."

"I don't like it when my doctor walks into the examination room, I'm there half naked, and he brings along another doctor, maybe a parade of doctors, who stand there gawking. It's not fair. It's humiliating and embarrassing. I hate it. He wouldn't treat Hillary Clinton like that!" Loss of privacy is painful for anyone. It's real on many levels, from the examining room to the large, impersonal waiting room, where your name, called out by the aide, reverberates noisily around the entire room and its occupants.

"Waiting is another hot-button issue. They should be able to schedule better than they do. Are we so unimportant?" You may have started with your doctor some years ago, and now you find there's a lot less time allowed for you than back then. The practice has enlarged, and the waits have lengthened.

I, too, hate waiting—anywhere—so I do whatever I can to minimize the time my patients wait to see me, but a physician's schedule is predictably unpredictable. Almost every day there are crises, beyond even the extra space in the day doctors do allow: a woman with a new diagnosis of breast cancer needs to talk about it ASAP, another patient must make her final decision about tamoxifen and has to review the pros and cons again, another is anxious, waiting for mammography results complicated by unexplained extra views—did the radiologist order more x-rays because he or she suspected a problem?

And then the interruptions during your appointment, especially the phone calls. It may seem rude; there you are in the middle of your talk time with your doctor when the phone rings, your conversation stops, and your doctor's attention is transferred to someone on the other end of the line. We can hope that only the most pressing calls get through, those that require immediate attention, such as a patient who is having a problem on the radiation table or in the recovery room, or it may be a return call from a doctor your doctor's been trying to reach for days to clarify a patient's therapy. Just remember, one day it could be your call that interrupts someone else, or your important questions that throw off the appointment schedule for patients after you.

So, other than taking a whole day off from work, or rearranging your child's entire carpool schedule, what do you do about the waiting? Try booking your appointment first thing in the morning, just after lunch, or at the end of the day, when appointments tend to go on time. Arriving early for your appointment may help if there's been a cancellation or if they're running ahead of schedule, but if all appointments are filled or they're running late, coming early may only add additional time to your waiting, especially to your perception of waiting a very long time. It may help to call the doctor's office before you leave home, to find out if appointments are running late, and by how much. Your doctor's appointment secretary should be a guide to the best time for the most streamlined visit.

If you have two doctors' appointments (or an x-ray appointment) on the same day, let the first doctor's secretary or nurse know about the other commitment so, if possible, you can be moved through without delay and on to your next appointment. Or if you're running late, call your next appointment to let them know of your delay.

If you feel you have waited unduly long, it is possible they have forgotten about you. Go up to the receptionist and be sure you have been booked in properly. Check back occasionally to be sure you are not forgotten. If you have been waiting an unavoidably long time, your doctor or his staff should do what they can to recognize your inconvenience. An apology can make you feel somewhat better; an offer of juice, use of the phone, a choice magazine, or access to music or TV can also ease the wait.

Some people get so annoyed with delays, or lack of attention, that they want to switch doctors. But continuity of care is essential, so if you find the level of care and communication to be good, don't let waiting be the sole criterion for making a change. Tell your doctor about your frustration.

Switching Doctors

Choosing to Switch

There are many reasons people decide to switch doctors. A study commissioned by the Commonwealth Fund of New York surveyed 2500 women and 1000 men about satisfaction with their doctors. Forty-one percent of the women had switched doctors because they were dissatisfied with their care, compared with 27 percent of the men. The women complained about being talked down to, not being listened to, and having symptoms summarily dismissed. (The main problem cited by both men and women was poor communication.)

Unfortunately, there are times when no matter how much effort you put into your relationship with your doctor, it doesn't work. You thought about what you wanted from your doctor and tried to communicate it, but it didn't sink in. Sophie's doctor was unbearably condescending and never picked up on her discontent. She finally gave up. "It was hard to make the break—it took me months—but I had to find someone more tuned to what I needed, to what worried me."

Linda had another reason for switching. "I couldn't get past his attitude. He was so pessimistic. You go to a doctor, feeling bad—and he makes you feel worse! Then he kept repeating it. Believe me, there's only one time you need to tell a patient a negative diagnosis. No one wants to hear it over and over. I'll be seeing my doctor the rest of my life; I deserve more. My new doctor told me I was going to have one lousy year, and then I'd get better. And that's what happened—six years ago."

Justine's father was a prominent physician, but, at forty-five, Justine was in charge of her own life. She left the doctor who'd been her primary physician when he told her he was planning to call her father and discuss her health with him. "It was such a patent violation of my right to privacy! My father was eighty years old; I was trying to protect him. I switched doctors immediately."

The husband of one patient made the decision to switch. "My wife didn't want chemo, and I agreed with her. And this pompous 'high-class' specialist says to me, 'Don't you love your wife?' I couldn't believe it! 'You haven't even looked at her report!' I told him. He hadn't. And when I mentioned going to the university hospital, he sneered, 'They don't know what the hell they're doing.' I couldn't wait to get out of that office, let alone get my wife out of his care." You may decide that your medical and emotional needs are different now from when you started with your original doctor. Can your current doctor meet your new needs? What matters most to you now?

You spend so much emotional energy investing yourself in your relationship with your doctor, it's difficult to wrench it away and find somebody new, but sometimes it's better to make a switch when you've identified a meaningful problem that won't go away or you need to address new priorities. It may feel better to take control and establish a better doctor-patient relationship.

Switching for Arbitrary Reasons

Are you being forced to switch physicians because your doctor is no longer a member of your insurance plan, or because you've just changed insurance companies and your doctor is not part of your new health plan—reasons that have nothing to do with the competence of, or your relationship with, your present physician? You may adore your doctor, but you can't get the necessary co-payment if your insurance has dropped him from its list, or he was never on it.

The structure of the medical insurance industry is changing

rapidly, attempting to provide excellent care and save money at the same time. Health care costs and quality are everyone's concern: consumers, insurance companies, doctors, hospitals, even the government. Insurance companies understand the desire people have to choose their doctors. Whether the preferred doctor appears on your list, however, depends on many factors: the time required to identify, recruit, and sign up particular doctors; and the time and facilities needed to complete necessary paperwork (which includes the financial conditions of contracts, for example). Doctors often participate in multiple plans, and popular doctors may find themselves besieged by multiple companies at any time. It can take them a lot of time and effort to sort out the details of joining one insurance company over another, which further limits their availability to patients. Or their practice may be so busy the doctor decides not to participate, in order to control the size of his or her practice and to limit paperwork and hassles.

Sometimes, a switch is necessary because you're moving out of town. You adore your medical team and would stick with them forever, but now you must find a new set of doctors. A few people keep their doctors, even when they move away; they have too much at stake and care too much for a doctor they trust implicitly to drop her because they no longer live nearby. They travel to their doctors a couple of times a year and it's no big deal. But even if such an arrangement works for you, don't neglect the need to have someone close to where you now live to take care of you. You certainly should have a primary care physician close at hand for ordinary and emergency health care needs.

Whatever the reason for switching—economic, political, or personal—it is frustrating, painful, and sad to disrupt a relationship that works; the move feels arbitrary and senseless. I have been disheartened by the loss of patients I care very much about from my practice because of "policy" reasons.

The Right Doctor for You

Most people take more time and care checking out a car they want to buy than the physician who will look after their health. If you find you must switch doctors or find a new one, take your time and take care. Rethink what it is you want in and from your physician. What is most important to you: a physician of outstanding reputation, a warm and understanding personality, crisp efficiency, patience, and fortitude? Sometimes you have to choose. "I knew he was the best in his field, but he was simply too cold and businesslike for me. I need someone I can turn to for support and encouragement, as well as good medical care." Gena went to a number of doctors before she found one who satisfied her primary requirements.

You are entitled to a doctor who treats you with respect and dignity, a doctor who shares information and decision making with you about your care. You need to be part of the process so that you can maintain control of your life. You want to look for a doctor whose style of decision making is most like your own. Communicate your preferences to your doctor, particularly to your referring physician, who connects you to the specialists you see off and on and helps you select who's best for you based on your needs and inclinations.

If you are moving, ask your current team if they know anyone in the area you're heading to. Medical specialists inhabit a small world: Doctors know each other from training, through the literature, from medical conferences, and from the media. And if they don't know anyone personally, there's always the medical grapevine they can turn to. There's also the directory that each specialty publishes, which lists doctors by location and provides information about training and experience. If you're using a physician referral service for the name of a doctor, don't expect unbiased information; the service may be one based at a particular hospital or one that includes only doctors who pay to be listed. Ask your friends and trusted neighbors for the names of doctors they recommend, especially if their medical experience is similar to your own. Remember, however, that many recommendations are made on the basis of bedside manner rather than clinical expertise.

If you're in any position to do so, inquire about a doctor who interests you among professionals who see her or him at work, and who have no vested interest in a recommendation: hospital nurses, interns, or residents.

What should you find out about your new physician? First, the medical qualifications: What medical school? What training hospital? What hospital does he or she admit patients to? How did you hear about this doctor? How old is he or she? You want someone young enough to be around for as long as you are, yet someone with enough experience to manage any complex issues your cancer care requires.

Interview your prospective doctor. Is communication good? Is he or she well trained, with expertise in the area that concerns you? Do you get a sense of warmth and respect? Any note of condescension or sexism? Is he or she willing to provide you with full information about your condition and related health issues? Is the office clean and cheerful? Is the examining room comfortable and adequate? Is the staff helpful, forthcoming, and competent? Is a nurse present during your physical exam?

Do you want a doctor who'll act as a partner in your care, or do you prefer the old-fashioned model of the doctor as authority figure? Some women prefer the traditional old-fashioned relationship with a white-haired male physician; others want a same-sex physician of similar age for the ease of communication and camaraderie they feel they should have in a modern patient-doctor relationship. (According to *The New England Journal of Medicine* and the *Journal of the American Medical Association,* women doctors also spend more time with their patients, listen more and interrupt less, and, finally, are more likely to discuss difficult issues.)

You want the right chemistry, the same attitude toward risk, treatment, and timing: Is this the point to hold back treatment, the moment for testing, or the time to try something new?

My own preference is for a physician who really enjoys being a physician, because such a person will continue to improve his or her skills and enjoy taking care of me. I want my physicians to be direct with me, and so I am straightforward with them and ask direct questions. I don't want them to withhold any information. Most physicians take their cue on this issue from their patients: If you want less candor than I do, let your physician know, so your reservations can be respected and you can be protected from total disclosure.

Follow your instincts; listen to your inner voice to find the doctor you'll like best. And keep listening, even after you make your choice—that intuitive sense of yours may be more helpful than you think. You make this decision with the hope that it will work out well, but your decision is not permanent or irreversible. If you've switched doctors, it's possible to switch again, or even to go back to your original doctor.

Once you've made your choice, arrange to have your full medical records mailed or faxed to your new physician. This transfer usually requires written permission. Call ahead to the radiology and pathology departments to have your radiographic studies and pathology slides ready, and set a time to collect them. You or a family member should pick up the studies and bring them to your new physician (you don't want them getting lost in the mail).

You'll be choosing a hospital affiliation when you choose your new doctor. The hospital you decide on may be determined by the treatment you'll require or by medical insurance regulations. Because you're starting fresh, you should think through what kind of hospital you prefer. Do you want a community hospital close to home, with a readily accessible cancer center staffed by physicians trained in university hospitals, practicing alone or in a small group without a large team of medical students and residents-in-training? Or would you rather go to a large university hospital teaching center with claims of state-of-the-art equipment, new treatments, and access to a wide number of research protocols? In a way, you can do both: you might choose a community cancer center with a university hospital affiliation for breast surgery, radiation and chemotherapy, and the main university hospital center for more complex procedures, such as a bone marrow transplant.

Whatever decisions you need to make, stand firm for your rights and your best interest. Medicine is turning around, and patients have become more informed and assertive, but both doctors and patients are losing autonomy to managed health care systems. You need to assume a more active role in your health care and work with your doctor as a partner to obtain the full measure of the care that you need and deserve.

Who Sees You, How Often, and Why

Once you've reaffirmed your relationship with your doctor or selected a new one, it's time to establish a new routine for long-term care. You may have been caught up in your cancer care to the exclusion of your other health needs. When were you last at the dentist? Gynecologist? Eye doctor? All of you should be reassessed and paid attention to now, with a "holistic" perspective—a look at the big picture—rather than the bits and pieces of your medical care.

Your gynecologic needs may have changed because of tamoxifen treatment (see Chapter 7), natural or chemotherapy-induced menopause (see Chapter 18), or treatment side effects that may have sexual repercussions (see Chapter 12). Your general medical care should resume with attention to physical fitness, stress reduction, nutrition, and weight control; minimizing the risks of heart disease, diabetes, high blood pressure, and osteoporosis; and monitoring the small risk of uterine, ovarian, or colon cancer.

It's important for you to ask your team of cancer care doctors about follow-up schedules, so you can establish some kind of control over your time. Continuing care from this team will command the most attention in the spectrum of your health picture for the first five to ten years after treatment ends, when the risk of recurrence and the chance of having lingering side effects from treatment remain highest.

Some women see a separate gynecologist; some get full medical care from their primary care doctor. Some of these choices are controlled by your medical insurance plan. Your relationship with your doctor is essential, but, as I've said, it's a relationship in transition, as medical care is changing drastically. We don't know what changes will come, and what medical care will look like for the individual in the years to come.

Any doctor who participated actively in your cancer care should continue to see you for routine checkups; that may include a surgeon, a medical oncologist (if chemotherapy or tamoxifen was part of your care), and a radiation oncologist (if you had radiation). Most doctors see you one month after their particular treatment is finished, and then they'll want you to be seen every three or four months thereafter, either by themselves or by another member of the cancer center team. So, your surgeon will see you one month after surgery, your medical oncologist one month after chemo, and your radiation oncologist one month after radiation is completed. After that, for example, you might see your surgeon in January, your medical oncologist in April, and your radiation oncologist in July; that pattern then repeats. By alternating doctors in this way, you can minimize your visits to doctors' offices. This rotation system works, however, only if communication among your doctors is cooperative and agreeable. The opportunity to maintain this kind of scheduling may be restricted by your HMO.

Some doctors may decline to share follow-up care. They schedule their patients for checkups every three to four months, independent of other team doctors' schedules. Occasionally, a doctor may sign off your case, staying involved only through reports sent on by the doctors providing active care. The more serious your cancer is and the more treatment you have received, the more frequently your doctors will want to see you.

By the end of three years, lingering side effects of treatment have usually subsided or at least stabilized. As your risk of recurrence decreases, so does the frequency of your office visits. You can probably schedule visits every four to six months.

As more years go by, the risk of recurrence diminishes further: After five years, you'll probably need only twice-yearly follow-ups. After eight to ten years, checkups once a year will probably do. The risk of recurrence is so low after ten years that many oncologists recommend having your primary care physician conduct your checkups. For quite a number of women, in fact, their primary care physician has handled all follow-up ever since their treatment was completed.

Your follow-up schedule is not written in stone. You can tailor it to your needs, the recommendations of your health care team, and your convenience. I have patients who don't want to graduate to longer intervals between appointments because they want the reassurance of continued close supervision. Other patients have to be convinced that they need to see *any* doctor on such a regular, frequent basis. Most patients find comfort and encouragement in these steady visits (allowing, of course, for the anxiety that comes before each visit).

As medical insurance companies establish new regulations to streamline cost, your visits to specialists may be restricted. To protect your access to your cancer care physicians, you and your primary care physician may need to act with persistence to have these follow-up visits covered.

Who's in Charge?

The multidiscipline cancer center team with combined follow-up is a great concept with much to recommend it, but you may also discover its potential disadvantage: the fragmentation of your medical care. "One doctor examines my uterus and does a Pap smear. Another does my radiation. Another does my blood work; another, my arthritis; another, diabetes; another, my eyes; another, chemo. I'm all over the place! Who sees me as a whole person and puts all these pieces together?"

As you wind through treatment and healing, it's important to have *one* doctor who exercises a holistic approach to your care, keeping track of your physical, emotional, and social needs. This doctor talks to your specialists and makes certain that everything necessary for your care is arranged and scheduled, and happens. If you run into any problems as you go along, this doctor can run interference for you. If you are in an HMO, your primary care doctor is the gatekeeper of your care and may be managing more of your medical services than if you are in a non-HMO format.

Although your cancer care doctor may assume the dominant role in your overall care while you're undergoing cancer therapy, the best person to oversee this holistic approach to your medical care before, during, and after treatment is your primary care physician. She or he is used to covering that big picture for you, to being your advocate with other doctors and with your medical insurance company. The two of you may have enjoyed a longstanding relationship that predated your cancer diagnosis, and seeing each other reinforces the prospect of your return to the routine of a normal life.

You can't assume good communication among your doctors; your primary care doctor may be uninformed of your current status. You can take a personal role in this communication. Make sure that each of your doctors calls and/or sends progress reports to the others, and also make sure that x-ray and pathology reports are sent to every one of your doctors. Call or send a note to keep your primary care doctor personally informed of your progress.

The Complexity of the Doctor-Patient Relationship

The doctor-patient relationship is a powerful and generally long-term relationship. Both of you want to make it the best it can be, which takes work and effort by each of you. But there's an intrinsic imbalance in the doctor-patient relationship no matter how wonderful the doctor, no matter how fine the communication. Your doctor is the expert and may have more access to your medical information than you do, as well as a deeper understanding of its medical significance. Tests are an example: your doctor usually gets results before you do, and you may need help to understand what the test results mean. Besides all this, you're there because of a threat to your health, whereas he or she presumably is well. And it's *your* health and life on the line.

Another inherent imbalance between you and your doctor is the time, anxiety, and expectations leading up to an appointment. Compare your preparation to see the doctor with your doctor's preparation to see you. When did you make your appointment for your visit to your doctor? Weeks or months in advance? Maybe the appointment had to be changed because of bad weather or an unexpected conflict in your doctor's schedule. The day arrives. You super-shower, shave armpits and legs. (I no longer worry about dressing up for my doctor as I once did; most of the time he sees me only in that blue paper "gown" anyway, so why bother.) Are your reasons for making the appointment still relevant? Are there complications that make the appointment a nightmare to get to, like a sleepless night or a sick child, a no-show baby-sitter, car trouble, traffic, parking hassle, diarrhea? Are you anxious? Worried about the mammogram? Convinced doom waits? The rest of the world looks so normal and calm while you sit waiting, feeling so tense. Meanwhile, your doctor reviews your chart, x-ray, and pathology results, talks to the nurse who has seen you first, and maybe gets to speak to your other doctors. He or she is focused and caring, but the work is not as time consuming or as personally stressful as the preparation you have undergone. And there's more imbalance: It's their schedule, not yours. They're dressed, you're not. They touch you, you don't touch them. You reveal important private information, they reveal only their names and phone numbers.

You probably carry other sensitive issues to your appointment. What's the state of your self-image, and how does it get mixed up in the doctor-patient relationship? How do you feel about yourself? "Of course your doctor likes seeing you," said one woman to her good-looking friend. "You're attractive and young. I'm neither. I sometimes think it must be a drag to have to take care of a lumpy old bag like me." You should not feel any less well treated or respected than any other patient. Your doctors care about you whether you are young, old, thin, fat, beautiful, or plain. Most doctors see below the surface, and that's exactly where their focus needs to be.

No one likes to disrupt a smooth relationship or to lose the doctor's concern and interest; many try hard to please their doctors, to present themselves as attractive, appealing, and engaging. One woman, determined to make an indelible impression on her surgeon—so he'd remember her forever and always look forward to seeing her—took a magic marker and drew a "smiley face" on her chest, with the mastectomy scar as a smiling mouth.

You may grow particularly fond of your doctor and show your gratitude with letters or gifts. It's also not uncommon to develop a crush on your doctor. "My doctor was a little too handsome for my comfort back when I started with him; he was an active part of my fantasy life. Then over the years he put on weight, lost some hair, got a little puffy; it came as a relief to me. I felt a lot more comfortable with him."

Anger can also get mixed into the relationship. Anger that generates from your cancer diagnosis, treatment, and long waits has to express itself somewhere, sometime. "Why me? What did I do wrong?" Sometimes it lashes out against the doctor or his staff. A trivial incident, a thoughtless remark, or an overlong wait triggers an explosion. If anger gets in the way of treatment or care, you need to look into it and work through it in some constructive way.

Given all the threats to a harmonious relationship, attention to a few formalities can enhance the doctor-patient relationship: how you greet each other, what you call each other, and how the scene is set.

Greetings and Discussion

The first time or anytime, whenever you meet with a doctor, you should expect eye contact and a greeting, and an introduction to anyone in attendance with your doctor. If your doctor wants to invite students or residents to observe, he or she should first ask whether it's acceptable to you. You should feel comfortable saying no if you find that having an audience is intrusive. In turn, you should introduce anyone who has accompanied you, indicating that person's relationship to you. Just as doctors occasionally forget to introduce themselves, patients sometimes forget to identify the person or people they're with. If introductions are not forthcoming, I will introduce myself to whoever is with my patient.

After the greeting, it's time to discuss the purpose of your visit and raise any concerns. I may be unsure of what you want me to say if someone is with you. I sometimes check with my patients privately about what they find acceptable to discuss in front of the person they're with, even if that person is a husband or partner. With important, delicate matters—sex, for instance—I can't assume that they will want to discuss it with anyone, including their partner—or me.

Lesbian patients may have an extra burden in their struggle with cancer: Their doctors may find themselves uncomfortable in their presence, unable to make eye contact and awkward in dealing with their patient's partner. The medical community is generally conservative, but it is committed to giving you the best care possible. You may want to let your doctor know you are gay and to introduce your partner to your medical team, especially if she is your primary caregiver. If you have decided to keep your family in the dark about your personal life, you may be even more grateful for the backup support of your physician, so it's worth the effort of bringing your doctor and your partner together as part of your health care team.

Doctors can forget to give you the consideration and respect you're entitled to. "I took one of my children to a doctor last year, and wewere sitting in the examination room together when a substitute doctor walked in studying the chart and proceeded to ask questions. Then he started examining my child—without a friendly word to either of us. No eye contact, not even a smile or a nod, much less a greeting, so I interrupted him, introduced my child and myself, asked him his name, and finally he realized how rude he'd been."

When I meet a new patient, I make a point of letting her know I've prepared for our meeting. "Even though we haven't met before today," I might say, "I feel I know you a little: I've talked with your other doctors, I've read your medical records, and I've studied your x-ray and pathology reports." Then I tell something about myself, information every patient has a right to know about her doctor: my background, my qualifications, my special interest in breast cancer, and how my office and practice operate. We move on from there.

What's in a Name?

Are you comfortable with how you and your doctor address each other? It's never too late to have this discussion. If your doctor calls you Ms. or Mrs., you can assume he wants to be called Doctor, but if an older or old-fashioned doctor calls you by your first name, that's probably not a signal for you to do likewise; misguided or not, this may simply be his way of showing he cares about you. He probably assumes that your use of Doctor is more reassuring to you as a sign of authority and professionalism. Meanwhile, you may not like being addressed by your first name; maybe you find it patronizing. Do you speak up, or let it pass?

Most physicians go by Doctor, although younger doctors tend to be less formal and may be comfortable being called by their given names. But if your doctor is fresh out of training, he may believe he needs the title "Doctor" to feel secure and to enhance the therapeutic relationship (particularly if he looks as young as your child or grandchild). I needed the boost of that title when I started out; now I have a surer sense of myself as a physician and I'm comfortable when my patients call me Marisa: I still address many as Ms. or Mrs., but every relationship has its own subtle protocol. I once suggested a patient call me by my first name, and she was appalled. "I would never call you Marisa! With all your education and your years of training!"

Take your cue from your doctor on how he or she wants to be addressed, or just ask what he or she prefers, and tell what you prefer to be called. Remember, each of you has the privilege of being addressed the way you wish.

Why all this fuss about names? I think it provides an opportunity for an open discussion on a relatively neutral subject as you get to know each other. You figure out what to call each other, and the process becomes one of the building-blocks of your doctor-patient relationship; a way to get comfortable, a chance to feel things out, to show that you care and respect each other's independence, dignity, responsibility, and professionalism, and to decide whether you would like working together for what can be many years into the future.

That Clean Touch

When I go to my doctor, the office, the table paper, the gown, the doorknobs, and the nurse's and the doctor's hands better be really clean or I'm out of there. I especially don't like my doctor fingering his nose, mouth, or mustache, then reaching over to shake my hand or examine me. It's important for me to see my doctor wash in front of me—I'm not there to swap germs. A doctor's examination room is a busy place, and a doctor's hands go unmentionable places.

You may not give much thought to this issue, but your doctors should and usually do. I keep my nails short, and I start off the physical examination of my patients by washing my hands in front of them, or by apologizing for cold hands because they've just been washed. This fuss about hand-washing, besides being a health measure, is a way of letting patients know they are important and a way to help set the scene before we get on to what we're both there for.

Your Visit
Draft Your Questions

Figure out what you want to know from your doctor, and how you want to work together. We're all different, and your doctor can't presume to know how you want to handle your medical affairs and what questions and concerns you may have unless you communicate them. Some of my patients tell me they've read everything there is on the subject of breast cancer, and they are active and informed about decisions in their care. Others rely more heavily on me for up-to-date information and what choices are available to them. In any one day, I may see thirty people with different styles of handling information and making decisions.

Prepare a list of what you think is important to discuss: a symptom (don't hide any), questions, concerns, your child's troubling comment, a family wedding. *No question is trivial or stupid.* If something is on your mind, put it on your list. Some questions may scare you. Putting them in writing may help you defuse their fearfulness. "When I wrote out the things I was worried about, they seemed a little less frightening." Have your list of questions organized and in hand so you can ask them with ease; write them out in large, clear print on a single piece of paper, so you can read your notes without fumbling or missing a question that's important to you. Avoid the scribbled bits of paper patients often bring in for reference; they struggle to decipher their scrawled questions and soon give up trying because they can't read their own writing. Make things as easy as possible. You may feel nervous, anxious, and under pressure—especially if you're preoccupied with a specific question or concern, like what's in your test results or a new pain in an odd spot—and everything you planned to ask about just goes out of your head.

One caution: Don't ask your questions in the middle of your physical exam. Few people can do two things well at once. On the other hand, you can't wait until your doctor's hand is on the doorknob. The best plan is to tell your doctor right off—before the physical exam begins—that you have a list of questions, so enough time can be allotted to answering them. Then, when the exam is over or you are sitting in the doctor's office, bring up your major concerns first, so your anxiety can be dissipated as soon as possible. If you feel time is running out as you go down your list, ask how and when you can get answers to the rest of your questions.

Never assume one doctor knows when another doctor orders a test, and don't assume any doctor knows exactly when it was scheduled or that you are anxiously waiting for test results. I was examining a patient, then talking to her about her treatment. As we finished up, I realized she hadn't been following anything I'd been telling her. "Is something wrong?" I asked. "What about my bone scan?" she replied. "Bone scan? What bone scan? I didn't know you had a bone scan." She had spent our whole time together with something else on her mind, tight with fear, consumed by a test ordered by the oncologist she had seen the week before.

Ask your doctor if there are any important questions you haven't brought up, if there's more you should know or think about that you haven't been aware of. Your doctor's role as a communicator is to explain complex concepts in understandable words and images, and to give you access to information like test results, new drugs, or new protocols on the horizon.

"The scariest part of cancer is the sense that you've lost all control over your life," Lillian observed. When you assert yourself with questions and suggestions and collect information important to your health, you get to plan your life and make things happen—even if it's only simple things. Taking an active role in your health care is really the only way to give yourself that vital sense of control and to stay as healthy as possible. It also makes it easier for your doctor to take care of you.

Awkward Questions—from You or from Your Doctor

The questions on your mind may be difficult, potentially painful, and awkward—but jump in anyway, even if you don't feel warmed up to the inquiry. Your questions will get answered and out of the way, leaving you able to concentrate on the agenda of the day, on what your doctor has to ask you and tell you.

Expect to stumble over some awkward subjects, some problem you might not want to ask about. ("Why am I having such itching—you know, *there*?") You know you should ask, but the words won't come. Everybody has experienced this awkwardness, this embarrassment. Don't hesitate; say what's on your mind. Rise to the challenge, gather your courage, bring up the subject, and force out the words. Ask your questions, so you can find the best answers. It's well worth the temporary agony of speaking up.

You may not have to take the initiative. Many of the same questions occur to other women affected by breast cancer, so your health care team may already be aware of your concerns. You might get lucky; occasionally a doctor will anticipate your questions and phrase them for you. "Are you experiencing menopausal symptoms, such as vaginal dryness? Any discomfort with intercourse? Is weight gain after treatment keeping you out of appealing clothes and making you feel sexless? Do hot flashes wake you through the night, so you feel exhausted and useless during the day? Is the fear of recurrence imprisoning you, keeping you from living your life? Are you seriously down in the dumps, unable to discuss how you feel because you can't or won't add to the burdens of your family?"

Once in a while, you run into a doctor who comes on like gangbusters, with questions that knock you off your feet. I can still remember being startled over twenty years ago by the gynecologist at my college student health service. She asked the same questions of every student she saw: "Do you masturbate? Do you have anal sex?" I think she hoped to let students know she was open-minded and nonjudgmental. I'm not sure she succeeded; many women were simply scared off. But other women may have welcomed the opportunity to talk about what was on their mind.

It's a good thing for a doctor to ask about your sex life. It can be an important part of your life that may be profoundly affected by your breast cancer experience. Most women want to talk about it, but won't bring it up unless asked. Three women who shared the same gynecologist were talking about their gynecologic exams and the questions they were asked. The first woman said, "So then he asked me whether I had any concerns or questions about my sex life." "He didn't! He's never asked *me*." "He's never asked me either. Why you, not us?" After they talked it over together, they decided it was because the first woman was the most outgoing and outspoken of the three.

Don't be surprised if your doctor doesn't ask personal questions. Doctors are not generally trained in this sensitive area of care. Also, they may not have the answers you need, or they may be without the insight and experience required to come up with practical suggestions. In a recent study by the Living Beyond Breast Cancer$_{SM}$ organization, 63 percent of the women wanted to discuss sexuality with their health care giver (doctor, nurse, social worker); only 15 percent had actually had this discussion. Health care givers were more likely to discuss sexuality with women having few, if any, problems. Least likely to ask for help were women suffering the most significant problems with sexuality. So you may not be able to count on your physicians for help with delicate issues. They may be warm and caring, terrific at giving medical explanations, but decidedly uncomfortable talking about anything too intimate; they may have their own hang-ups and communication problems. If you're getting a lot from a particular doctor, you're not likely to trade that doctor in, but there should be someone on your team who can handle these issues for you: the nurse, your primary care physician, your gynecologist, the hospital social worker, or the support group therapist. Ask your doctor to direct you to others who can address your concerns.

There may be questions you don't want answers to. Not everyone wants to know all there is to know about this disease; some in particular don't want to know about their prognosis—especially if it's grim. In fact, very few of my patients ever ask. Respect your own limits regarding information.

A Second Set of Ears

To hear, understand, and retain as much information as possible during your visit to your doctor, bring someone along with you: your husband, partner, a close family member, or friend. Remember how distressed and confused you may have felt after that initial diagnosis, and how much of what your doctor told you, you forgot almost immediately? It can still happen. You can't fully process everything you hear when you're anxious, and being nervous or frightened can interfere with your ability to remember the information you're being given. You may need someone at your elbow who'll help you remember all that your doctor has to tell you in a short space of time.

It's very helpful to have that second set of ears when you're trying to catch and digest so much material important to your health, and bringing someone with you allows for shared reception and interpretation of information; together you can watch the doctor's face, listen to the tone of his or her voice, and catch any subliminal message. If you can't find someone to bring with you, consider using a tape recorder so you can replay and rehear what you may have missed the first time. But first make sure your doctor has no objection: Doctors may assume that the appearance of a tape recorder suggests you're preparing a lawsuit. If you explain your purpose, you should be able to defuse such an assumption.

Listening, Not Just for Answers

Many women try not to ask too many questions, no matter how badly they want the information, because they anticipate a brush-off or rejection from an overloaded, harried, or arrogant physician. (Patients don't want to be labeled a pain in the neck.) At the heart of this issue is the fact that patients are generally not encouraged to ask questions. Don't let yourself fall into this mind-set. You are paying for the doctor's services and are entitled to have your concerns addressed.

You might not have specific questions that need to be answered. You might just need a doctor to listen to the concerns you've been turning over in your head and to give you some kind of feedback. As you talk with your doctor, you realize it's the listening that matters. A doctor who listens is providing the ultimate in care: empathy, support, understanding. That listening may be the "answer" you've been looking for.

Before You Go Out the Door

Before you leave your doctor's office, take a moment to ask yourself these questions: Did my doctor listen to me? Did he or she answer all my questions? Did I understand what I was told? If not, let your doctor know.

Maybe you have more questions than the length of your appointment allows for answers. Don't let unresolved issues gnaw away at you. Be direct: "I know time is running short, but I still have questions. Do you have more time now, should we talk later by phone, should I make another appointment with you, or can you recommend someone else I might talk to?"

At the end of the visit to my doctor, I like some kind of physical contact: a pat on the shoulder, a handshake, or a hug. Whether you have been seated across from each other, separated by a desk, or side by side, your visit to your doctor is an intimate exchange. Your body has been bared, and you have revealed things about yourself you may have told no one else. That parting moment of physical contact connects the two of you spiritually, and signifies your importance as an individual, not just as a patient file or a health care number. Remember, it's a privilege for doctors to take care of you. And you probably feel privileged to have the care of good physicians. When you're happy with your doctor and your care, let your doctor know it. Positive feedback will enhance the quality of your relationship and your future health care.

Just One "Quick" Question

Occasionally I get a phone call from someone I know—or don't know—who doesn't want to come in for a comprehensive evaluation, but who wants to ask "one simple, quick question": "Should I take tamoxifen?" or "Should I get my silicone implant removed?" Such straightforward questions inevitably require complex answers that cannot be handled by phone, questions that involve many gray areas and ambiguities—and more than one right answer.

A whole range of detailed information is essential to supply thoughtful, responsible assistance if you're asking about tamoxifen, for instance: family history, stage of tumor, hormone receptor status of tumor, medical history (such as blood clots, uterine cancer, hysterectomy, or allergies), current history, and symptoms. In addition, a physical exam is necessary, plus lab and radiographic results. A doctor needs to review all of this information before giving a thoughtful answer.

Perhaps you're calling because you need a prescription filled or refilled. It's best to have the doctor who originally prescribed the medication renew the prescription for you. Patients often think any one of their doctors can renew a prescription for them: just a quick request. But a prescription is given for very specific reasons, and only the doctor who originally prescribed the medication for you should order your refill.

When you call your doctor for a refill, have your prescription or old bottle right in front of you, ready to read off the drug's name, amount given, and other information. Include the name and phone number of the pharmacy you want your doctor's office to call to fill your prescription. Know the pharmacy's hours, so that if you reach your doctor in the early morning, evening, or on a weekend, you are not asking him or her to call after it has closed. And even if you are a longtime, well-known patient of your doctor's, don't expect him or her to recall your specific allergies or medications. These are important details you can't expect anyone to know offhand, so automatically remind your doctor about any restrictions you have for medication and which medications you are presently taking. And if you have been prescribed a new drug, ask about drug-to-drug reactions. Supplying this information will help you get the best care possible.

When Should I, May I, Call?

How do you decide, after treatment is over, when it's important or simply okay to call your doctor with a question or concern? You should report any new, persistent, or possibly progressive symptoms such as fever, arm swelling, back pain, headaches, stress, or progressive weight gain. Ask those nagging questions that trouble your peace of mind. Although you may be seeing much less of your doctors than in the recent past, they are there for you when you feel you need them.

Second Opinions

If you decide, or your physician decides, to call in someone beyond your immediate health care team, that's asking for a second opinion. Second opinions are sought to enlarge the scope of information on which to base your care. The second opinion can offer additional information that corroborates what you've already been told, thus giving you welcome reassurance and security. You may also acquire a totally new perspective on the decision you are trying to make. A difference of opinion can be disconcerting and confusing but, at the same time, valuable.

Doctors should know and accept their limitations and be able to call someone else in for help or confirmation. They should not feel threatened when you feel you need more information before making a crucial decision. One health care professional can't take care of *all* your needs, not in today's world.

"My doctor told me I should have both breasts removed. I didn't feel I needed my breasts, and I didn't think it would make a difference to my husband. I was ready to go ahead, but my husband said, 'Let's just get a second opinion.' I told this new doctor I didn't need my breasts. 'Look at Nancy Reagan,' I said. He told me, 'You're not Nancy Reagan. You're not built like her, and you're not seventy-two years old. I recommend lumpectomy and radiation.' I went with his treatment after we talked it over, and I've never regretted it."

There is always enough time to get the information you need, even a third opinion if that's what's called for. (Some women get more than three opinions.) Linda got three differing opinions—and she became absolutely confused. "I thought they'd all agree, but they didn't. I found that very disturbing. I felt the doctors should have spoken to each other about my care and created a solid front. Each said what he felt was best, but it was left to me to sort through the advice and tie it all up." It's not uncommon to have a couple of different opinions without a clear consensus. There can be several correct ways of interpreting a medical problem. (It's not as though you're a car and there's just one way to fix you.)

The final word on a treatment decision is yours. If you are beyond your initial therapy, you may be deciding whether to have silicone implants removed, whether you should start tamoxifen, or whether to go ahead with the reconstruction you originally were unsure about. To that end, you need all the information and expert advice you can collect, even if it's confusing at first.

How to Work with Your Doctors When the Data Are Unclear

We all know that medicine is an inexact science, and sometimes a decision must be made based on insufficient data, without clear-cut answers. So how do you work with your doctors to settle on a course of action? How do you decide what's best for you? Should you start taking tamoxifen three years after you've finished your treatment for breast cancer? What is the healthiest diet for your needs? Will cutting fat to 20 percent of your caloric intake reduce your risk of recurrence? Is hormone replacement therapy safe for you? Should you remove your silicone implant?

You need to work with your doctors: Find the best information available (see the resource section at the back of this book) and come to the best decision possible, guided by your managing doctor's best medical judgment, your knowledge of your body, and your personal needs and wishes.

Your primary care physician can be especially helpful here, with the least investment in your specialists' presentations. She or he can facilitate discussion among consultants with differing opinions, suggest questions you should ask, and give you a perspective on choices and values and long-term considerations.

Listen to all information, gather all points of view (including those from family members closest to you), and think about each one carefully. Then find someone with whom to bounce around ideas. Make up a balance sheet of various topics: tamoxifen, for instance. Have one column listing which benefits from tamoxifen apply to you, and another column stating which side effects apply to you. Circle the factors that matter most. Finally, get back to your managing physician with your information and hammer out the details of your treatment decision together.

4

You and Other Health Professionals

> The tech who administered my radiation was the most wonderful person in the world. She tried to tell me one joke at least each time I saw her. But one time when I was feeling blue, she told me I needed to cry—and she cried along with me.

You've probably already met or worked with a number of the members of your health care team besides your doctor. These nurses, physician's assistants, technicians who administer your chemo- and radiation therapy, social workers, nutritionists, physical therapists, psychologists, chaplains, and secretaries are as much a lifeline and resource as your physician, and working with them effectively can do much for your outlook and welfare as you move toward recovery.

Nurses

Nurses do most of the frontline work in the hospital, delivering your chemotherapy, providing care before and after surgery and radiation, and working with your physicians. They're often the most accessible and attentive to your questions and concerns. "I was a grouch, but the nurses were gentle, soft-spoken, and very kind to me—and they were always ready to listen." Nurses can be your most helpful navigators within the system, identifying your needs and guiding you to solutions. But with cost-cutting what it is, hospital stays are short and the nursing staff has been drastically trimmed, along with the services they provide. Some jobs that were once the responsibility of registered nurses have now been passed on to nurses' aides, and, moving in the other direction, nurse practitioners have stepped into the shoes of primary caregivers; nurse practitioners may be managing many of your primary health care issues, working along with, or independent of, your doctor.

When you enter hospital inpatient care, you meet nurses in the operating room, recovery room, and, of course, in your hospital room, and you may get input from your nurses on which doctor to see. Nurses work as a team with your doctors in an outpatient setting as well—with your surgeon, radiation oncologist, and medical oncologist, in genetic clinics, and with your primary care physician. "If I had things on my mind, I'd ask the office nurse, and if she said it was okay, I could stop worrying."

A nurse practitioner may be the first person you see in medical and surgical practices. For example, in a surgeon's practice, a nurse practitioner may see you independently to check how your wound is healing, manage your drain, and change your dressings. Nurses in medical oncologists' offices draw blood, start your IV or access your port, administer the prescribed chemotherapy and follow you through treatment, help you manage side effects, and see you when you return to the doctor after treatment. A nurse may also assist you in a genetics testing program.

Visiting nurse services are evolving to expand in-home nursing assistance, much of which is covered by insurance. Oncology nurses are joining regular home care nurses in providing in-home nursing services, such as administering chemotherapy, growth factors, blood transfusions, and intravenous medication, and staying on with patients for an observation period after treatment. "My oncology nurse always made me laugh, made me feel so good I didn't mind the treatment; I felt I was being taken care of by a good friend." The pool of oncology nurses is growing, and now there is the Oncology Nursing Society, a professional organization of nurses who specialize in treating cancer patients.

Physician's Assistants

Physician's assistants (PAs) are trained to assist the physician with a full range of medical procedures. PAs have diverse backgrounds: Some received certification after a two-year program; others were first army paramedics or nurses who received further training in this specialty.

Physician's assistants generally work in individual medical or surgical practices and, depending on their particular background and experience, will have more or less responsibility and involvement in patient care. They assist the doctor by obtaining your initial history and performing a physical, arranging prescription refills, and finding answers to your questions.

You will probably appreciate the quick service and ready accessibility of the PAs, particularly when your doctor is occupied with another patient or is tied up in a meeting. The PA will facilitate your connection to your doctor, either by phone or in person, and smooth out the details when you come for an appointment. If, for instance, you've come in about your bone scan, the PA will have pulled your old films, obtained your newest films along with the report, and have it all lying on the doctor's desk when you arrive for your evaluation. The process of care becomes much more efficient, and you end up with more quality time with your doctor. In addition, here is one more person on your team who cares about you, and who may be the one most available to help you when you're seized with a burning question and can't reach your doctor.

Radiation Therapy Technologists

"The techs were great—people who talked to you rather than each other." Radiation therapy takes place every day for weeks, and it's the radiation therapy technologists who get to know you, who help you onto the table, position you, give you that daily treatment, and then help you off and out.

Radiation technologists do a lot more for you than turning a machine on and off. They work closely with your doctor during the initial planning simulation that maps out the fields to be radiated, and then they treat those designated areas when you come in each day. They see you often, and can really get close to you. "My tech was absolutely wonderful. She made a potentially frightening experience one I actually looked forward to. Our chats and the support she gave me were invaluable. She had the ability to cut any situation down to size for me, and I will always be grateful for the sense of well-being she gave me."

If the tech doesn't think you're feeling or looking well, or you know you're not feeling right but you're not scheduled to see your doctor, your tech will let the doctor know so you can be evaluated while you are still on the premises. A lot of patients truly miss this connection and support when their treatment finally stops.

Social Workers

Hospital cutbacks may have compromised or even curtailed your access to a social worker, especially for follow-up assistance. The social workers at the hospitals where I work are now doing at least twice the work they signed on for.

Social workers handle the complex logistics of situations you might otherwise find overwhelming, making health care delivery as accessible and manageable as possible. They help arrange insurance coverage for home-care nursing, medications at discount, food supplements such as Ensure, wigs, transportation to and from hospitals or doctors' offices, coordination of free services and resources, community services, and hospice. They may also help settle bills and arrange for medical assistance. "My social worker was outstanding. I don't think I could have managed my treatment if she hadn't helped arrange the day-to-day details." Social workers also lead support groups or provide individual counseling, and often work to ease family stress in a more relaxed setting. They work through the hospital and through in-home care services, such as hospice.

Nutritionists

A nutritionist may be assigned to help with your health care, particularly if you are having a problem gaining or losing weight. Traditional nutritionists are generally hospital based, and few patients actually get to meet them. You can request their assistance, but you won't get cutting-edge alternative dietary advice from most of them, because they have a conventional scientific background, and their focus is on helping you achieve a balanced healthful diet. Most nonhospital, private nutritionists specialize in healthful eating and weight control. It's hard to find nutritionists who specialize in cancer prevention, although a few work in innovative centers that attempt to combine state-of-the-art cancer therapy with the latest nutritional treatment, such as the Block Medical Center in Evanston, Illinois. Others provide an alternative nutritional and vitamin approach entirely separate from cancer treatment services. "I have a nutritionist with an alternative background, and she's been very encouraging. She gives me tips for a much healthier lifestyle."

Finding a reputable and effective nutritionist is no easy task. Ask for suggestions from The Wellness Community, local breast cancer organizations, your doctor, your nurse, and members of your support group. Make an appointment with a nutritionist and ask about his or her qualifications and approach to your care. Ask how this approach will be integrated with your conventional therapy, how much it will cost, and how the results will be assessed, and when. Watch out for the nutritionist who makes grandiose claims, promising results for an endless list of diseases or enormous benefits for exactly your kind of cancer. Be cautious if he or she constantly criticizes conventional medicine or insists that you pursue nutritional therapies to the exclusion of other treatments. Avoid high-cost therapies that come from a bottle instead of the vegetable stand. And don't be a slave to a complicated, time-consuming, costly, and rigid nutritional regimen.

Physical Therapists

Physical therapists provide postoperative care for women who have had breast and lymph node surgery. After lymph node resection, you may be unable to raise your arms enough to complete your prescribed course of breast radiation therapy; physical therapy can improve your arm mobility and reduce tenderness and pain.

A physical therapist can teach you how to use your arms to recover your range of motion and strength, how to reintroduce exercise, and how to manage pain. Most problems can be resolved after a few weeks of treatment that can include stretches, exercises, massage, and water therapy. "My physical therapist was supportive and encouraging. She kept telling me, 'Everything will be all right. Everything will work again.' I got individual instructions, slowly, and it was a real boost." Physical therapists also help with prevention and management of arm edema (see Chapter 10).

Psychologists

You're most likely to come in contact with a psychologist if you join a support group. Trained in the science of human behavior, usually with a master's degree, psychologists are qualified facilitators of support groups as well as provide individual therapy.

Dealing with breast cancer requires adjustment to new physical and emotional conditions and new ways of looking at your life. A support group can help you deal with this situation (see Chapter 2), but sometimes you need more help; individual counseling might work better for you. Most health insurance plans provide minimal, if any, coverage for psychotherapy, pointing to the absence of conclusive data proving its benefit. Generally, HMOs pay only for crisis care, or about ten sessions of therapy over a one- or two-year period. Co-payments are high; limitations on fees encourage the use of psychologists rather than psychiatrists. (Psychiatrists are physicians with advanced training in mental disease; their fees are usually higher than those of psychologists.)

Chaplains

Most hospitals have a chaplain on staff, who qualifies in a broad sense as a health care provider. Many women who have breast cancer seriously question their faith in God at some point. "How could God have let this happen to me?" And they are angry that their body has betrayed them, allowing cancer cells to destroy their well-being. "Is there a spiritual meaning to all this?" they ask. "Was this some kind of test from God?" A chaplain can help you work out these spiritual questions, to reconcile these conflicting feelings and gain better insight and perspective.

As outpatient care supplants inpatient service, chaplains have expanded their role to circling through the emergency room and checking with patients who come and go within twenty-four hours. Chaplains traditionally visit patients before they go for surgery, and they respond to suggestions from medical and other hospital staff members to visit patients who are in particular need of spiritual counseling. A visit from the hospital chaplain doesn't mean you're going to die. Most chaplains drop by to check things out, but don't push themselves on patients who aren't interested in their services. Chaplain services are supposed to be nondenominational.

If you spend more than a day or two in the hospital, you may particularly welcome a visit from someone who isn't there to take your blood or blood pressure, but who just wants to talk and provide comfort and support. The more you learn about healing and the spirit, the more you may value the opportunity to speak to a hospital chaplain when you're in such a highly stressed situation. It may be the first step in gathering some form of support to help you recover from the breast cancer experience. Any way you want to look at it, prayer enhances healing.

Secretaries

Don't forget the secretaries, the essential communicators for your doctors, nurses, and technologists. They take phone messages; coordinate procedures, tests, and visits; and facilitate treatment. Before you arrive for your appointment, they make sure your file is complete. If your x-rays are missing, they spend time tracking them down. If your appointment runs late, they call your next obligation. They do the paperwork and billing, communicate with your medical insurance company, check the referral process from your primary care doctor to your specialists, and make sure all forms have been properly filled out. In many quiet, unseen ways, they smooth your passage through treatment and beyond.

Getting Along with Members of Your Team

These other members of your health team can make your treatment experience tolerable, outstanding, or a disaster. Generally speaking, anyone who goes into these professions does so because she or he cares about people, so it's infrequently that you bump into someone who turns you off or upsets you. But it happens, and if it happens to you, don't let it go by without trying to set things straight.

Of course you want everyone to like you and enjoy taking care of you—and you're probably afraid of alienating *anyone* who is in a position to help you (and who, you fear, might sabotage your care). What a bind! I tell my patients I want to hear about anything that bothers them. I've listened to many accounts of difficult interactions, and assumed an important role in working things out. Most problems can be fixed, and confidence restored between patient and caregiver. Usually the problem resulted from some misunderstanding or miscommunication.

If you feel prepared to speak up yourself, do so. "When you spoke to me so sharply, you really upset me. I'm not used to being spoken to that way." You may be nervous doing it, but you'll feel good about yourself afterward. If you don't feel comfortable handling the problem directly, speak to your physician, the charge nurse, or the hospital's patient ombudsman or patient-relations person. Every hospital or office practice has some way of responding to patients' concerns and resolving conflicts; a patient-relations representative will help you get attention, better care, a switch in your caregiver, or maybe just an apology.

Most patients tell me only good things about the health staff support people. "The techs always listen." "That nurse brought me flowers and she hardly knew me!" A smile and a warm thank-you are always appreciated, and can make someone's day brighter and better.

When people are particularly helpful or kind, I like to do something thoughtful to acknowledge what they have done. It doesn't have to be much, just something that says thank-you in a personal and meaningful way, such as bringing bagels or doughnuts now and then when you come in for treatment. More significant is a word or a note to a superior—the head nurse, the head tech, or, even better, the president of the hospital. Letters count big time: They can help a worker feel better about her job and can even help with a raise or promotion.

5

Tests: Peer, Poke, Prod

I wasn't looking for surprises or trouble; I just wanted to keep watch over my health, have the routine mammogram my doctor told me to get. Something worried somebody, because I had to have more pictures, then come back for a biopsy. I thought that would be like a needle stick—but it was a real operation. I should have been warned about that, but I can't really complain. What they took out was benign, and I'm okay.

Tests can be nerve-racking and a nuisance, but they are an indispensable part of your diagnostic evaluation and continuing care. Mammography is the most important tool we have to detect early evidence of breast cancer. About one third of breast cancers are found by mammography alone, one third are palpable lumps also seen on mammography, and one third are found by physical examination alone (not seen on mammography). Most of the lumps found by touch are found by the women themselves or by their partners.

High-magnification mammograms, ultrasound, magnetic resonance imaging (MRI), bone scans, computed axial tomography (CAT) scans, and positron emission tomography (PET) scans may all be part of your follow-up treatment. If a finding is abnormal, you may need a biopsy as well. You'll also need blood tests and other studies periodically.

You may be skeptical of all these tests and possibly angry that we have nothing better with which to detect the presence of cancer, particularly if your breast cancer never showed up on mammography. But as more money is funneled into breast cancer research, a simple, more accurate, and inexpensive test to detect the earliest signs of breast cancer will be developed. Until then, we have to use the best tests currently available. I'll review them here.

Mammography

Background

Mammography, or x-ray photography of the breast, has been in active use as a diagnostic tool for breast cancer for only about thirty years. It wasn't till the 1960s that mammography's usefulness as a screening device for women with no breast cancer signs or symptoms was recognized. Not till the 1970s, with reduced radiation and exposure time, did it gain general acceptance and use.

Mammography is used to detect breast cancer tumors as early as possible (even before they can be found by physical examination), when breast cancer is most curable. It is also effective for evaluating a palpable mass in the breast.

Mammography does not prevent breast cancer, but, by finding breast cancer as early as possible, it does save lives. It lowers the death rate from breast cancer by 35 percent in women over fifty, and recent studies suggest it may lower the death rate for women between forty and fifty by 25 to 35 percent. Controversy still clouds the issue of whether women between forty and fifty should have mammograms every year or every other year. But leading experts, the National Cancer Institute, the American Cancer Society, and the American College of Radiology (ACR) now recommend annual mammograms for women after age forty, because the reduction in death rate means real lives saved.

Technique

Film screen mammography (the technique used in most centers today) involves minimal radiation exposure, about a quarter of a rad, and takes only a matter of seconds for each x-ray picture. A skilled technologist positions and compresses the breast between two plates. Then an extremely specialized camera takes two pictures of each breast from two directions (north–south, east–west). Only mildly uncomfortable for most women, mammography can be painful for some. But the compression of the breast, which is what causes the discomfort, is necessary to flatten it and reduce the thickness of the breast so the x-ray beam can visualize as few layers of overlapping tissues as possible.

If you have had breast cancer surgery, it's helpful to have the technologist mark both ends of your scars with BBs. These small metal balls, taped on the skin, show up on the film and indicate where treatment-induced scar tissue now lies. Your scar helps define the surgical bed where the breast cancer used to be—the site with the highest risk of recurrence.

Digital mammography technique is identical to film screen mammography, except that instead of recording the image of the breast on film, the image is recorded directly into a computer. Once the image is registered within the computer, it can be manipulated and enhanced in many ways. If there is a suspicious area of asymmetry or increased density or calcification, the computer can take a closer look at the area, without having to take more breast pictures. This technique is both more expensive and less available than routine mammography.

Site

You should have mammography only at a center that is accredited by the ACR. Quality is a critical issue. The ACR has guidelines that set standards not only for the doctors who read the films, but also for the technicians, reports, mammography machines, and even film-developing materials. If, after a full review, quality standards are met, the site becomes ACR approved.

Mammography can be performed in a mobile unit, in a free-standing center, or in a traditional hospital setting. The quality of mammographic equipment generally depends more on its age than on where it is located. Choose your mammography center carefully. Call the National Cancer Institute (800-4-CANCER) or the American College of Radiology (800-227-5463) for the nearest certified mammography provider.

Evaluation

Mammogram films can be read just after they have been developed, or at a later time and place. In a center with a radiologist present, films are reviewed while you wait to make sure the entire breast has been pictured and that anything unusual or suspicious can be further pictured or evaluated, and you are usually spared having to come back at a later time for more pictures. Further evaluation of a potential abnormality can be done with magnified mammogram images or ultrasound.

Some centers arrange to have two radiologists read each evaluation study separately and sequentially, to reduce the possibility of missing a lesion. Two readings of each study improve the accuracy of the interpretation, picking up 10 to 15 percent more cancers than only one reading. It's unlikely that films will be double-read while you wait;

the second reading is generally done at a later time just prior to writing the official report.

The digital mammography computerized image of the breast is manipulated for optimal analysis and interpretation. For instance, images can be enlarged or magnified, contrast can be varied, and particular areas can be highlighted. The computerized images can be read both by a radiologist and by a Computer-Aided Diagnosis program; the two interpretations are integrated within the report. It is not yet known how the live radiologist compares in accuracy to the computer; we don't have the data—the technology is too new. We do know that regular film screen mammograms first read by a radiologist and then later digitalized into the computer as a "second opinion" constitute a sensitive technique with a low false-negative rate (that's when the test says everything's okay, when in fact something is wrong). The computer misses very little, but it also overinterprets or exaggerates breast changes that are likely to be benign (that's called low specificity, high false-positive rate). Please stay tuned: Studies are now under way to define the effectiveness of computerized digital mammography. Finally, the computerized image can be transmitted electronically to another, distant location (anywhere in the world) for interpretation or for an interactive consultation between two radiologists. However, this technology is not yet widely available.

If at all possible, I prefer an on-site radiologist because of the adequacy and accuracy of the study, attention to scars, and faster test results—especially for women who have had a previous breast biopsy (even if it was benign), who have a personal or family history of breast cancer, or who have just discovered a lump in their breast.

Mammography After Reconstruction

Some doctors recommend that you have a mammogram every six months, until the effects of treatment have settled and your results have stabilized. At the least, you'll need a mammogram once a year.

Most doctors believe mammography of a breast reconstructed from grafted tissue is not clinically useful, because essentially no breast tissue is present. There are times, nonetheless, when mammography under these circumstances may be helpful: if a woman is at high risk for local recurrence where the breast used to be, if manual palpation of the tissues is difficult, or if there is a questionable finding. I have seen several recurrent breast cancers detected this way in women who have had TRAM reconstruction. (See Chapter 6.) Be aware that reconstructed tissue can form small calcifications, visible on mammography, which usually represent benign fat necrosis. (Some fat cells die after the transfer procedure, forming calcifications.) Fat necrosis can also manifest as palpable lumps.

Occasionally, a woman who has had a very large lumpectomy may be left with significant distortion of the breast. She may choose to have the missing area reconstructed with transplanted tissue, preceded or followed by radiation to the remaining breast tissue. Mammographic interpretation after this type of combined treatment can be quite tricky. Once a baseline mammogram has been established, however, and treatment effects have "cooled," mammograms usually become easier to interpret.

Women who have had a mastectomy and reconstruction with saline or silicone implants don't need mammograms of the affected site because essentially no residual breast tissue remains and the implant, which appears as an opaque white oval, obscures visualization of the surrounding tissues. An implant, however, does not interfere significantly with manual palpation of the area at risk, because the implant is out of the way, inserted behind both the muscle and the at-risk soft tissues of the chest.

Ultrasound

Ultrasound is a diagnostic tool that produces high-frequency sound waves that travel through the breast and are transformed into images appearing on a monitor. Ultrasound can detect many breast abnormalities, determining size, shape, consistency, and location. It is complementary to mammography, allowing further interpretation of what was first seen on mammography, to determine if the lesion is solid (such as a benign fibroadenoma or cancer) or fluid filled (such as a benign cyst).

Ultrasound would be the first method of radiographic evaluation for a woman under thirty with a palpable breast lump. Mammograms are difficult to interpret in younger women, because younger women's breasts tend to be glandular rather than fatty, and gland tissue appears densely white on x-ray, much like a cancerous tumor. (Locating an abnormality in such an x-ray is like locating a polar bear in a snowstorm.) Most breast lumps in young women are benign cysts or clumps of normal glandular tissue.

If a biopsy is ordered, ultrasound can be employed to guide biopsy needles precisely to suspicious spots in the breast.

Ultrasound is not a substitute for a screening mammogram; its value as a general screening test for breast cancer is unproven.

Chest X-rays

Chest x-rays are most commonly ordered for medical reasons not directly related to breast cancer, such as pneumonia, asthma, heart disease, diabetes, lung cancer, or asbestos exposure. A simple x-ray (two views: front to back and side to side) produces a picture of the entire chest. Its specific role for women with breast cancer is to evaluate the small possibility that breast cancer may have spread to the lungs, and to assess the heart and lungs prior to general anesthesia or chemotherapy.

In women with metastatic disease to the lung, a chest x-ray is used to follow the status of the disease's response to treatment.

Chest x-rays may also be used for women who sustain a fever during chemotherapy, to evaluate the possible presence of pneumonia (infection of the lung). If a woman who has had radiation therapy within the past few months experiences new shortness of breath, with or without a cough, a chest x-ray may be ordered to see if there is any radiation-caused inflammation or scarring of the lung.

The chest x-ray is no longer used as a routine screening test for lung cancer or tuberculosis. Screening chest x-rays for lung cancer do not improve survival, and the incidence of tuberculosis is minimal.

Bone Scans

Bone scans are obtained by injecting radioactive material into the blood system, where it is taken up by bone-making cells. Areas of intense bone activity (common in both cancer and arthritis) appear as dark patches on radiation-sensitive monitors. The greater the bone cell activity, the darker the image. If cancer is present, dark patches are visible around the cancerous spots where bone cells are busy making new bone to patch the holes cancer has created. Any part of the bone can be affected with cancer.

If arthritis (inflammation of the joint) is present, radioactive material shows up on bone surfaces of joints. Bone scan abnormalities from cancer can usually be distinguished from arthritis on the basis of location, but arthritis and cancer are hard to distinguish from one another in scans of the spine (which is made up of many bones and joints), so changes in the spine may require additional studies and evaluation.

A baseline bone scan study is often done at initial diagnosis and staging for women who have invasive breast cancer. There is no need for yearly bone scans in the absence of symptoms. The exam is expensive and time consuming, and it doesn't improve the quality of life or length of survival. (If bone metastases were to occur, finding them a little earlier by bone scan rather than waiting for active symptoms does not improve outcome.) But for a woman experiencing persistent back or leg pain, a repeat bone scan that shows no change from the baseline study can prove reassuring. Back pain is a common complaint for a great many people, but for the woman who has had breast cancer, it can create anxiety and immediately awaken the fear of recurrence.

Bone scans are unnecessary for women with noninvasive breast cancer.

Magnetic Resonance Imaging

Magnetic resonance imaging (MRI) is a powerful diagnostic tool that uses magnetic fields, not radiation, to create images of the body. You lie on a table and are moved in and out of a doughnut-shaped structure. The machine makes a thumping sound, and confinement within the doughnut can be claustrophobic for some people. (Some facilities have an open MRI machine to avoid this problem.) A magnetic field is pulsed on and off around the part of the body under study. When it is on, the cells are excited and start spinning; when it is off, the cells relax, giving off a special signal that is received by an amplifier and then translated into an image. The area to be studied can be better distinguished from normal surrounding tissues by injecting the contrast agent gadolinium.

The value of MRI for breast cancer detection remains undefined. Some doctors believe MRI can distinguish a breast cancer from normal breast gland tissue better than other techniques. But MRI is expensive, and it requires highly specialized equipment and highly refined expertise to interpret the findings, available in few MRI centers. Even with the best MRI facilities and experts to read the test, there is usually a broad range of findings, many of uncertain significance, called "unidentified bright objects" (UBOs). Only with a laborious process of breast imaging and biopsy, followed by careful clinical, radiographic, and pathologic correlations, can we learn which UBOs require further biopsy and which can be left alone.

It's therefore unlikely that MRI will be used as a general screening tool for breast cancer. It may, however, prove useful in evaluating a woman who has a palpable mass not visible with ultrasound or mammography, or it may be helpful in assessing a lesion in the densely glandular breast of a young woman, where it's very difficult to analyze the area by any other imaging method. It may in fact become an important screening test in women who are at high risk for cancer, such as young women with an abnormal breast cancer gene.

MRI scanning is particularly useful in detecting leakage from a silicone-filled breast implant. Silicone gel has its own characteristic appearance on MRI, easily distinguished from surrounding normal breast and chest wall tissues.

MRI can also be used to evaluate other parts of the body. A woman who has progressive back pain, or who develops a new weakness or numbness in the arms or legs (not just hands or feet), can have an MRI scan done of her back to evaluate the possible presence of a tumor in the backbone surrounding the spinal cord. The scan can also be used to assess the possibility of brain metastasis.

Computerized Axial Tomography

Computerized axial tomography, or CAT scan, is x-ray imagery of consecutive cross sections of the body, which allows detailed study of a specific area. As for an MRI, you lie on a moving table, passing through a doughnut-shaped machine that creates a composite, synthesized image of the part of the body being studied.

CAT scans are not used routinely to evaluate breast conditions. In a woman with a large breast cancer, a surgeon may order a CAT scan to assess whether the cancer is removable by mastectomy or if it is unresectable because of invasion into the chest wall.

CAT scans are used to evaluate the liver, spine, or any other particular area in detail. If a woman has progressive headaches or double vision, CAT scans may be used to rule out metastases in the brain. If a woman has known metastatic disease, CAT scans of the head, chest, and abdomen may be performed to assess the extent of metastatic disease prior to treatment, and periodically during treatment to evaluate response.

PET Scans

A positron emission tomography (PET) scan is one of the newest breast cancer diagnostic techniques, and it is still in the experimental phase. The patient is injected with a small amount of radioactive material that is taken up by metabolically active cells, which are characteristic of brisk cancer proliferation. Areas of high metabolic activity, suspect for cancer, are identified by their bright appearance. Once localized, they can be further evaluated with other techniques.

Early results of PET scanning in women with breast cancer show a number of important possibilities, in particular an early assessment of a tumor's viability after radiation or chemotherapy, and cancer involvement of axillary lymph nodes, without extensive surgical dissection.

PET scans, in clinical use for only a few years, are available in only a very few centers. This is an expensive, sophisticated test that requires exceptional expertise, and whose value as a diagnostic tool has not been consistently established. It is also not reimbursable by most medical insurance plans.

Blood Tests

Blood tests can assess the health of different organs and systems in your body. Blood tests include blood cell counts, blood chemistries, and blood cancer markers.

Blood Cell Counts

A full lineup of immune cells that defend your body against foreign invaders can be measured with blood cell counts. Immune cells can be significantly reduced by chemotherapy and, to a lesser extent, by localized radiation therapy. These cells are therefore checked before each chemotherapy cycle to make sure your body is able to tolerate the next dose of treatment. The cells may also be checked during a course of radiation, depending on how large an area is treated and whether chemotherapy is given at the same time. If your immune cells are significantly reduced, growth factors can be given to boost levels. (Neupogen is an example.)

Other blood cells that can be measured are your red blood cells— the cells that carry oxygen from the lungs to your body's tissues. Measurements of hemoglobin and hematocrit are a way of quantifying your blood's oxygen-carrying capacity. These indices reflect the amount and concentration of the complex protein molecules in the red blood cells that transport oxygen from your lungs to your tissues. The number of platelets in your blood can also be counted. (Platelets are involved in the formation of clots to prevent bleeding.) All these components can be reduced by cancer therapy, blood loss, and chronic illness. All blood cell counts are therefore closely monitored during chemotherapy. You may need blood transfusions or growth factors such as epogen/Procrit to increase your counts.

Blood Chemistries

Blood chemistries are used to evaluate the overall function of the liver by measuring the levels of liver enzymes (special proteins that facilitate vital chemical reactions) and bilirubin (a substance that helps break down fat). Other blood chemistry levels are also important: Your potassium, chloride, and urea nitrogen levels reflect the health of both the liver and the kidneys; calcium levels reflect your bone and kidney health; and blood sugar tests are used to follow people with diabetes and people who are taking steroids.

Cancer Markers

If cancer is present and it is the type that produces a specific substance (usually a protein) that can be measured in the blood, that substance can become a "marker" for cancer. CEA, CA 15.3, and TRU-QUANT are examples of such measurable proteins.

Some doctors consistently rely on markers as an early indicator of disease progression or recurrence, in order to find a local, curable tumor, or to assess response to chemotherapy. The clinical usefulness of these cancer markers, however, has some limitations. A marker test that registers normal does not prove that you are cancer free, nor does an elevated test mean that you positively have progression or recurrence of cancer. Using markers to find metastatic cancer earlier has not yet translated into a survival benefit.

Biopsy

Biopsies are done for palpable lesions or for any lesion that looks suspicious on a radiographic study, palpable or not. Only about 20 percent of biopsies turn out to be malignant, which might suggest that many of the biopsies we do are unnecessary. In this country, patients and physicians are unwilling to ignore a questionable image, because missing a breast cancer, or delaying the diagnosis of a breast cancer, is unacceptable, especially because a biopsy can be a relatively simple procedure. (It can, however, cost the woman who undergoes this form of breast surgery considerable anxiety, apart from economic cost.) In Sweden, where medical cost accounting is much stricter than it is here, 80 percent of biopsies turn out to be malignant because only the most suspect lesions are biopsied.

Various techniques are used to biopsy tissue. A surgeon tries to make a tissue diagnosis with the least invasive procedure. *Needle biopsy* of palpable lesions is the very least invasive and can be done in the doctor's office. Using a hollow-center needle, the surgeon obtains material from the area in question for microscopic analysis. Results are generally available in twenty-four hours. *Incisional biopsy* involves taking a small piece of tissue from a lump for sectioning and examination. This procedure is done if the needle biopsy is inconclusive and if the lump, mammographic change, or suspicious rash is too extensive or too big to be removed, or to be removed easily. The disadvantage of both needle biopsy and incisional biopsy is a possible inconclusive result because of sampling error; the advantage is a fast result. *Excisional biopsy* is an attempt to remove the entire lump of tissue. This is the surest way to establish the diagnosis without sampling error. If the lump is completely removed, the biopsy also has therapeutic value and can give you peace of mind. Both incisional and excisional biopsies can be done in an outpatient surgery center.

Needle localization guides a biopsy of a nonpalpable lesion detected by mammography, so the surgeon can find it and remove it. A long, thin needle is placed in the lesion with mammographic or ultrasound guidance. When the needle reaches the lump, a collapsible hook at the end of the needle keeps the needle in place until the surgery is accomplished. (Local anesthesia can be used to reduce the discomfort.) X-rays are done of the removed tissue to verify that the abnormal area seen on the original x-rays is within the excised tissue specimen. *Stereotactic needle biopsy* involves multiple core biopsies of a nonpalpable lesion using a complex localizing technology and a hollow-center needle.

Tissue removed by the various types of biopsy is then examined with a microscope for cancer cells.

Biopsies are not medical emergencies and can be scheduled at your earliest convenience. But for peace of mind, most women want their biopsies done yesterday. Before proceeding with a biopsy, your doctor should review the mammogram in question with you, show you the area of interest, discuss how and why the biopsy is to be performed, answer any of your questions, and arrange for you to sign any consent forms required.

Test Results

Results While You Wait

Everyone wants to get test results immediately. But when your doctor orders a test, the nurse or staff in the lab or radiology department does the scheduling; your doctor isn't likely to know exactly when the test actually gets done and when the results are available until the report comes into the office three to seven days later (depending on the facility and the kind of test ordered). Meanwhile, you're probably thinking your doctor has the news and isn't getting back to you.

Each center has its own policy regarding presentation of mammography results, good news or not. Some tell you all results on the spot; other centers will not reveal any information directly to you, no matter how you insist.

It may be possible to get the results of your mammogram right away at a center that has a radiologist present to review your study. If your test is negative (that is, it shows no abnormality), you're given the information and you go home. If your films are suspect, however, you may or may not be informed at the time; you might just be told you'll be hearing from your physician. (But you may already suspect something because of the extra views you've been called back for.)

In general, the best person to give you your mammography results is the doctor who recently examined your breasts and ordered the study. This doctor knows you best. Some radiologists regularly perform both the mammogram and the physical exam, in which case an immediate reading of your study is appropriate. Many women want an instant interpretation of their mammogram by the reading radiologist even if there are no physical examination correlations. They don't want to wait till their physical exams can be assessed or their referring physician notified, but it can be very awkward for one doctor to tell another doctor's patient any news, particularly bad news.

When I get a mammogram, I need to know my results right away, and I selected my mammography center based on its medical reputation for quality *and* its commitment to immediate communication of results. Linda felt the same way: "I don't wait anymore. I was such a good girl in the beginning: 'Yes sir, no sir,' I'd spend a week in agony. I finally became assertive enough to get what I wanted. I had this mammogram, and my doctor says to me, 'We'll tell you as soon as the results come in.' 'No, now. I'm not leaving. I don't need to wait for a written report.' And he looks, and he tells me the results!" If you are the kind of person who must have results quickly to prevent anxiety, choose a high-quality center that will accommodate your wishes. Unless your mammography center has an explicit policy to the contrary, as long as there is a radiologist on-site who can read your mammogram, your demand for immediate results can usually be met.

If you have come in for a mammogram without a doctor's referral, the delivery of test results can be more complicated. An experienced radiologist regularly has this dilemma: "If a woman has no referring physician, it may be hard to reach her after she leaves. I may be the only doctor at hand who can tell her the results and recommend further evaluation. She has a right to the information and she does need to know it."

Regardless of who orders the mammogram, who does it, and who reads it, some immediate feedback is needed if you are called back for extra views. Ask to speak to the radiologist who will be reading your mammogram so you aren't left to go home feeling puzzled and anxious.

Results at a Later Time

Not every result can be determined immediately, and often the information gained is limited without radiologic interpretation joined with full knowledge of your medical background and physical examination findings. That can mean two physicians connecting to discuss results, bringing together whatever information is necessary to make an accurate interpretation, and more delay. Agony or not, sometimes you can't be spared that wait. The likelihood is that it won't take a whole week.

Some doctors have a standing policy requiring all patients to come in for all results, good or bad, so the request "Come in to my office" is routine, not the signal of doom. But if you want results as soon as possible and your doctor has too busy a schedule to allow you to come in on the spot, you may opt for the results-by-phone system—whether the news is good or bad.

To expedite the process, call your doctor when you've completed the test; leave a specific message stating exactly what you are calling about: what test was done, when it was done, where it was done, where you will be, providing all your phone numbers and when and till how late at night, to call. In this way, your doctor can get back to you and give you the information you want as soon as it's in hand. You may also want to specify just what information can be passed on to you through a third party if you miss the call and someone else takes it for you, or, if you are out, what information may be left for you on your answering machine.

Save yourself stress and phone-tag hassle. Make an appointment for that phone call, realistically allowing a time frame between, say, one and three o'clock, arranging in advance that if you don't hear from your doctor by three o'clock, *you will call him or her back*. This way, you won't be stranded waiting, and you can plan to have someone around when you get the call—just in case. Usually, test results are easily presented and discussed over the phone, but occasionally they are going to be complex, or possibly unfavorable.

Your doctor may not be able to get back to you right away because she or he may not yet have connected with the radiologist who read the test, or with the laboratory that conducted the blood test or pathology analysis. Many centers insist that the radiologist who establishes the finding must pass it on directly to the referring physician, to avoid any slippage, misplacement, or loss of information—but it may be hard to make that connection. Doctors are busy and often are unavailable at the moment of a call, and information can lie idle. If your mammogram is unremarkable, your doctor may insert the report directly into your record without calling you with the results, assuming you would expect a call only if something abnormal were found. Make it clear to your doctor that you want to hear any and all results.

Some states now require that your mammogram report be sent directly to you. These reports can be more confusing than helpful. For instance: "Your mammogram showed no evidence of cancer," followed one sentence later by "Remember that a mammogram does not entirely exclude all cancer. Although mammography is the most sensitive tool available for the detection of breast cancer, it is not perfect and may fail to detect cancer in 10 to 15 percent of cases. If you have a persistent lump or other problem in one of your breasts, you should consult your physician for further evaluation." This language is designed to cover all possibilities, including protecting the reporting institution from being sued, but the report often leaves you worried and upset, and still dependent on your doctor's explanation.

You might also receive a report that suggests a potential problem: "Your mammogram revealed findings that require evaluation. It is important that you follow up on this recommendation with your physician." In fact, the findings may be quite benign, related to past surgery and treatment, but until you make contact with your physician you could be going crazy with anxiety, particularly if the report arrives at a time when you can't reach your doctor.

You should make sure that the results of every test (positive or negative) have been secured and passed on to the physician who will act on those results. Once in a great while, test results get lost and no one is aware of the loss. So it's a good idea for you to keep track of your records yourself.

Access to Medical Records: For Doctors and Yourself

You have a legal right to all of your medical records. Only you can authorize the release of records between hospitals or from a hospital to an individual. A personal letter, note, or signed form is required.

Continuity of care is crucial. All new films should be compared with prior ones, which are generally stored at the site where they were taken. Both old and new films should be stored at one center. If you change centers, arrange to have your mammography file moved with you. Some women maintain their own file of mammograms in their home. Copies, that is; most hospitals keep the original mammograms.

If you are seeking a second (or third) opinion on your care, mammogram, or other tests, you will want the consulting physician to be able to go over your history, reports, films, and records. You may want to carry your records yourself to the consultant if the consulting doctor is out of state, or if you made a last-minute appointment and need to be sure the consultant gets to see your past films and reports, or if you worry about the mail not making it on time. Most doctors want to see the x-ray reports and the actual films, so get both, or authorize the transfer of both via secured mailing. In general, copied films are fine, but when it comes to a mammogram, the originals are the best way to evaluate subtle changes in the breast. Getting your hands on those originals may involve a test of your patience and persistence. Remember, they are films of *you* and you have paid for them. You have every right to them.

You are probably the best agent to cut through red tape and delay, and to collect all essential information. Clarify how, when, and where to get the material you want, and be sure you get the *complete* file. Make an appointment to pick up your records: "Thank you for getting them together for me. I will be there at two o'clock, promptly." You may need to assert yourself and be unnaturally persistent. Do what you have to do. Don't worry about being Ms. Nice Gal.

Keep in mind that "the best patients are the worst patients," according to Claire Fagin, Dean Emerita of the University of Pennsylvania School of Nursing. "Nudge, nudge, nudge. Don't sit back and accept anything that fails to satisfy you. Speak up, protect your interests." No one else is as concerned as you are about your well-being. The old days of being talked down to and told what to do, and what's best for you, while you meekly accept it all, afraid to ask any questions, are over.

6

After Mastectomy: Re-creating a Breast— With or Without Surgery

> I went through life looking terrible in clothes and feeling horribly self-conscious about my huge breasts. So when I had to have a mastectomy, I agreed only on condition that I could have reconstruction and reduction of the other breast at the same time. I had the TRAM flap, and between that tummy tuck and waking up with reasonably sized breasts—even though somewhat uneven—I made the best of a bad deal.

Stop and think: How important is it to you to re-create your breast? Must it be there all the time, or can you live with "off-and-on" alternatives? Do you feel you need reconstruction to seem whole again? Must it be now? Sort out your reasons and rationales, and consider advantages and disadvantages. What are your personal priorities? What are the medical priorities and considerations?

Whatever your age, marital status, or sexual activity or orientation, and whether you work outside or inside the home, you can't predict how you will react to the loss of a breast. You can't predict how you will feel about re-creating a breast. Betty had bilateral mastectomies and rejected reconstruction; she was in her mid-thirties. Evelyn was in her late seventies when she had a mastectomy and decided on an implant: "My bosom was my friend; I had to replace that side with a buddy for the other."

Prosthesis

"I was pretty flat-chested, but I'll tell you, it's amazing how the smallest breast turns into a mountain when there's nothing there next to it. I had to put something in my bra right away so I could feel normal again: a use at last for those stupid shoulder pads I always take out of my clothes. Slip 'em in, slip 'em out—just like my contacts. I went back to work, and no one could tell a thing. That was very important for me."

The beauty of a prosthesis is how fast it fills the void. Literally. Often it's only a temporary filler, but it makes such a difference if you're someone who's just suffered the loss of part of yourself. And after so much trauma and so many decision-making responsibilities, it's a relief to be able to slip into underwear and appear as you did before. "I wanted to be with my friends and co-workers and not think they were eyeing my chest, wondering what had happened to me when I was out for cancer treatment."

Not every woman is convinced two breasts are necessary to feel complete. Betty, who had the double mastectomies and no reconstruction, had no plans to shop for a prosthesis. "This is the way I looked the first fourteen years of my life. I can handle it. But if I change my mind, or decide to wear a sexy dress from my former life, I can stick something into a bra or buy falsies."

When Ruth Handler, inventor of the Barbie doll, was looking for a prosthesis in the seventies, her doctor told her to stuff some stockings into her bra. That wasn't good enough for Mrs. Handler: She ended up inventing the first lifelike, natural-feeling artificial breast, called Nearly Me. "And I trained fitters to do a really good job. Not like those saleswomen in the seventies, who would hand you something over the top of the dressing room door!"

Reach to Recovery, a program of the American Cancer Society, connects with breast cancer patients soon after surgery. Support comes from a woman who's already been through this and is surviving and functioning; she brings along an information packet complete with a puffy temporary breast replacement. A list of shops and services is included: You can choose among surgical supply stores, pharmacies, custom lingerie clothes shops (with the assistance of a trained fitter), or a private home service (usually at no extra cost). At a time when you're entitled to extra comfort and convenience, the opportunity to have personal service in the privacy of your own home is a marvelous treat. You can try out various samples under an assortment of your own clothes, from lingerie to sweaters to low-cut evening gowns.

Special bathing suits and lingerie have been designed for breast cancer survivors and are available from Land's End, Sears, Nordstrom, or JC Penney catalogs, as well as small shops and department stores. The clothing comes with a pocket to hold the prosthesis, or you can have pockets sewn into the bras or suits you already own. (Average cost for the service is under twenty dollars.) "The pockets are great! I don't worry anymore about diving in and coming up to watch my breast filler floating off among the waves."

Prostheses come in many shapes, sizes, and materials: silicone gel, foam, or fiberfill interior, weighted or not, with the ideal product having the shape, weight, balance, and motion—and simulated nipple—of the natural breast on the other side. They don't always come with instructions, however: "You have it in backward!" Lynn was told, months after she had begun using hers. Bobbie couldn't get over how well they worked for her: "I can try on clothes in Loehmann's big open dressing room and nobody knows it's not me in that bra."

Ready-made products are matched to your natural side (one company offers eighty-six sizes). One product comes with adhesive patches that attach to the upper edge of your breast area, allowing you to go bra-less if you so desire. The adhesive patches last about one week, and then you replace them. Our expert advises caution applying adhesive to what may be particularly sensitive postsurgery skin, but most women have no problem. (External silicone prostheses pose no known health threat.)

You'll probably want to buy two styles of prostheses. A lightweight model (polyfill or foam) is recommended for the initial postsurgery recovery period and is useful for informal leisure activities thereafter, especially during warm weather and swimming. (The product is machine washable.) A lifelike silicone product (hand washable) is more aesthetically pleasing and women prefer it for more formal social occasions, including love-making. Two shapes are offered: asymmetrical (one for the left side, one for the right) and symmetrical or pear-shaped, worn sideways to fill out the side, or straight up for center fullness and cleavage.

If you're really prepared to splurge (and you may have to, to pay for this style that few insurers cover), you can buy a custom-made breast prosthesis, individually constructed and cast to match the natural contours of your body and your other breast. One company refers to it as "external breast reconstruction."

You may find the weight of the lifelike prosthesis—which is designed to replicate actual breast weight—intrusive and fatiguing, but the balanced weight it provides does help keep your shoulders even and your posture straight.

Prices of prostheses range from choices under $100, to high-quality products between $200 and $500 (size is not a factor). (A custom-made model is considerably more expensive.) They last from two to five years. Salt water, pool water, and hot tubs will damage silicone products.

If you're applying for health insurance money to pay for a prosthesis, you may jeopardize the possibility of payment for surgical reconstruction at a future date. Some insurance plans won't pay for both. Be sure to check with your insurance company to find out exactly what it will cover for your recovery and rehabilitation. Most coverage allows for the cost of two special brassieres (with prostheses pockets) a year and a new prosthesis every two years.

It's important to obtain a doctor's prescription for your prosthesis in order to be reimbursed by your health insurer. Be prepared to defend your request. Money for health care is getting tighter. But don't be discouraged: You can usually get this cost partially or completely covered if you are persistent.

Summer will test how happy you are with your choices. Revealing clothes make you conscious of what's missing. Heat causes discomfort when nonporous synthetic material presses up against your skin. Beach time and swimming challenge prosthesis-embellished bathing suits. My patients say summer is when they're pushed to think about reconstruction.

Reconstruction

"I was fed up with searching about every morning for pieces of my body, to stuff into a brassiere, that I never had to bother with before the mastectomy. I wanted to make my body as normal as possible and that's why I decided on reconstruction. My husband tried to talk me out of it: 'It doesn't matter to me,' he said. 'But it matters to me!' I told him. 'I'm doing it for me!' And I did, and I love it."

Why Reconstruction?

What do you want from reconstruction; what are your expectations? "I want to be able to wear my favorite clothes, have them hang right. Mostly I don't want an empty side reminding me of my cancer history every time I get dressed." Another woman's hope: "I'm dating and I don't want the world to know I've had breast cancer; I want to look sexy, maybe show a little cleavage."

Joan, an aspiring opera singer, has to wear seductive costumes. "I might be able to get away with a prosthesis, but I don't want to worry about reaching for high C in an embrace with the tenor—and have the damn thing pop out. It happened to another soprano I know. I don't want anyone knowing my business, especially one of those lecherous tenors."

Lily was set against double surgery: mastectomy and then a reconstruction operation. "A prosthesis will do me fine." But her husband said: "I know you too well. You're not going to be happy walking around with a double D breast on one side and nothing on the other. Face the tough issues now and figure you'll have a longer time enjoying the new you."

Your reasons for reconstruction may not suit everyone. June's support group jumped on her when she suggested she was considering reconstruction to please a man. "No way! Guys come and go. Do it for yourself or don't do it!" For some women, though, doing it for a lover may be reason enough.

Seventy-five percent of women who have mastectomies have reconstruction. Roughly half of these women decide on implants. Most of the rest choose the TRAM flap, described below. If women are offered the choice, almost all ask for immediate reconstruction.

First Steps

If you have had a breast removed, or you are about to, as part of your breast cancer treatment, you or your physician will raise the possibility of breast reconstruction. Even if you can't bear the thought of further surgery, you shouldn't dismiss altogether the idea of reconstruction until you've given it some careful consideration. At the very least, you'll want to read about what reconstruction offers and entails.

It took a while for Gena, tired of looking for spare parts to stuff into her bra, to make up her mind about reconstruction: "I hadn't thought about it before the mastectomy—the whole business of my disease overwhelmed me, so I couldn't think about my options at the time."

Before you proceed, you need to do a little investigation, a "reality check." Find out what your medical insurance company will pay for. Some companies will pay for the entire procedure, even if it's years after the mastectomy. Other companies will pay only for reconstructing the removed breast, not additional "nonessential" procedures like reducing the other breast to achieve symmetry.

Obviously, you must also find out exactly what your plastic surgeon thinks needs to be done and why, including immediate and delayed procedures. For example, a possible sequence is right breast reconstruction from TRAM flap, with left breast reduction, followed at some later time by nipple reconstruction.

If you meet resistance from your insurance carrier, be prepared to mount a strong case in advance of your surgery, with your doctor's support. Persistence will pay off, with additional pressure, if necessary, coming from your state or federal representative. (See Chapter 26.)

Medical Priorities

"It's never too late to get breast reconstruction," says Dr. Gordon Schwartz, a prominent Philadelphia breast cancer surgeon. Rosa decided on reconstruction at age sixty-nine, fourteen years after her mastectomy. (She was tremendously pleased with her new body.) "Give yourself time to recover from the trauma and treatment of a life-threatening disease before going on to another major procedure," says another cancer surgeon.

If you are diagnosed with early-stage breast cancer and choose or need a mastectomy, immediate reconstruction is fine. Two separate surgical teams are necessary for these two different operations; such a procedure requires complex coordination and may result in scheduling delays.

But if your diagnosis is intermediate or advanced stage, it's likely that you will require prompt chemotherapy or radiation, or both, after mastectomy. It is therefore advisable to delay reconstruction until treatment is finished (six months to a year). By that time, your needs and desires, your shape, and any weight gain from chemotherapy, all will have stabilized and you'll be at a much better point to start anew.

If you were diagnosed with locally advanced cancer or inflammatory breast cancer, you should not have immediate reconstruction, because the extra plastic surgery may require additional healing time that would delay necessary chemotherapy and radiation. Also, implanted tissue distorts the relationships among the tissues of the chest wall region that needs radiation, the region that must be carefully followed because of a high risk of recurrence. A tissue expander alone, however, does not delay recovery or significantly alter normal anatomy when first put in place, compared to autologous procedures (procedures that use the patient's own tissue). Radiation also will temporarily—and sometimes permanently—stiffen whatever tissues are treated, including transplanted tissue—another reason to delay reconstruction.

Every woman is different, and medical advice varies from one end of the spectrum to the other on the issue of immediate or delayed reconstruction. You will want to get opinions from each of the oncologists on your team to help you make your decision.

The fact, though, is that you may be adamant. Despite advice from doctors, family, and friends, you may be determined to have reconstruction as soon as you can get your plastic surgeon to fix a date, preferably to coincide with the time of your mastectomy. You may want to wake up with something like the shape you had before. "I want to go into that operating room asleep, have the doctors do what they must, wake up, and have it all over, with *something* sitting on my chest. If I can't have tissue reconstruction, I want that expander in place and on its way, because it'll be six months before I'm where I hope to be."

Immediate reconstruction may be fine for most women, but despite how strong you may feel about this, I think it should not be done in any woman who needs to start chemotherapy soon after her surgery—particularly if she has a large tumor, a significant number of affected lymph nodes, or any skin involvement.

Options

Implants: saline (salt water) or silicone gel filled; tissue transfers from the back, belly, or buttock, each with or without implants; smooth surface or nipples (tattooed or made from your own transplanted tissue). A confusion of choices that sort themselves out under the guidance of your doctors and advice from friends who have had experience with some of these procedures.

Implants

Implants involve the least amount of surgery; slim, small-breasted women tend to do best with implants. Some women can have immediate placement of a permanent saline-filled or silicone-gel-filled implant, but most women require some expansion of the skin that remains after mastectomy in order to accommodate the permanent implant.

To stretch the skin, a balloon-type device called a tissue expander (it's a silicone bag) is inserted, or implanted, under the chest muscle. It is gradually expanded with the injection of saline at regular intervals until the predetermined size is reached. Skin and soft tissue stretch to achieve the desired appearance. (Think of how pregnancy slowly stretches the skin of the belly.) The expander is actually hyperinflated: the tissue is stretched beyond the desired size to achieve a natural droop. This hyperinflation can create significant discomfort, and occasionally flatten an area of your rib cage.

The process of expansion takes about six months. At the end of the process, the expanding device is replaced with a permanent saline-filled or silicone-gel-filled implant. (Despite the controversy over its safety, silicone is still used by some women because it is most like the normal breast weight and consistency; it is available only to women who enroll in an ongoing study of its safety.) Or, if a permanent expander has been used, it is filled with saline and the port (a metal or plastic plug, valve, or coil part of the implant, through which the saline is injected) is removed. Other fluids, such as peanut and soybean oils, can be safely absorbed by the body if they leak from the implant; they are currently being tested for possible use.

Once an implant is in place, your body makes scar tissue that encapsulates the implant. Ninety-five percent of the capsules are soft to firm. Five percent of women form hard capsules that can be painful and distort the breast. Radiation therapy to the breast area increases the risk of scar tissue around the implant. Massage and exercises that move the implant up, down, and side to side, may reduce the risk of hard capsule formation. An implant placed behind the chest muscle is less prone to hard scarring. If you develop a hard capsule, frequent massage and exercises may help, but surgical correction may be necessary.

The chance of your breast implant leaking increases over time; most implants that have been in place for ten to fifteen years have some leakage, usually insignificant. Leakage of a silicone-filled implant is detectable by loss of volume or by a magnetic resonance imaging (MRI) scan. A leaking silicone implant should be removed.

After fifteen years, Elizabeth found that her implants were leaking, although her breasts hadn't lost their shape. Their replacement meant another trying experience, another recovery period, but six weeks later Elizabeth was back to her exhausting normal routine. "I'm as good as new. I'll be satisfied with another fifteen years."

You could have trouble keeping your implant in the right position. It may have a tendency to move upward, sometimes and you may need to massage it down into place, repeatedly.

There has been a lot of controversy about the use of silicone-filled implants. Some women claim they have had adverse effects from leakage of the silicone fluid, and they've sued the makers of the implants. A class-action suit was brought against the manufacturers, which was settled out of court shortly before the publication of studies (one a fifteen-year review, another involving 120,000 nurses) indicating there were no differences in the incidences of certain autoimmune diseases (arthritis, lupus) between women with and those without the silicone implants. Most surgeons and oncologists are satisfied that today's silicone implants are safe, but the litigation and resultant caution have almost completely eliminated their use.

Autologous Procedures

Other surgical reconstruction options involve the movement of the patient's own tissue—a so-called autologous procedure—from one area of the body to the chest, to re-create the breast or breasts that were removed (either minutes, weeks, months, or years earlier). Tissue can be taken from the abdomen, the back, or the buttock, either as a detached piece or as a flap connected to its own blood supply, then sewn into place in the opening where the breast was removed (which is reopened if the reconstruction was delayed).

The TRAM flap (named for the transverse rectus abdominus muscle) is one of these procedures, and the most popular of all reconstruction choices, especially for women with excess belly fat or stretched-out postpregnancy abdomens, who are pleased with what amounts to a fringe-benefit tummy tuck. But the TRAM is not feasible for thin women who don't have enough tissue, for those who smoke and have compromised blood vessels, or for those who have multiple surgical scars on the abdomen. (Cesarean-section scars ordinarily are not a problem.)

An ellipse of skin, fat, and muscle is taken from the lower half of the abdomen and slid up through a tunnel under the skin to the breast area, with blood vessels still attached when possible. Body organs are undisturbed. The ellipse of tissue is shaped into a breast and sewn into place. If blood vessels have been cut, they are reattached by microscopic surgery to blood vessels in the chest area. The procedure takes about three hours.

Most of the women I've taken care of are pleased to have a flat belly from the tummy tuck that goes along with the TRAM procedure. Your tummy tuck scar and your refashioned "belly button" (navel) may take some getting used to, however. The tummy tuck incision is horizontal, located midway between the top of your pubic hair and your navel, and it is long, extending from hipbone to hipbone. Your surgeon may need to create a new navel because after the abdominal area is reshaped, your natural navel may be stretched, distorted, or in the wrong place.

When reconstruction is performed after a double mastectomy, a single piece of tissue is removed from the abdomen, provided there is adequate tissue. It is divided in half, and each half is placed in position, in paired openings on the chest, allowing for the closest symmetry of the two new breasts. In a less common condition, if you had a breast lump removed that resulted in significant deformity, you might want to consider having the area reconstructed with tissue transplanted from your abdomen or side.

The use of the thick layer of tissue from the abdomen allows for clever remodeling into a natural-looking breast replacement. This new breast can be augmented with an implant behind the body tissue if a larger breast is required or desired.

The consistency or touch of abdominal tissue most resembles a natural breast, so it is the preferred source for most autologous (using the patient's own tissue) procedures. This newly transferred tissue may feel most natural to the touch of the toucher, but you probably won't get much sensation from that touching. The area usually remains numb because the nerves are cut when the tissue is moved.

Tissue from the abdomen can be harvested only once, so if you had the abdominal flap done for a single breast mastectomy, and at some future time you need a mastectomy of the second breast, tissue can be drawn from the side of your back.

The latissimus dorsi flap refers to the back muscle that is used for this tissue transfer procedure: below the shoulder and behind the armpit. An implant is almost always required in addition to the tissue, depending on the desired size of the reconstructed breast, because there is so little body fat in this part of the back. This procedure has enjoyed considerable popularity with surgeons. The flap is easily slipped to the front through a short tunnel in the skin, with excellent results and few complications. But the color and texture of the transferred back skin are different from those of breast skin, and it does result in some asymmetry of the back, although there's usually no compromise in back function or strength.

The buttock crease is still another source of transferable tissue for breast reconstruction. The transplanted tissue will have its blood supply microscopically connected to blood vessels on the chest. An implant may or may not be required. The scar is concealed in the buttock crease.

The buttock surgery is technically much more difficult because the blood supply must be completely disconnected, then reconnected to a new blood supply, requiring the use of a microscope. The procedure can take up to twelve hours. If the reattached blood vessels nourishing the reconstructed breast tissue are compromised in any way, part or all of the transferred tissue may not survive, and additional surgery may be necessary. Buttock crease surgery may be the only option for women who are not candidates for TRAM or latissimus dorsi procedures because of inadequate tissue on the back, belly, or side.

Achieving Symmetry

Symmetry is the ideal goal of any reconstructive breast surgery. Weight gain, one factor among many, has a major effect on symmetry. Whereas the TRAM flap breast gains weight with the rest of the body (although it may gain at a different rate than regular breast tissue and there may be some strain or discomfort along the scar), in women with an implant, the natural breast gains but the implanted side does not.

The effect most difficult to achieve is the natural droop of a normal breast; it's simpler to raise a drooping breast than to match it, particularly with implant reconstruction. The natural breast can be reduced and lifted to help it resemble the perky new reconstructed breast. Over time, however, the natural breast may droop or sag, while the reconstructed breast continues to hold its upward tilt. Fine in a bra, a bummer in the buff.

Asymmetry of some kind is commonplace. Because the close match of one side to the other is what every woman hopes for, your surgeon may recommend surgical adjustment of the unaffected breast to equalize size, shape, position, or placement. If you give permission for this additional surgery, this adjustment can be made while you're under anesthesia for breast reconstruction or some time after, when the size of the reconstructed breast has stabilized. This may be your opportunity for cosmetic surgery. If ever—in your pre-cancer, normal life—you considered breast reduction or enlargement, this is the moment to capture something positive from a difficult time. (Before you go ahead with this additional surgery, be sure to find out who will pay for it, your medical insurance company or you.)

"I was reborn," said Lily. "Ten years after a lumpectomy I had to have a mastectomy, and so I decided on the TRAM flap and the doctor suggested I have reduction of the other side. Well, for years I'd thought about breast reduction—from a size double D—but I never could get up the courage for elective surgery. You could call this a bonus: I lost my potbelly and I got two young breasts. I can wear any bathing suit I like, and I look great! As for symmetry, my breasts were never exactly equal before—how many women's are? I put them in a bra and no one can really tell the difference."

At the conclusion of the tissue-transfer operation, the new breast will be somewhat larger than the natural breast; as the reconstruction site heals, swelling will subside and the breasts tend to equalize. If this doesn't settle out to your satisfaction, your surgeon can extract fat (by liposuction) to reduce the size of the reconstructed breast.

Risk and Disappointment

For all your surgeon's efforts, there is no guarantee that you will be 100 percent satisfied with the results of reconstruction. Your breasts may not live up to your expectations, in size, position, angle, or balance. They may not be as soft or natural-feeling as you had hoped.

And you are not likely to have normal sensation in the transplanted tissue. Ask your surgeon to show you photographs of the full range of reconstruction results, not just the showcase chests. Some images may shake your resolve. Ask yourself again, "What are my expectations? What are realistic results?"

All surgery involves risk. Breast reconstruction involves slightly more than a 5 percent risk of one or a combination of the following: infection, bleeding, pain, hernia, implant rupture, tissue breakdown.

The TRAM flap and buttock transfer are the more complex of the autologous procedures; they take longer and carry the most risk, the worst being the possibility of flap failure, or a breakdown of the transferred tissue because the blood supply is not adequate. It happens in about 5 percent of breast reconstruction cases, generally an unacceptable rate for surgeons for any procedure, but one that cannot seem to be lowered for these procedures.

If tissue breakdown occurs, the dead tissue needs to be trimmed away. The open area needs to be closed, either by natural regrowth of normal tissue, which can take time, or with surgical repair.

The TRAM abdominal incision and removal of the muscle does weaken your abdomen, making sit-ups difficult. But it's possible to overcome this difficulty. A patient of mine who had had a TRAM flap procedure was a belly dancer. After an adjustment of her costume to cover her incision, she was able to continue her customary gyrations. Occasionally, there may be other problems: hernia (when a small portion of the intestines bulges out through a weakened area of the abdominal wall) or persistent pain or discomfort where the muscle was removed and along the incision. Surgical revision of the hernia may be necessary; persistent pain needs to be evaluated.

Transplanted tissue can form lumps, "fat necrosis," that may or may not go away. They are most common along the suture line and usually don't affect your appearance. You feel them, and they may show up on a mammogram as lumps or as small calcifications. Feeling lumps can be worrisome, and some may need to be surgically removed to prove they are not cancerous.

As I mentioned, implants have a small risk of riding up the chest, as muscle activity squeezes the implant up or out of place over time, and they occasionally leak fluid. A silicone leak can usually be detected by an MRI scan or sometimes by regular x-ray; it shows up as an opaque shape. A saline leak is undetectable (unless the implant collapses) and is probably harmless. Underinflated implants can feel wrinkled beneath the skin.

In perhaps 20 percent of cases, hard scar tissue capsules form around the implant, which makes the implant stiff and smaller. Radiation to the chest wall over the implant area can increase the risk of scar capsule formation. A friend gave Bag Balm to Annamarie to massage into her scar, to help soften it. "For a moment I thought I was back on the farm, but I think in fact it helped."

Whatever surgical procedure you settle on, there will be scars. They do fade and recede in time in most women, but they don't go away. They are generally located out of sight, even in a bathing suit or low-cut gown.

There's always that matter of expectations; they don't always coincide with reality. When Annamarie had expanders replaced with permanent implants, she had a hard time getting adjusted to the firm, standout, high breasts that sat on her chest, "kind of like being an adolescent again, getting used to my surprising new breasts." She warned her friends: "If you hug me, you're going to bounce off!" She talked to her plastic surgeon, but he didn't really respond to what she was saying. He had great hands for surgery but wasn't good with words, she realized. So she saw another surgeon and asked her, "What should I look like?" This doctor told Annamarie that over time her breasts would develop a more natural sag, scarring that accounted for some stiffness would probably soften, and—just in case she was interested—those stand-up breasts were what many models and show-biz women would consider a happy result. Her husband told her she had a better shape now than she had before, but that didn't altogether please Annamarie. Still, she decided to give herself time to get adjusted to her new look.

Decided and Determined

Despite these cautions, the potential relief of feeling and appearing normal again is enough to convince a large number of women to go ahead with reconstruction as soon as possible. "It's a giant step toward putting the disease and my cancer experience behind me. I'm willing to take my chances on a good-enough result." That was one patient's emphatic conclusion to a discussion of options. Every one of her friends tried to talk Andrea out of still another bout of surgery. "Why go through another complicated operation, plus all that controversy about implants. Stick with a prosthesis," her sister told her. "But I couldn't wait for that reconstruction. I had gone on a trip to the Greek islands for sun and swimming—and the airline lost my luggage with my specially adapted bathing suit. I knew then I had to have the freedom reconstruction brings. I love my new breast almost as much as my old one."

TABLE 5.1. Reconstruction Options

Procedure	Timing	Length of operation	Eligibility	Relative cost	Pros	Cons
Implant alone	Immediate (only for small implant) or delayed (when skin must be expanded first to accommodate a larger implant)	1 hour	Only for small or medium breasts	Low	Simple, no extra scars, fast placement, immediate final results, unlikely to delay radiation and chemotherapy	Doesn't have natural breast consistency; can dislodge, wrinkle, leak, encapsulate, cause pain
Tissue expander implant (one that can be converted to a permanent implant, or one that is later replaced by a permanent implant)	Immediate or delayed	1 hour	Only for small or medium breasts	Low to moderate	Simple, no extra scars, fast placement, doesn't delay radiation and chemotherapy, an option for smokers	Delayed final results: implant requires multiple port injections; second surgery required if expander is replaced by permanent implant; doesn't have breast consistency; can dislodge, wrinkle, leak, encapsulate, cause pain

Procedure	Timing	Length of operation	Eligibility	Relative cost	Pros	Cons
TRAM flap	Immediate or delayed	3–8 hours, depending on surgical skills, whether blood supply remains intact or needs to be reattached with microsurgery	Depends on belly size; not for smokers or anyone with a history of diabetes, vascular disease, or multiple abdominal surgeries	High	Feels the most like a natural breast, nothing artificial, tummy tuck can be used to create most breast sizes	Extra scars; longer surgery; longer convalescence postpones radiation and chemotherapy; can cause fat necrosis, hernia, persistent breast and belly pain, abdominal weakness; can be done only once

Procedure	Timing	Length of operation	Eligibility	Relative cost	Pros	Cons
Latissimus dorsi	Immediate or delayed	3–6 hours	Small to medium breast size, side or back tissue permitting; not for smokers	High	Simpler operation than TRAM, excellent tissue viability, feels like natural breast tissue, nothing artificial; alternative for women with multiple abdominal surgeries	Skin texture may be different from chest area skin; convalescence longer than implant but shorter than TRAM; can cause fat necrosis; may cause discomfort, limit vigorous back and shoulder activity; can be done only once; healing may delay radiation and chemotherapy

Procedure	Timing	Length of operation	Eligibility	Relative cost	Pros	Cons
Buttock area	Immediate; delayed better because of length of surgery	9–12 hours	Depends on size of buttock or hip, not for smokers or diabetics	Very high	Feels like natural breast, nothing artificial, bigger breast sizes possible, can be done more than once, alternative for women with multiple abdominal surgeries, minimal effect on function	Long operation with more perioperative complications, higher risk of tissue breakdown; can be done only by plastic surgeon skilled in microvascular techniques; can cause fat necrosis; could delay radiation and chemo; pain and discomfort while sitting

Nipple Replacement

There's still the issue of nipples. What are your choices? You can do nothing. You can apply polyurethane, removable nipples; in a semi-erect mode, these rubbery tips are surprisingly lifelike in texture and color. You can tattoo a look-alike. Or, you can go for nipple reconstruction from transplanted tissue. Fake or real, flat or "stick-out."

Nipple and areola reconstruction can use tissue taken from the labia (the skin folds of the vulva, at the entrance to the vagina). (Ouch!) As in most tissue transfer, the reconstructed nipple has very little sensation. (Sensation in the vulvar area is usually unaffected.) The vulvar surgery and nipple reconstruction can be done on an out-patient basis in under two hours, under local anesthesia. All hair folli-cles are removed before it is formed into a nipple. You can usually drive the day after surgery; vulvar discomfort lasts about a week.

Tissue can also be taken from the inside of the thigh (the skin gets darker as you move from the knee toward the labia), or from local chest wall skin flaps. The skin may darken naturally, or tattooing can provide custom-color to match your other nipple in a twenty-minute office visit. The color may need to be altered at a later visit. Avoid using part of your existing natural nipple to create a new nipple on the other side, because then both nipples will be numb. One of my pa-tients was very upset to lose sensation in her nipples—they had been so much a part of her sexual pleasure.

Nipple replacement isn't scheduled till at least two months after breast reconstruction, to allow for swelling on the reconstruction to recede, any lumpiness to dissipate, and the breast to settle into its "nat-ural" sag so the nipple can be properly sited.

"I thought about tissue transfer for areola and nipple. It was going to come from the inside of my thigh—but I have hairy thighs and I didn't want hairy nipples! Tattooing worked fine for me, especially when they made me a real stick-out nipple from nearby skin."

7

Tamoxifen Therapy: Is It for You?

> I thought chemotherapy was the last step. Now you tell me about tamoxifen. Doesn't it go on for years? Aren't there side effects? Isn't it expensive? Do I really, honestly, need it? Will my treatment never end!

Just when you think you have your life in hand, the disease is behind you, treatment is over, and all major decisions have been settled, your doctor tells you about tamoxifen (also known as Nolvadex).

"What is this 'tamoxifen'?" Maybe the name is new to you, but it's currently as familiar as aspirin to many women around the world. Tamoxifen has become the most commonly used medication to fight breast cancer. Millions of women have taken it after the diagnosis of breast cancer, and thousands take it as participants in clinical studies: more than 500,000 women are on it in the United States today; each year 80,000 more will join their ranks.

Tamoxifen is a miracle drug to a lot of people, doctors as well as breast cancer survivors, but a significant number of these women reap its benefits while feeling less than thrilled by its side effects. Just about every woman who takes the drug still has some questions about it. In the fourteen major conferences our Living Beyond Breast Cancer_{SM} organization has presented, tamoxifen has been the most popular topic by far.

Tamoxifen Appears on the Scene

A major goal of breast cancer therapy is to reduce or eliminate the ovaries' production of estrogen and its stimulation of breast cancer cells. In the past, this type of therapy could be accomplished only by surgical removal of the ovaries (oophorectomy) or x-ray treatment of the ovaries. And it was done only for women with breast cancer that had spread to lymph nodes or other parts of the body (metastasis). Tamoxifen appeared on the scene about twenty years ago as an effective alternative to these invasive procedures. Here was hope in a pill, a new and powerful weapon against the progression of metastatic breast cancer.

Encouraged by its effectiveness against metastatic breast cancer, researchers set up studies to test the benefit of tamoxifen for breast cancer patients *without* metastases or lymph node involvement. Tamoxifen was found to substantially reduce the *recurrence* of breast cancer. After this breakthrough discovery, further studies established tamoxifen's ability to prevent formation of *new* breast cancers in the other, unaffected breast. Now the NSABP (National Surgical Adjuvant Breast and Bowel Project) Breast Cancer Prevention Study is under way to determine whether tamoxifen can *prevent* breast cancer from ever starting in women who have certain risk factors but no personal history of breast cancer.

How Tamoxifen Works

Tamoxifen is actually a very, very weak estrogen. Normal estrogen is a powerful sex hormone manufactured by a woman's ovaries. It travels through the bloodstream until it finds an estrogen receptor (located in normal cells and cancer cells all over the body) into which it fits, much as a key fits into a lock. (A receptor is a specific protein molecule that acts like a locked switch for a particular activity within the cell; if the complementary molecule key comes along—i.e. estrogen, serotonin, antigen—and locks into place with the receptor, the switch is turned and the activity starts up.) Once in the receptor, estrogen sends a signal to the nucleus (the "headquarters") of the cell; this activates the cell's DNA (the genetic blueprint that determines the cell's function), which in turn stimulates the cell's growth and proliferation.

When you take tamoxifen, it passes into your bloodstream, joining all kinds of hormones, nutrients, oxygen, and other molecules, and circulates through the tissues of your body. If breast cancer cells are present, tamoxifen flows around them as well. If these cancer cells have estrogen receptors (about two-thirds of cells do, and the number of receptors on a cell's surface can vary considerably), tamoxifen slips into the receptor "locks," instead of the body's natural estrogen. Because tamoxifen is such a weak estrogen, its estrogen signals fail to stimulate cell growth, and because it has stolen the place away from more powerful estrogen, it blocks estrogen-stimulated cancer growth and proliferation. In this way, tamoxifen acts like an anti-estrogen. Breast cancer expert Dr. Lisa Weissmann likes to tell her patients that it's as if breast cancer cells can grow only if you feed them steak (normal estrogen), and tamoxifen is like feeding them watery soup.

Tamoxifen may also displace natural estrogen in the receptors of healthy breast cells, thereby suppressing growth activity and possibly preventing abnormal growth and the development of a totally new breast cancer. (Refer to Chapter 28 for an explanation of how normal cells become cancerous.)

Dominated by tamoxifen, deprived of normal estrogen stimulation, the cancer cells shrivel and wither like deflated balloons. As long as tamoxifen is hogging all the estrogen receptors, the cancer cells remain dormant and relatively harmless. After a long period of this suspended animation, the cancer cells may die.

Tamoxifen does not work against all breast cancers. And in some cases it works only for a while—years, in some instances—and then loses its effectiveness. In a few cases, breast cancer cells may learn to adapt to the presence of tamoxifen and possibly learn to survive on it. For a person with this kind of breast cancer, it may be therapeutic to stop taking tamoxifen.

Will Tamoxifen Work for You? Benefits and Side Effects

Whether your tumor will respond to tamoxifen depends largely on what is learned in the laboratory about the presence of estrogen receptors in the cancer cells that have been removed from your breast. The more receptors present on those cells, the more likely it is that tamoxifen will work against your particular cancer. About 60 percent of breast cancers are estrogen-receptor positive, "positive" meaning a significant number of receptors are present on the cancer cells. If the number of receptors is low, tamoxifen may have some effect, but probably only a minimal one; if receptors are absent, or "negative," tamoxifen has little or no benefit.

A few women may not get hormone receptor results from their tissue biopsy because the tumor was too small to permit adequate testing; these small tumors, however, commonly behave as though they were estrogen-receptor positive.

Some women may have breast cancers that are both receptor positive and receptor negative, meaning that their breast cancer is made up of different kinds of cells. Their cancers may have a mixed response to tamoxifen.

Benefits

Preventing Recurrence

The primary reason for taking tamoxifen is to fight the breast cancer you've already been diagnosed with. For women with early-stage breast cancer without known metastases, tamoxifen is used to prevent recurrence of the disease in the breast, lymph nodes, or beyond.

How your breast cancer responds to tamoxifen depends not only on the presence of estrogen receptors, but also on your menopausal status at the time of diagnosis. In postmenopausal women whose cancers were estrogen-receptor positive, tamoxifen can result in a 30 to 40 percent reduction in recurrence rate. In postmenopausal women who were estrogen-receptor negative, the advantage drops to 5 to 10 percent.

Tamoxifen is generally recommended for most postmenopausal women with breast cancer, unless they have a very "favorable" tumor (for example, the tumor measures less than one centimeter and doesn't look "angry" or aggressive under the microscope). Postmenopausal women who have extensive lymph node involvement or other unfavorable findings may need chemotherapy and tamoxifen.

The value of tamoxifen for premenopausal women is not quite as significant as it is for postmenopausal women. For premenopausal women who are estrogen-receptor positive, there is about a 20 to 30 percent reduction in recurrence with tamoxifen; in premenopausal women who are estrogen-receptor negative, there is no apparent benefit.

Most premenopausal women with breast cancer are advised to receive chemotherapy, unless they have an extremely small or otherwise "favorable" cancer. Premenopausal women who have an estrogen-receptor positive cancer but otherwise unfavorable findings may take tamoxifen after they've completed chemotherapy. (But it's still not clear if tamoxifen gives any additional protection beyond what has already been achieved with chemotherapy.) If a woman with these cancer features refuses chemotherapy, she can take tamoxifen as an alternative, but it is about 10 percent less effective than chemotherapy. Premenopausal women with receptor-negative tumors require chemotherapy, because the absence of receptors is "unfavorable," and tamoxifen exerts its effect through the estrogen receptors: If they are absent, tamoxifen has no place to work.

New data are emerging that may help answer some tough questions, such as whether women under fifty whose tumors are estrogen-receptor positive and lymph node negative have comparable results from chemotherapy alone, tamoxifen alone, or removal of the ovaries alone, and whether there's any benefit to adding tamoxifen after chemotherapy.

Halting the Progression of Metastatic Disease

Tamoxifen has been used to treat women whose breast cancer has already metastasized, and it has been found to be effective, in many cases halting the progression of the disease. It can often induce remission. Postmenopausal women with metastatic disease tend to have a more dramatic response to tamoxifen than premenopausal women. Regardless of their menopausal status, women with hormone-receptor positive tumors have up to a 75 percent response rate; tumors that are receptor negative have a lower response rate of about 15 percent. If you are a woman with metastatic disease and negative receptors, tamoxifen can still be worth trying, because you could be one of the 15 percent who gets a good response—without the more significant side effects of chemotherapy.

Reducing Your Risk of Cancer in the Other Breast

Tamoxifen reduces the possibility of a new cancer in the unaffected breast by about 50 percent. Women who have had breast cancer in one breast are at increased risk of getting cancer in the other breast compared with women without a history of breast cancer. The risk increases by one percent per year; within ten years your risk would be 10 percent: tamoxifen can halve this risk.

Reducing Osteoporosis

Tamoxifen, because it is a very weak estrogen, seems to help prevent the bone loss that occurs after menopause, much as estrogen replacement therapy does. Postmenopausal women may have transient increased bone density, followed by stabilization. Premenopausal women may have transient bone loss, followed by stabilization.

Lowering Cholesterol Levels

The other important, although secondary, beneficial consequence of taking tamoxifen is the reduction of heart disease and stroke by lowering the level of LDL (low density lipoproteins, the "bad" cholesterol). Women taking tamoxifen have fewer heart attacks and strokes, benefits normally associated with postmenopausal estrogen therapy. "It's lowered my cholesterol level—from 250 to 158. My blood pressure is down, too. I like that!" Joanne added. She felt that these advantages, for someone with a strong family history of both breast cancer and heart disease, made tamoxifen especially attractive.

The noncancer benefits of tamoxifen are real, but its ability to lower cholesterol and preserve bone density has not yet been shown to lead to survival benefits. Early studies showed that among women on tamoxifen, there were fewer deaths from heart disease, but a recent randomized study did not show that there were fewer heart attacks.

Side Effects

Tamoxifen's unwanted side effects depend on (1) whether you have any personal history of blood clots or endometrial cancer, (2) your susceptibility to hot flashes associated with menopause, (3) your tendency to gain weight, and (4) your vulnerability to depression. Add to these the cost of the medication, the fact that some women have real trouble sticking to the routine of taking a daily dose of pills, and many women's philosophical objection to taking any regular medication except perhaps for vitamins.

Although most side effects are not life threatening, the lesser side effects may diminish your quality of life, sometimes to a considerable degree.

Blood Clots

One potentially serious side effect of tamoxifen is blood clots, also known as thrombosis. The most common place for a clot to form is in the leg veins. These clots are dangerous because they can break loose, travel to the lung, and clog a vital blood vessel; this is called a pulmonary embolism. If you have had any history of blood clots, tamoxifen will probably not be an option for you. The possibility of pulmonary embolism is 1 percent, meaning that it's likely to affect one woman in a hundred taking tamoxifen. Tamoxifen can also cause inflammation of a blood vessel. Call your doctor if you notice any new swelling, redness, discomfort, or warmth in your legs.

Endometrial Cancer and Other Uterine Effects

Another serious risk associated with tamoxifen treatment is cancer of the lining of the uterus (endometrial cancer). Regardless of tamoxifen use, women affected by breast cancer are at increased risk of developing endometrial cancer; tamoxifen, however, does make this slightly higher risk a little higher still. Here, the risk is two women in a thousand, and there are usually—but not always—clear warning signs of trouble, as I'll note later. The longer a woman takes tamoxifen, the higher her risk of developing a tamoxifen-induced endometrial cancer. (But the risk is still low, even for women taking tamoxifen for ten years.) If an endometrial cancer is diagnosed within the first two years of taking tamoxifen, the cancer was most likely there before treatment with the drug began.

Endometrial cancer—related or unrelated to tamoxifen use—can usually be detected in the early stages, and it is usually curable with surgery. See your doctor if you have any unexpected vaginal bleeding or discharge. You should also have a gynecologic exam every six months. The routine Pap smear, however, is not adequate for detecting endometrial cancer, because it assesses the health of the cervix only. Ultrasound testing or a uterine tissue sample obtained by biopsy are the most effective ways of evaluating the endometrium, but experts from large, internationally known cancer centers believe that there is no benefit to routine endometrial ultrasounds and biopsies unless you have symptoms. Discuss this issue with your doctor.

If you have had a hysterectomy (removal of the uterus) because of endometrial cancer, tamoxifen may be contraindicated for your treatment of breast cancer. If, however, you have had a hysterectomy for a benign cause, such as fibroids, endometrial hyperplasia (an overgrowth of normal endometrial cells), or endometrial polyps (fingerlike projections made up of normal cells), you don't have to worry about endometrial cancer.

Tamoxifen can stimulate the benign changes in the endometrium mentioned previously, and it can also exacerbate underlying endometriosis, in which normal endometrial cells grow outside the uterus in the belly cavity, on the ovaries, or on the bladder.

Tamoxifen can also affect the uterus wall, which can lead to uneven thickening of the muscle and supportive tissues within the wall. Fibroids, ball-like overgrowths of these tissues, can result, or there can be lumpy bumpiness in one area or throughout the uterine wall. These changes can confuse ultrasound assessment of the endometrium. The ultrasound study can show a thickened or uneven endometrium, when in reality the change is in the underlying uterine wall. No increase in uterine wall cancers has been observed in women taking tamoxifen.

The benefits of tamoxifen as a breast cancer preventive still outweigh the risk of its contributing to development of an endometrial cancer.

Hot Flashes

Tamoxifen can produce menopausal side effects that include vaginal dryness, mood changes, and hot flashes. These sudden flushes can plague you, make you miserable, and undermine your quality of life, but they do not endanger your life. Most women find hot flashes the worst side effect from tamoxifen. About half the women on tamoxifen are affected by them. Leslie: "I'll be sitting at a meeting, flushed and perspiring. It's damned embarrassing, as well as uncomfortable. Almost as bad is waking up in the middle of the night with those sweats." Annamarie was unusual in her view of hot flashes: "I've always been cold. Tamoxifen gives me a buzz through my whole body and warms me up. I love the feeling."

You may find that a regular course of exercise helps moderate the problem. In most cases, women and their bodies adjust to tamoxifen; others grow to tolerate the problem, expecting it to diminish over time, and over a number of months it usually does. One tip is to figure out how long it takes between taking the dose and the appearance of the hot flash, decide what time of day is the least inconvenient for you to have a hot flash, and time your medication accordingly. You may find that taking both doses together (10 mg twice) results in hot flashes a few hours later, and you can control the timing for the least inconvenience. (See Chapter 18.)

In the uncommon situation where severe hot flashes persist despite reasonable solutions and tamoxifen therapy is strongly indicated, talk with your doctor about two possibilities: (1) start with 5 milligrams of tamoxifen and slowly increase the dose up to 20 milligrams daily, or (2) try a short-term course of low-dose hormone therapy to ease the transition period. The course should be short term (no more than a few months) because the estrogens in hormone therapy are not known to be safe for women with breast cancer.

Premature Menopause and Fertility Issues

The menopausal symptoms brought on by tamoxifen tend to be more intense in premenopausal women than in older women. Tina, thirty-five, stayed on tamoxifen for two years, but the hot flashes and other menopausal symptoms, the fear of side effects, and the stress of feeling so out of step with normal women her age finally were too much for her. "I gave it up. I want to try some alternatives, be a little kinder to my body, and enjoy my thirty-something age a while longer." Tamoxifen alone does not produce permanent premature menopause. But the closer you are in age to menopause, the more likely you are to slide into menopause a little sooner if you are taking tamoxifen.

If you are on tamoxifen and are premenopausal, you may still be fertile. If you do not want to get pregnant, you must use a barrier form of birth control. (Oral contraceptives contain estrogens, which, as I have noted, are not known to be safe for women who have had breast cancer.) It's also important to stick to your daily dose schedule of tamoxifen; if tamoxifen is taken intermittently, it can actually stimulate the ovaries like a fertility drug. If you want to get pregnant, stop the tamoxifen before you start trying, because the drug should not be taken during any stage of pregnancy. However, if you do get pregnant while on tamoxifen and you want to keep the pregnancy, stop the tamoxifen and don't drive yourself crazy worrying about the effect a month or so of tamoxifen might have had on the baby. There are no reported birth defects in people attributable to tamoxifen.

Vaginal Changes

You may have noticed a watery or malodorous discharge, dryness, irregular periods, or thinning of the vaginal wall while on tamoxifen. As many women note an increase in vaginal discharge (an estrogen-like effect) as report dryness (an anti-estrogen effect). Infrequently, intercourse may become painful, which can diminish your sexual activity or bring it to a halt. Discuss any changes with your physician, and consult Chapter 12 about coping with vaginal dryness and atrophy. Again, any new pattern of vaginal bleeding requires immediate medical attention to rule out cancerous change of the endometrium.

Nausea and Vomiting

Reported by about 10 percent of the women on tamoxifen, this problem generally resolves itself in a couple of weeks. It's uncommon to have it last more than a few months. This can be another unpleasant experience, even if it poses no danger.

Weight Gain

Chemotherapy, and the steroids that are given with it, cause weight gain in many women, and that weight gain may be perpetuated by tamoxifen. Many women feel strongly that tamoxifen makes them gain weight and that it makes it nearly impossible to lose weight. For these women, the tendency to gain seems to continue as long as they are on tamoxifen. One woman after another tells me about this unending battle with weight gain. "I put on twenty-five pounds, and it's real hard to get it off. It's been three years and I'm still trying!" It's not known why this weight gain occurs. Perhaps tamoxifen affects your metabolism and the way you process calories.

A major national study showed that women taking a placebo (fake tamoxifen in a sugar pill) were just as likely to gain weight as women taking tamoxifen, although other, smaller studies suggest that there is a tamoxifen effect on these symptoms. There are many concomitant reasons why women taking tamoxifen may gain weight. They may be less physically active, eating as much as ever—or more (and with reduced caloric needs because of menopausal changes), struggling with a wounded self-image, and fighting depression. More studies on tamoxifen's side effects are necessary for a final determination on the weight gain issue.

If you haven't gained weight in the first six months of tamoxifen use, you're probably not going to have the problem. A few women experience weight *loss,* and some women who have gained weight do manage to lose it over time.

Mood Swings and Depression

It is not certain that moodiness or depression in women on tamoxifen can be attributed to tamoxifen alone. The same national study (the NSABP mentioned before) also found that depression (based on the researchers' method of measurement) was not more common in women taking tamoxifen than in women taking the sugar pill. In my own practice, I've observed that women with the tendency to mood swings and depression can experience more profound "downs" while on tamoxifen. But trying to get your life back together after breast cancer can cause depression in the most well-adjusted woman. Whatever the cause, depression that doesn't go away should not be ignored. It should be evaluated and treated. Depression's relationship to tamoxifen should be explored. Depending on its severity, depression can be addressed with psychotherapy, medication, or both. Temporary discontinuation or reduction of tamoxifen dosage can be tried, but this doesn't usually eliminate the depression. It may be worth trying if other therapies are not effective and your oncologist says it's okay. Some women on tamoxifen have reported anxiety attacks; if such attacks are persistent, medication or short-term counseling is advised.

Loss of Energy

You may experience loss of energy with tamoxifen in the same way that you may experience loss of energy with menopause. In both situations, there is less estrogen effect. Estrogen seems to provide the "go-go juice" for some women, enabling them to get through the daily demands of busy schedules. Betsy, on tamoxifen for just a few months, said she had to talk herself into getting up off the sofa and out of the house to walk the short block to the beach. "The only other time I felt like such a cow was when I went on birth control pills. I'm determined to move myself around. I've always been someone who gets things done, and I'm not giving up on that image and expectation of myself. If I can't shake this lethargy, I may stop taking tamoxifen." (Eventually Betsy did stop taking tamoxifen and got back her zip.)

Hair and Nail Thinning

This problem is unlikely to happen to you but it can be distressing if it does, especially if it follows loss of your hair from chemotherapy (see

Chapter 9). Tamoxifen-induced hair loss behaves like postmenopausal low-estrogen-related hair loss, which tends to level off with time. It usually responds to minoxidil (Rogaine), but these treatments are expensive and time consuming to apply. For nail thinning, use moisturizing cream on your hands and avoid vigorous manicures. Watch for any signs of infection and follow the do's and don'ts of arm edema care for the affected side (see Chapter 10).

Memory Loss

You may experience memory loss on tamoxifen. Other factors in your life can also contribute to memory loss, such as depression, stress, sleep deprivation, medication, or medical problems. There has been no proven association between memory loss and tamoxifen. But given the number of women who report memory loss at our conferences and in my practice and the connection between reduced estrogen levels and memory loss, I'm convinced that some direct connection exists between tamoxifen and memory loss in some women.

Any sign of memory loss can be unnerving. Vivian would not abandon her use of tamoxifen, but she had to get better control of her life. She solved the problem for herself by keeping a detailed daily calendar. "I write down everything, the minute I think of it. It's a nuisance, but it keeps me sane." If you believe you have memory loss related to your use of tamoxifen, discuss it with your physician. The manufacturer of tamoxifen, Zeneca, will respond to any information you send them. This reported side effect is under study at this time.

Vision Changes

Eye problems are another potential, but rare, side effect of tamoxifen. Years ago, when much higher doses of tamoxifen were in use, a number of patients reported blurred vision in one or both eyes; their doctors found signs of damage in the cornea and retina (structures of the eye). Today's dosages carry an extremely low risk of visual distortions, which are almost always fully reversible if tamoxifen is discontinued.

There are no strict guidelines on follow-up eye exams for women on tamoxifen; some, but not all, oncologists recommend examinations every twelve months. Any change of vision should be evaluated immediately. You will need to have your pupils dilated during the exam so that the eye doctor can get a good view of early, subtle changes. An ophthalmologist or optometrist specially trained to detect retinal changes can handle this exam. Again, studies of this issue are ongoing.

Liver Cancer

Studies to date show that liver cancer is not a risk. Liver cancer has been associated with high doses of tamoxifen in rats, but Dr. Walter

Troll, an early investigator of tamoxifen's influence and the husband of a breast cancer survivor, says you can get liver cancer from this medication only if you have a tail and are a rat. (Mice do not get liver cancer from tamoxifen.) Says Dr. Troll, "My wife is a very nice person—she doesn't have a tail, and she's on tamoxifen."

Dosage, Cost, Source

If tamoxifen is prescribed for you, you'll usually start taking it after surgery or chemotherapy. It then takes several weeks to build up the desired level in your body.

There is only one kind of tamoxifen, but it goes by several names: tamoxifen citrate is its full chemical name; tamoxifen is its short chemical name; Nolvadex is its brand name. At this time, there is no generic available. All tamoxifen is manufactured by Zeneca Pharmaceuticals. Zeneca sells tamoxifen as Nolvadex; through an agreement between Barr Pharmaceuticals and Zeneca, Barr is able to sell tamoxifen as tamoxifen citrate. Nolvadex has a woman's face on the surface of the pill; tamoxifen citrate is plain. Tamoxifen citrate costs about 10 percent less than Nolvadex. Both tamoxifen citrate and Nolvadex can be purchased through the American Association of Retired Persons (AARP) at a discount even if you're not a member (call 800-456-2277). You may be able to receive a discount at a drugstore if you are a senior citizen. In an informal survey, I priced a one-month supply of Nolvadex and tamoxifen citrate at a small local drugstore, at a large drugstore chain, and through the AARP. At these three places, the cost of Nolvadex was $221, $210, and $168, respectively; tamoxifen citrate was $187, $188, and $150, respectively. Built into the extra cost of Nolvadex is Zeneca's cost to discover and develop the drug.

A generic form of tamoxifen is expected in the year 2001, at which time the price will drop considerably. If you are experiencing financial hardship, your doctor can fill out a special form from Zeneca, and, if you qualify, you can get the medication free.

Dosage is 20 mg a day, in two 10-mg pills or a single 20-mg tablet. It's just as effective to take both 10-mg pills at one time, rather than one in the morning and one at night. You don't have to time tamoxifen with meals. An occasional missed pill is not a cause for concern. Marty had been worried about that point when she came to our recent conference. "I had to get up so early to get to this tamoxifen workshop, I forgot to take my pill." She got reassuring information and a big, empathetic laugh.

Women with metastatic breast cancer who are disease free on tamoxifen are generally encouraged to continue tamoxifen as long as the disease is in remission. If cancer recurs and progresses while they're on tamoxifen, they should discontinue the medication and try another therapy.

Ongoing studies will further define the duration of therapy appropriate for every woman.

The Bottom Line:
Should *You* Take Tamoxifen?

Tamoxifen isn't a perfect treatment, but it can produce remarkable results with fewer side effects than chemotherapy. There are factors you must sort out, and pros and cons you must weigh, before you start tamoxifen therapy. You and your oncologist will go over the issues, balancing the potential benefits with the potential side effects, for your unique situation.

The magnitude of tamoxifen's benefit to you depends on (1) the likelihood of recurrence for you—and that depends on the particular characteristics of your breast cancer, (2) whether you are pre- or postmenopausal at the time of diagnosis, (3) whether your cancer is estrogen receptor positive or not, (4) whether you have already had chemotherapy, (5) your risk of developing a new breast cancer, (6) significant medical problems that could prove a greater threat to your life than breast cancer, and (7) your risk of heart disease and osteoporosis.

If your risk of recurrence is 40 percent and tamoxifen can reduce it to 20 percent, that's a significant benefit. If your risk is 15 percent and tamoxifen can reduce it to 10 percent, is that an improvement worth your taking tamoxifen? Were there no serious side effects to consider, the answer would be easy, but you have to balance the magnitude of the benefit against the 1 percent risk of endometrial cancer and the 1 percent risk of pulmonary embolism. How do you weigh one danger against another? And how do you weigh in the secondary benefits: reduced risk of cancer in the other breast, protection for your bones, and a lower risk of strokes and heart attacks?

Lily was working on these issues. "Both my parents died of heart problems, so I think about which way I'm going to die—someday far in the future, I hope. I think it makes sense for me to go on tamoxifen even if the breast cancer benefits are minimal. Tamoxifen will help my heart, and maybe I won't get osteoporosis. Always worth looking at the bright side, right?"

You also need to factor your age and general medical condition into your decision making. If you are eighty, with a small tumor, then the potential long-term benefits may not be worth the immediate side effects. If you are sixty-five, with an equally small tumor but with serious diabetes and heart disease, the threat of your medical problems may be greater than the threat of your cancer, and the long-term benefit of tamoxifen may be outweighed by the short-term side effects. If however, you are a sixty-five-year-old woman in good health with a 2.5-centimeter tumor that is estrogen-receptor positive, tamoxifen can offer important, compelling benefits that are likely to outweigh the side effects. If you are forty and have just completed chemotherapy for a hormone-receptor positive tumor with lymph nodes involved, tamoxifen may provide additional long-term protection against recurrence. If your receptors are negative, however, tamoxifen's ability to reduce recurrence is marginal, in which case you might conclude that the potential side effects are not worth the gamble.

If you have finished chemotherapy, you are premenopausal, and you want to have children, you may be struggling with the decision to take tamoxifen. There are several considerations: (1) tamoxifen taken after chemotherapy in premenopausal women has no proven additional benefit (which doesn't preclude a *potential* benefit in a particular individual); (2) most doctors suggest waiting two years after breast cancer treatment before starting a family, to get through the highest risk period for recurrence; and (3) you should not be on tamoxifen when you are trying to get pregnant. If you and your doctor together decide that you should take tamoxifen, it is reasonable to take it for two years and then reevaluate your family-planning options.

Whether to take tamoxifen or not is a tough decision for you if you have a breast cancer that is a mix of receptor-positive cells and receptor-negative cells. Two years after chemotherapy, Lela began tamoxifen. "I had been told I was estrogen negative and not a candidate for tamoxifen therapy, but I never take things at face value and I always put up a fight, though it took me a while after my treatment ended to get my old feisty self back together. I made them take another receptor test and that time I was found to be estrogen-receptor positive—so they agreed to give me tamoxifen. I feel back in control, and safer about my future." The original results were not a mistake; the test results depend on which cells are sampled. Lela's first receptor test had sampled cells from a field of estrogen-receptor-negative cells; the later test established the presence of estrogen-receptor-positive cells in a different area of the tumor. A mixture of positive and negative cells within a tumor can lead to the kind of confusion Lela experienced. In this situation, tamoxifen may prove effective only against the estrogen-receptor-positive component of the tumor.

There's also the question of benefit from initiating tamoxifen years after primary treatment. Some women ask whether they can start tamoxifen a year or more after the end of primary treatment. The answer to this question depends on what type and stage of breast cancer you have had, how far out from treatment you are (one month, one year, ten years), what treatment you've had, and your general medical condition. Although there is only a small window for starting chemotherapy, there may be benefits, even though diminished, from tamoxifen therapy whenever it is started. But there are no definitive data as yet.

If you have metastatic breast cancer that is hormone receptor positive, tamoxifen can be an important part of your treatment, whether or not you have had chemotherapy. If you had inflammatory breast cancer, or more than four to ten lymph nodes involved—both of which are associated with a very high risk of occult metastases—and your hormone receptors were positive, taking tamoxifen after chemotherapy is likely to benefit you.

Ambivalence and uncertainty are the norm for most of the women in my practice who are considering tamoxifen. "It's like betting on a horse race," said a speaker at one of our conferences. You weigh the odds, the percentages, the risks, the benefits—and you try to come up with a decision. Angela wanted everything possible to prevent a recurrence, even if the exact benefit for her was unclear. "It's my life insurance," she said. "I will do whatever I can to keep the cancer from coming back."

How Long Do You Stay on Tamoxifen?

How long do you stay on tamoxifen? We don't know. We *do* know that two years are better than one, and that five years may be better than two. The benefit of taking tamoxifen for five years lasts longer than five years. Women who have been on tamoxifen for five years are thought to be over the most at-risk time period for cancer recurrence. There are women who have been on tamoxifen, without threatening side effects, for ten years, some even longer. There are doctors who believe tamoxifen should be taken indefinitely, perhaps for life. Studies published in 1996 strongly suggest that five years is optimal for women without lymph node involvement, and that in fact the use of the drug beyond five years may provide no additional benefit and may pose an increased risk for endometrial cancer.

You continue to reduce your risk of breast cancer recurrence as well as that of cancer in the other, healthy breast at least as long as you're taking tamoxifen. Data show that tamoxifen can have a lasting effect against the breast cancer even after you stop the drug.

Tamoxifen's ability to keep your bones strong and lower cholesterol lasts only as long as you take the drug. And these health benefits haven't yet translated into extended life from fewer heart attacks and fewer complications from osteoporosis. In a large national study (the NSABP B-14), women who took tamoxifen for ten years had no fewer heart attacks or fractures from osteoporosis than women who took it for five years. It will take more studies to learn about these long-term health issues.

You'll need to be reassessed periodically to determine the balance of benefits versus side effects, and the optimal duration of therapy. Some women are determined to take the drug indefinitely, prepared to deal with the side effects because of the benefits they perceive. Other women worry about the risks posed by tamoxifen use and want no share of the down side; they want as short a period of treatment as possible. Most oncologists would not prescribe tamoxifen beyond five years for women who had had no lymph node involvement in the original diagnosis. Women who have significant lymph node involvement, with over four to ten involved nodes, have a significant risk of occult (hidden) metastatic disease; some doctors may treat them as if they already had metastatic disease and prescribe an indefinite course of tamoxifen.

Tamoxifen is a powerful drug when used appropriately. You and your doctor have to work with your best combined judgment, using the limited data, his or her medical expertise, and your preferences. Medicine has a lot of gray areas. There are few perfect answers to many of your important questions. But you and your physician should be able to come up with a thoughtful and responsible solution to the question of whether *you* should be taking tamoxifen, and if so, for how long.

THREE

Coping with Lingering Side Effects of Treatment

8

Fatigue and Loss of Energy

I hate the word tired. I was bone-tired all the time. It wasn't until a year after the chemo that the fatigue went away.

"The fatigue was indescribable." And that's a big part of the problem: You can't point to a place and say, See? here it is. "Nobody understands how dreadful you feel—I lay in bed all day, nauseated and out of sorts, unable to concentrate on anything for more than a few minutes at a time." Nothing shows, and after months—sometimes years—of living with this condition, some of the people around you begin to think it's all in your head. Even *you* may begin to think so. But fatigue is real.

If you're in the midst of treatment, your body is in a war against cancer; it needs all its resources to fight the disease, so it shuts down your energy for other activities that would divert your strength from the battle. Fatigue is a result.

If you've finished treatment, the fatigue may be trailing you. The effects of treatment linger, you're trying to catch up with everything that you had to put on the back burner, and you're trying to meet expectations of "normal" when you're not yet yourself. The reality of your diagnosis may only now be sinking in. Even more fatigue.

What will it take to get you to stop for a moment and pay attention to the way you're feeling? Are you used to being a dynamo? Do you think you have to be Superwoman, pushing your career and covering the home front, too? "I didn't miss a day's work!" Well, maybe you should have. Maybe you haven't been kind enough to yourself. Maybe your body is saying, Stop!

Give yourself a break; listen to your body. "My job right now is to take my chemo and let go of the other things that deplete my energy."

"I have no sick leave left, so I'm borrowing cash against my Visa credit to take a little more time to recover."

Is It Fatigue?

Fatigue can be confused with tiredness. You get *tired* from exertion, from arduous or long-sustained effort—running a marathon, running errands all day, or running your home and your kids' lives. When you're tired, it's usually after a day's activity, then you get some sleep, and the next day you feel better. Fatigue is less precise, less cause-and-effect. Fatigue is a daily lack of energy, a kind of weakness or inertia that pervades your whole body, even a loss of interest in people and the things you normally like to do.

Where Does Fatigue Come From?

If you've been treated for breast cancer, your fatigue may be chronic. It comes from worry, diagnosis, treatment, other medical conditions, and all that baggage—and it hangs on. It's a total lack of energy: "I wanted to keep going—but I couldn't do anything for a year." You don't feel normal; you don't feel good. "My mind keeps making appointments my body can't keep."

There's also the emotional stress. Traveling to the hospital every day of the week for up to twelve weeks—of course that's going to wear you out, physically and emotionally. "We missed only one day of treatment, through the whole of that ice-and-snowstorm-filled winter. There were so many days I wanted to stay home, but my husband would say, 'Come on, you can do it.' " Physical exhaustion blends with low spirits, and you wind up with fatigue. Paradoxically it may hit hardest during the easiest part of treatment, or when treatment is all over, just when you're relaxed enough to think about how you're doing.

Medical Problems

Fatigue often follows surgery, disrupting your body's rhythm and usually lasting longer than you expected. Fatigue associated with radiation tends to accumulate over the course of radiation and can last an extended period of time. Fatigue after chemotherapy may be greatest when your immune cell counts are at their lowest, but it may have no correlation with this blood count.

If you're suffering from anemia, you'll also suffer fatigue. Anemia is a deficiency of red blood cells or hemoglobin (which contains iron, which picks up oxygen in your lungs and delivers it to the cells and tissues of your body). The result is that the amount of oxygen that reaches the cells of your body is reduced. Because your body needs oxygen for any activity, you have less energy. Normal hemoglobin is about 13 grams per deciliter; if yours is significantly below that, especially if it's under 10, you should have an evaluation for the cause, and treatment.

Chemotherapy can lower blood counts and cause irritation of your mucous membranes, sometimes resulting in bleeding, which in turn can cause anemia. Chemotherapy can also foster fever and infections, which can cause prolonged fatigue, especially from urinary tract infections or lung infections such as pneumonia.

If your thyroid gland is underactive (i.e., you have hypothyroidism), your metabolism slows down and your body doesn't burn up food fast enough to give you the energy you need to be as active and interested in life as you should be. Hypothyroidism is a fairly common condition in general, and if you had radiation to the lymph nodes at the base of your neck (the supraclavicular lymph node area, directly in front of the thyroid gland), you are more likely to develop hypothyroidism, which may explain your fatigue. Nausea and pain—and pain medication—may sap your energy.

Other factors associated with breast cancer and treatment that contribute to fatigue might be changes in your eating pattern, appetite, or diet, increased weight, diminished activity and lack of exercise, premature menopause, and sleep problems. You may find yourself eating more to ease nausea, or putting on weight as a side effect of treatment, and suddenly you're twenty pounds past your tolerance point and your self-image sinks through the floor. Not surprisingly, you then tend to be less active, and you may give up all efforts at exercise—and going out and meeting your friends. ("Like I need people saying, 'Oh, you've put on a little weight.' ") Lack of activity sets in motion a cycle: the less you move, the less you feel like moving. (See Chapter 14.)

Hot flashes are another insult, seeming especially unfair if you have been thrust into early menopause by your breast cancer treatment or you had to discontinue hormone replacement therapy after your breast cancer diagnosis. When hot flashes wake you up in the middle of the night, they can cost you a good night's rest. If you are on steroids as part of your breast cancer treatment regimen, your sleep may be affected. Even if you are getting more than eight hours of sleep a night, you may not be getting adequate rest, because steroids interfere with deep, restful sleep. Steroids can also weaken muscles, particularly in the hip and shoulder areas. You may not be able to change your medication, but knowing where the fatigue and weakness come from may help you cope.

Emotional Stress

The breast cancer experience is itself enough to drain all energy from the toughest woman. There's uncertainty, from the moment you think you have something to worry about, to your initial visit to your doctor when the weight of the breast cancer diagnosis is laid on you, to the tests, waiting, results, and treatment, and then more tests. And always the questions Will this work? What next? Each test is another question, followed by an answer that raises another question. And the fear and anxiety of recurrence never leave. "It's like hanging your life up on the line and watching it dry out." Absolutely exhausting.

Many ordinary stresses seem—or are—worse now: your job, your marriage, your children, your financial situation. Any of these problems can wear you out.

If you suffer from fatigue, you may also be vulnerable to depression. Your doctors should have prepared you for the fatigue phenomenon so that you know what to expect and know how normal this abnormal feeling is. But if they haven't, not knowing why you feel washed out week after week can make you or anyone depressed. On the other hand, depression may come first. It may be a side effect of the breast cancer experience, or you may have a natural tendency to depression. Perhaps tamoxifen is tipping your depression deeper. Fatigue may be a major symptom of your depression.

Practical Help

So what do you do? Unfortunately, there's no magic pill that will cure fatigue. But I do have some suggestions and guidelines that have helped my patients.

Listen to Your Body

First and foremost is a Zen-like suggestion. Fatigue *is,* so accept it, don't fight it. Fatigue is a sign to you that your body needs to recover. Go along with those signals. Accept the changed you. Stop trying to do more than you need to. Develop distraction techniques. Sit. Meditate. Listen to your breathing. Stop and enjoy the sunset, or the moonrise. Rest and recover. Stop running away from fatigue, "move into it, explore it," and gain control of it. Maybe this sounds too mellow for you, but the idea of listening to your body is very important. (See Chapter 19.)

Medical Solutions

Most of the medical causes of fatigue are treatable. Your doctor will check the medical conditions that may be contributing to your fatigue. If your doctor doesn't respond well to your concern about these problems, find a doctor who will. You must assert yourself if you know you've reached your limit and you need help.

Low immune cell counts improve with time off from treatment, good nutrition, and growth factors such as Neupogen. Infections are effectively treated with the appropriate antibiotics. Anemia caused by the inadequate production of red blood cells can be treated with iron if the cause is iron deficiency, or with Procrit or Epogen if the problem is the slow cell production associated with chronic illness. Treatment of a bleeding polyp in the colon or uterus, or management of a stomach ulcer, can reduce blood loss. Blood transfusions can increase your blood counts immediately. Hypothyroidism is easy to diagnose and remedy: a blood test, results within a week, and one pill a day does the trick with no side effects. The treatment of depression is essential, by individual therapy and/or medications.

Reestablish a Reasonable Routine

Establish a more disciplined routine in your life to help you pull yourself back into normality. Dr. Barbara Piper, who specializes in fatigue research, suggests keeping a daily index of your fatigue to identify a pattern of when it's worst and when it's least troubling. Then block out your week with activities during the times you have the most energy, and rest periods when your energy is lowest.

Get a handle on what is stressing you most—job, family, money—and try to figure out how to make things better. But don't let handling this stress, stress you further. If you haven't yet learned that it's okay to ask for help, now is the time to find that out. (See Chapters 2 and 4.)

Control your uncertainty: Address the questions you have about your illness and treatment, and find answers to those that have tangible answers. Then write down the unanswerable questions on a nice piece of stationery and stick it in a drawer: *off your mind*. (See Chapter 3.)

More Down-to-Earth Advice

Get Moving

More down-to-earth things you can do: Get moving. Exercise—a little bit at first. Amble along your favorite street; walk to the house of a nearby friend. Then work up to a pattern you can live with: three times a week, half an hour a session. Try out a gym. You might love strolling on a treadmill. Or swimming: water therapy. Or Nordic Track: "I got on that Nordic Track, first to music, then to silence—and I got to feeling great." Exercise may not thrill you at first, but almost everyone who gets into the groove finds it does wonders. You'll find you sleep much better on the days you exercise. Exercise reduces hot flashes, making it less likely that they will wake you up at night. Every therapist who treats fatigue prescribes some form of exercise.

Drink lots of water to keep your bowels moving and kidneys flushed, but not too close to bedtime (you don't want to lose sleep getting up to pee). Eat well, especially low-fat foods, nothing too heavy—meaning smaller portions and less rich food (with an occasional chocolate exception, of course).

Rest

If you are fatigued during the day, try to catch catnaps—but watch out for long naps. You'll pay for them. You'll be wide awake in the middle of the night, wondering why you can't sleep. A wise family doctor I work with, Dr. Su Kenderdine, says if you must take a nap in the daytime, set your alarm for no more than thirty minutes. You'll get some rest, but you won't fall into deep sleep, which would compete with deep sleep at night. If you wake up groggy from your nap, you are waking from deep sleep; you've napped too long.

Try to keep to a regular routine. Eat your evening meal as early as possible before you go to sleep. Avoid all caffeine after five o'clock in the afternoon, or after twelve noon if you're especially sensitive. I even have to watch those decaffeinated versions of coffee and tea after twelve noon (some have more caffeine than you think), so I stick to "sleepytime" versions or warm milk with honey. Sodas—Coke, Pepsi, Mountain Dew, Jolt—all have a lot of caffeine along with the bubbles. Chocolate, especially dark, keeps some people up. Alcohol may help you fall asleep, but ultimately it makes you more tired because it interferes with deep sleep—you wake up too easily and too early.

To help you fall asleep at night, read the dullest book you can find, or a soothing book you've read before, or try a sweet, old-fashioned children's book like *The Five Little Peppers*. Counting backward from a hundred helps some, including Dr. Art Ulene and me. Count sheep if that works for you.

Let's not forget sex and the role it may have in sleep. A *Consumer Reports* survey of its readers found that sex was the second-best remedy for sleep problems. (First was prescription sleep medication.) But maybe sex keeps you up, instead of putting you to sleep (uh-oh), or maybe your partner chooses inconvenient times to rouse you: You finally fall asleep at eleven o'clock, and your partner is rubbing up against you at one in the morning, when you need to be at work by seven. I suggest you bring in a little discipline along with the foreplay. Avoid nights when you have to get up early for work, and have sex at a time that works for both of you. I've told more than one patient who really needed her rest to hang a "Do Not Disturb" or "Don't Even Dream About Waking Me" sign over the bed.

Dr. Kenderdine suggests that if you have trouble sleeping, you should keep away from bed, unless you want sleep or sex. Bedtime is lights out, go to sleep. Keep your room dark and quiet. Don't use your bed for watching TV or reading or listening to music. If you're trying to sleep and you can't, don't toss and turn for more than twenty minutes. Get out of bed and do something decidedly unpleasant or boring for half an hour: Read a dull book, balance your checkbook, or clean the bathroom. It's negative reinforcement (I call it punishment), and it may get you back into the mood for sleeping. Shortly before bedtime, avoid exercise, talking on the phone, or watching the news (murder, rape, and highway accidents are not soothing bedtime stories)—anything that is too stimulating. (Exercise *early* in the evening can help you sleep.) Instead, massage your neck or legs, or take a warm bath, try ear plugs to cut off the outside world, daydream, meditate, or visualize. Imagine yourself in a gondola on the Grand Canal, swimming off the Florida coast, or sunning naked on a Cape Cod sand dune. (Listen to the birds, sniff the salt air, and watch the clouds pass overhead.)

Acetaminophen (Tylenol) or ibuprofen (Advil) might be enough to help you get to sleep, especially if hot flashes are keeping you up or waking you up. If transient anxiety is responsible for your sleeping problems, ask your doctor about Ativan. If anxiety is more an everyday problem, see if your doctor thinks Elavil, Pamelor, or Serzone might help. If your insomnia is nonspecific, occasional use of something like Ambien can be helpful, but follow doctor's orders and don't take it more than two times a week or your body will get used to it and it will lose its effectiveness. If your problem is waking up in the middle of the night, Ambien won't do you much good because it's short-acting: It helps to put you to sleep, but not to keep you asleep. Some doctors think clonazepam (Klonopin) is a better choice because it's long-acting; however, longer-acting pills can leave you groggy in the morning. (Most of these medications can be obtained only with your doctor's prescription and should only be taken with your doctor's approval.) Never borrow pills from a family member or friend.

Distribute Household Chores

If you've been reluctant to ask for help with chores you find especially burdensome, move past that resistance. As independent as you may have been before, now is the time to ask something back from those around you, especially if you're trying to keep up with your job as well as your household. Your family may be looking for ways to help you. Friends are always willing to pick up something from the grocery for you. Cash in now on the goodwill and friendship you've built up in the past. If it makes you feel any better, write out promissory notes for return favors when you finally feel more like yourself.

Give up unfinished business that means little to you. Then do something you enjoy unequivocally. One expert suggests you focus on just one good thing. "I made a list of things that make me feel good, and when I'm feeling bad, I pick something from the list." Do what you want to do, not what others think you should. That includes saving your energy for the people you really care about.

How Long Will This Go On?

There is no time limit to how long fatigue may last. My rule of thumb is that it takes at least as long as the time from diagnosis through the end of treatment. If diagnosis and surgery took two months, followed by six months of chemo, it will take at least eight months for the fatigue to go away. Complete recovery from major surgery often takes six months. But fatigue related to breast cancer treatment has been known to go on for years, with all efforts helping to decrease, but not eliminating, the problem.

The suggestions in this chapter will help you take charge of your life so you can live it fully. If you've done all you can and you are still fatigued, keep up your anti-fatigue program and try to accept the fatigue and your reduced energy level as one aspect of the breast cancer experience. You're stuck with it for now, but keep control by going with the flow, capitalizing on what energy you do have at this moment.

9

Hair Loss: Terrible but Temporary

Nothing was as bad as losing my hair. My best friend called me when I was feeling so blue about it. "We're going out to get you a wig." "I can't—it's a really bad day for me." "Look, getting a wig is one of the worst things you can do—so why screw up a *good* day? I'm coming over, and we'll screw up the rest of a bad day!"

No other side effect of breast cancer treatment seems to be more disturbing than hair loss. For many women, it's worse than losing a breast. Hair loss is so visible—so much a part of your image, how you appear to others and the reflection you see every time you look in the mirror, *you*. And you look so transformed, bald. It's the final insult, on top of the gray skin, the look of exhaustion, and the weight gain. "It's hard enough to have cancer and feel bad, but to have to look bad, too!" It's so traumatic—but it's also temporary.

Bobby was beside herself when she went bald. "What if it doesn't grow back?" she asked her doctor. "Then you'll be the first one." It took six months—first fuzz, then real lush hair, curly, too. Bobby had always wanted curly hair, and here it was. "I was ecstatic. I figured this was my reward—but I felt like an impostor."

Nancy's two-year-old daughter had a much harder time. She loved sitting on her mother's lap and playing with her mother's hair, and she was terribly upset when it started to fall out. "I got a wig very quickly after that, and Nora was placated. But when she'd wake up in the middle of the night, I'd have to pull the wig on—half asleep and in the dark—before going in to see to her."

Why and How It Happens

Chemotherapy affects all rapidly growing cells, which include the cells that make hair. Within a few weeks of starting chemotherapy, you may lose some or all of your hair. Some drugs affect only the hair on your head; others cause the loss of eyebrows and eyelashes, pubic hair, hair on your legs, or hair on and under your arms. The extent of hair loss depends on which drugs are used, and for how long.

Adriamycin (the A of CAF) causes complete hair loss on the head in all women who take it, usually in the first few weeks of receiving the drug. Some women also lose lashes and brows. Methotrexate (the M of CMF) can cause thinning of hair in many women, but no hair loss in some; complete hair loss from methotrexate is uncommon. Cytoxan and 5-fluorouracil are commonly associated with hair loss, usually minimal, but occasionally some women may have more significant loss. Taxol usually causes complete hair loss in all areas: head, brows, lashes, pubic area, legs, and arms. Radiation therapy to the whole brain (used to treat cancer metastatic to the brain) causes complete hair loss on the head in all women (eyebrows may be spared). Tamoxifen can cause some thinning of your hair, but not baldness.

Loss may be gradual or dramatic: clumps in your hair brush, handfuls in the drain of your shower or on your pillow. No matter how forewarned you may be, it's always a terrible shock.

When Will Your Hair Grow Back?

How soon your hair grows back depends on how fast it normally grows. A few weeks after chemotherapy is finished, you'll see soft fuzz; by a month, your hair will have started to grow in. At six weeks, you may have an inch of hair, which will continue to grow at its normal rate. Your new hair may be just like your old hair, or it may be thicker and curlier, or straighter, than your original hair, and it may be a different color. Gerry's hair used to be straight and wispy, and then grew back curly and thick. "Your hair looks so good!" said a friend. "Where'd you have it done?" "Paoli Hospital."

If you had hair loss after whole brain radiation for brain metastases, it can take four to six months before you regrow an inch of hair. Your new hair will probably be thinner than it had been and you may have a small bald spot along the top of your head. You might want to hold on to the wig or head gear to spruce up for special occasions.

Very, very rarely, permanent baldness occurs after many years of chemotherapy: Your hair follicles get "burned out" and they shut down. Thinning of your hair from tamoxifen usually levels off after the first year, but in some women the tendency continues as long as they are taking the drug. Using Rogaine or minoxidil is a safe and effective approach to tamoxifen-induced hair loss, but it's a daily messy chore and it's expensive. One of my patients followed the daily ritual for years, but she got tired of it and stopped. Her hair loss has stabilized, and she now has a full head of hair, although she says it's not as thick and lush as it used to be.

In the Meantime

Until your hair returns—and it will—you have a choice of cover-ups, or you can decide to go bold and bald. One young woman at a Living Beyond Breast Cancer$_{SM}$ conference went for the bare-head look, with great makeup and big, bold earrings. She was stunning. Most women, however, want to find some way to disguise their bareness—and keep warm. Then, it's a matter of what you're most comfortable with: a wig, a scarf, a hat, or a baseball cap.

Wigs: "I bought two wigs—but I couldn't get used to either one." Evelyn was despondent until her own hair was back in full. Betty: "I was philosophical about losing my hair and I found a great wig that fooled everybody into thinking it was all my own hair." Which one of these women speaks for you?

One woman became a wig sales specialist after her own experience with breast cancer, mastectomy, and hair loss. "Within four weeks, I lost a major part of my body and all my hair, including eyebrows and eyelashes. I was at my lowest. I know how important a beautiful wig can be."

If you have lead time, it's less troubling to select a wig before you lose all your hair, because you can get used to wearing the wig in short trial sessions before you need to wear it all the time. It's also a good idea to have your hair cut short before chemotherapy begins. With a becoming cut (many women look better with short hair), you'll see how short hair can work for you. A short-haired wig is easier to wear and to care for, and if your hair is already short, you'll have an easier time living with temporary hair that's a similar length. Shorter is also cooler, an important consideration, because wigs usually feel hot in the summertime. Besides, if you can get used to yourself in short hair, you won't have to wait as long for your hair to grow back and to feel like yourself again. And it's a lot less traumatic to lose short clumps of hair than long ones.

"When my hair started to go," Florrie said, "my husband shaved off all of his. Then he put on a Howard Stern wig and we horsed around and had a few laughs." Annamarie's husband cajoled her into shaving her head bald, once she started to shed clumps of her hair. "Let's both shave it off!" That sparked a lot of conehead jokes. Annamarie did get a wig, exactly like her own hair, and none of her friends realized the difference. "But as soon as one hair grew back I got rid of the wig." When her hair was about an inch long her husband told her, "You look so much better with short hair." "I kept it that way, but I did try dyeing it. It had been ash blond before and it grew back gray with blond streaks. I wanted it brown. I dyed it, and it came out purple. I kept it purple for a while—life was kind of wild, so why not a wild hair color?"

"My friend Jane had begun to lose her hair long before she ever got breast cancer, so when she lost it all after chemotherapy, she felt she had a proper excuse for getting a really good wig. It was beautiful, she was beautiful—and she looked ten years younger."

Breast cancer organizations often have a list of wig specialists in the area, or your hairdresser may be able to suggest a wig sales place, or you can ask friends or your doctor or a health center. Some wig specialists will come to your home, if you are concerned about privacy.

Wigs come in all styles and colors. You can order a wig made of real hair, but it could cost you between $800 and $1500, or more, and it requires more care than you give your own hair. Most women choose synthetic: It looks and feels good, needs very little attention and care, and costs much less ($30 to $500). The cheapest and most popular catalog for wigs: Paula Young (800-343-9695).

A really good wig isn't cheap, but it may be what you should buy—and your health insurance may pay for it. You want to buy a good-enough wig, one that doesn't have an obvious part line and won't get matted or look silly. I'm sure you've seen some bad toupees; you don't want a wig with that kind of look. You also want to be sure it isn't scratchy against your scalp (most wigs are designed for women who have some hair). Ask your doctor for a prescription for an "extracranial prosthesis" (a.k.a. a wig) that you can submit to your health insurance company. Not every company will reimburse you, but *try*. It is, after all, a remedy for a treatment side effect. (Antinausea medication is covered as a side effect remedy; a wig should be handled in the same manner. See the Claims section in Chapter 26.) Some American Cancer Society branches offer free wigs.

Although you may wear your wig almost every day, most women use a wig for less than a year, so it's not necessary to buy something that will last forever. Alternating occasionally with a turban can help keep the wig looking fresh. (You can fashion your own wig stand with two sixty-four-ounce plastic soda bottles: Cut them in half, discard the tops, face the cut edges of the bottoms together, and force one inside another to get a football-shaped stand.)

Wigs are formed on an open-weave mesh that allows for ventilation, and they are fitted with adjustable tapes along the temple, or by elastic and Velcro around the ears. They wash easily (every two weeks is recommended). You can set them with sprays or gels. The only thing you have to worry about is heat. Stay away from hot ovens, hair dryers, and curling irons. "The front of my wig was all singed when I got too close taking a pizza out of the oven." The lesson? Order out.

Color is probably the most important issue in choosing a wig. Select a somewhat lighter color than your own hair for two reasons. Your skin color may be off during chemotherapy—grayish, greenish, or yellowish—so you don't want to call attention to these off colors in your skin. (Less contrast is generally more flattering under these circumstances.) The other reason is that wig hair is usually thicker than your own hair, so while the shade may be the same as your hair color, the wig will appear darker.

You might want to turn the wig-thing into something that gives you a smile or two: Try a new color, a new length, a new style. You might as well find something upbeat in this experience. Mary Beth had always toyed with being a blonde, so she bought a high-styled blond wig, and she liked it so much she dyed her own hair blond after it grew back. Deena had had a similar thought, but her daughter Jill stopped her cold; she wanted her mother to look exactly as she had before the cancer therapy, and the only way to come near accomplishing that was for Deena to buy a wig just like her natural hair. Deena capitulated, and it calmed her daughter's distress. Jill did have a sense of humor: She gave her mom the magnet toy with iron filings enclosed with a bald-headed face under plastic; you can move the filings around to style the "hair." "Thanks for getting the wig for my sake," Jill said. "Here's hair *you* can control."

Scarves: Head scarves suit some women more than a wig. "I knew my hair would be coming back, and I was just more comfortable in a scarf. I didn't let anyone see me bald, my husband in particular. I figured he'd had enough to deal with, and I guess I was worried he'd find me unappealing. I wore beautiful scarves and earrings and made myself up, something I never normally did. It made me feel much better about myself."

You can learn to tie scarves in clever, creative ways. Top the scarf with a dramatic hat, and it needn't look anything like a disguise for lost hair.

Turbans: Turbans fit close to your entire head, unlike hats, which tend to sit on the upper part of your head; unlike scarves, they don't need tying or adjusting—you just pull them on. Turbans may fit like a simple cloche or sport a twist, or they may have pleated folds of fabric such as terry cloth, jersey, or felt. They're easy to put on and take off, many are washable, and they're cheap ($5 to $100). Some come with an attached fringe of hair along the top like bangs. Elsie wore a turban alternately with a wig. "I wear the turban to sleep, for warmth. Apart from how it looks, a bald head gets cold at night." (The Paula Young catalog also offers a full line of attractive, inexpensive turbans.)

Hats: Deena went to work in hats. (She was never comfortable with her wig.) Her co-workers started wearing hats to work too, to help make her feel better. When Jeannie lost her hair, she bought a supply of baseball caps, snug-fitting and funky, and wore one of them to work each day. After the first day, everyone in her office showed up in caps, and wore them every day after that, until Jeannie gave hers up when her hair grew back.

Makeup: If you lose your eyebrows and eyelashes, you may want to try makeup to restore the balance in your features. Some women normally shave off their natural eyebrows to paint on eyebrows they believe are more becoming in shape and color. If you compare early photos of Greta Garbo with later ones, you'll see the dramatic change in her eyebrows, and how much more beautiful she looked with the graceful arches Hollywood gave her, which became part of her personal signature.

Thumb through a good fashion magazine to come up with possibilities. Then take a little time in front of a mirror and practice your technique with shapes you like. Feather in strokes along your brow with slightly different colored eyebrow pencils to give it the most natural look, or ask for help at your beauty parlor. As for eyelashes, you can try eye shadow to give the effect of contrast and drama around your eyes, or, if you really miss your eyelashes, you can buy false ones. (Think of Liza Minnelli or Dolly Parton.)

10

Arm Lymphedema: Prevention and Management

I was a model twenty years ago, when I had a mastectomy. I got a prosthesis and continued modeling—until the arm edema. I did everything I could to beat the edema, but I finally just had to learn to live with it. I've always loved clothes, and I'm still what you'd call glamorous. I can't wear designer clothes, but I can sell them. My customers at Neiman Marcus tell me I'm the best.

How Arm Lymphedema Happens

Lymphedema of the arm is an accumulation of lymph fluid in the soft tissues of the arm with accompanying swelling. (Think of it as a plumbing problem.) Blood travels from your heart to your arm within arteries and capillaries (the small blood vessels that connect arteries to veins). As the blood percolates through the capillaries, oxygen, nutrients, and a clear, colorless fluid called lymphatic fluid pass through the capillary walls into the tissues of your arm. The veins carry the depleted blood back to the heart and lungs, and another type of vessel, thin-walled lymphatic channels, carry excess lymphatic fluid from the tissues back into circulation via the thoracic duct.

Lymphatic fluid is propelled up your arm by muscles of the arm and contractions in the wall of the lymphatic channels; valves within these lymph vessels keep fluid moving in a forward direction. The lymphatic channels pass through bean-shaped structures called *lymph nodes* (located in the arm, neck, groin, and other regions), which filter out bacteria, cellular debris, and toxic substances from the lymphatic fluid. The trapped debris is broken down and excreted from the body.

Lymphatic fluid has lots of nutrients in it, and as it ebbs back into circulation it is an easy target for bacteria that may find their way past the protection of the skin through something as seemingly innocent as a torn cuticle or splinter. These bacteria can then cause infection, which results in increased blood flow to fight the bacteria, and more lymphatic fluid accumulating and needing to be drained away.

Veins and lymphatic channels can handle the normal load of fluid, but if the lymph nodes under your arm have been removed, the drainage of lymphatic fluid is partially disrupted. When increased blood flow to the arm occurs because of an infection, a burn, or even a bug bite, the larger quantity of returning lymphatic fluid can sometimes back up and accumulate in the spaces between the cells of the soft tissues of your arm—skin, fat, muscle, nerves, blood and lymphatic vessels, and connective tissue. Swelling results from this buildup of lymphatic fluid and is called arm lymphedema.

Lymphedema can affect the whole arm or only a limited portion, such as the hand, the wrist area, the area below the elbow, or, much less often, only the area above the elbow. Some women experience mild lymphedema, which is hardly noticeable, and others experience severe lymphedema, resulting in discomfort and disability.

Fallout from Lymphedema

Fortunately, lymphedema affects relatively few women after lymph node surgery, but if you suffer with the problem, you may find it alters your self-image, interferes with your routine activities and what clothes you can wear, and serves as a troubling reminder of the disease you thought you had overcome. Your arm may feel heavy as lead, an appendage that is you and is not you. It may look swollen and unattractive. Adding insult to injury is the continuous medical care and expense that attends this unpleasant condition.

Severe cases of lymphedema, which can cause thickening of the skin, stiffness and hardness of the arm, and leakage of fluid from minor injuries, are unusual. Most cases are neither disabling nor unduly uncomfortable. Although episodes of lymphedema may be transient, once an episode occurs, the condition tends to persist or recur, sometimes varying in degree. The episode may resolve spontaneously or it may resolve only if the precipitating cause is treatable, and if it is treated quickly. Episodes may last for days or weeks. If your edema lasts for months, it's likely to be permanent.

Breast Cancer and Lymphedema

If you have had lymph node dissection (with mastectomy or lumpectomy), lymph node irradiation, or systemic chemotherapy, you have a 5 to 25 percent risk of developing a swollen arm at some time in the future. The more treatment you have, the higher your risk of lymphedema. The risk is the same after a mastectomy with lymph node dissection as it is after a lumpectomy with lymph node dissection, with radiation treatment confined to the breast.

It can happen just weeks after surgery or years after initial cancer treatment. It can be precipitated by trauma or infection, or it can be tripped without any obvious cause. Occasionally, lymphedema can be caused simply by extensive breast cancer in the lymph nodes, unrelated to treatment. In rare circumstances, backed-up fluid in the arm is caused by a blood clot in the axillary (underarm) vein. Being overweight puts you more at risk for edema; posttreatment weight gain can precipitate its onset. Too high a temperature in a hot tub, or too long a time in a hot tub, may also trigger lymphedema. Flying in an airplane can trigger or aggravate lymphedema because of the changes in air pressure.

The longer you are free of lymphedema, the greater your chance of avoiding it altogether, because your body has probably learned how to reroute any excess buildup of lymphatic fluid. On the other hand, the more lymphedema you have and the longer you have it, the harder it is to reduce your arm back to its original size.

How Do You Prevent Lymphedema?

Prevention is the best tool against arm lymphedema. Familiarize yourself with warnings and precautions, and incorporate these guidelines and a heightened awareness into your lifestyle. Current methods of breast cancer treatment minimize the risk of lymphedema. But if you had a radical mastectomy many years ago, you may have experienced arm edema or you may still be at risk for the condition, so prevention is very much in your interest. Even the safest and most effective therapy may only stall or modulate the condition. If any trauma occurs, immediate care is essential.

Skin care is your first line of defense. The skin acts as a barrier to infection, thus any breach of this barrier can spell trouble. Burns, chafing, dryness, cuticle injury (such as hangnails), cracks, cuts, splinters, and insect bites are immediate risks for infection.

Learn to recognize the signs of infection: fever, redness, swelling, warmth, or tenderness in the at-risk arm. Infection and inflammation can escalate quickly. Call your doctor as soon as you suspect infection. You may need to start antibiotics immediately with any early sign of trouble. Patients who already have edema or who have diabetes (with or without edema present) need antibiotics after just the smallest of injuries—even without any sign of trouble.

These are the preventive guidelines I recommend to my patients:

- **Do** moisturize your skin frequently and regularly, with lotions such as Moisturel, Eucerin, Vasoline Intensive Care, or your own favorite brand, to make your skin supple and prevent it from cracking.
- **Do** keep your hand and arm extra-clean, but don't use harsh soaps such as Ivory (despite Ivory's advertised image as a gentle soap) or Dial. Use Dove instead.
- **Do** use rubber gloves when you wash dishes or hand-wash clothes.
- **Do** wear protective gloves when you garden or do outside chores.
- **Do** wear oven mitts when handling hot foods.
- **Do** use an electric razor instead of a safety razor.
- **Do** use insect repellents that don't dry out the skin, such as Avon's Skin So Soft, which actually moisturizes the skin. Avoid brands that contain a significant amount of alcohol. (Any ingredient that ends in "ol" is a type of alcohol.)
- **Do** apply antibiotic ointment to any insect bites or torn cuticles (as long as you are not allergic to its contents).
- **Do** protect your arm from sunburn with sunscreen, minimum SPF 15, although SPF 30 is preferable.
- **Do** use a thimble when you sew.
- **Do** rest your arm in an elevated position.
- **Do** control your blood sugars very carefully if you have diabetes, to minimize the danger of small blood vessel damage and infection.
- **Do** wear compression bandages on the affected arm when flying in airplanes (if you already have arm edema).
- **Don't** take unusually hot baths or showers.
- **Don't** go from extreme hot to cold water temperatures when you bathe or wash dishes.
- **Don't** go into high-heat hot tubs, saunas, or steam baths.
- **Don't** carry heavy objects with your at-risk arm, especially with the arm hanging downward.
- **Don't** wear heavy shoulder bags on the affected side.
- **Don't** wear clothing with tight sleeves or that restrains movement.
- **Don't** wear your watch or other jewelry on your affected hand or arm.

- **Don't** use a heavy breast prosthesis after mastectomy. (It may put excessive pressure on alternative routes of lymphatic drainage that are already doing double duty; find a lightweight model or make one yourself.)
- **Don't** drink much alcohol and **don't** smoke. (Smoking constricts the small blood vessels, adversely affecting the flow of fluids in the arm and alcohol causes blood vessels to dilate and leak extra fluid into the tissues.)
- **Don't** get manicures that cut or overstress the skin around the nails.
- **Don't** permit blood pressure testing on your at-risk arm.
- **Don't** permit any piercing of the skin for injections, blood draws, or vaccinations on the at-risk arm. (Don't trust anyone, not even your personal physician, to remember which is your at-risk arm.) If you have had breast cancer in both breasts, blood should be drawn from your nondominant arm.

You may have had breast cancer in both breasts and need to protect both your arms against arm edema. If you are in this position and need to have your blood pressure measured or blood drawn, present your nondominant arm. (If you are right-handed, use your left arm for the procedure.) In an emergency (e.g., a car accident), however, if an IV needs to be started, let them do what they need to do to establish an intravenous line as soon as possible.

How Do You Manage Lymphedema?

You can usually control lymphedema with good care and adherence to basic guidelines. Your physician and nurse are more likely to take your symptoms seriously and follow your progress through various treatments attentively if he or she regularly measures the circumference of your arm and compares it with your unaffected arm, documenting the measurements over time.

The health care professionals who specialize in the management of arm edema problems are physical medicine doctors (physiatrists) and physical therapists. But don't assume that anyone in these specialties is an expert to be trusted. Ask about experience and references before you let anyone work on your edema problem. Most metropolitan areas have physical therapists whose practice is dedicated to managing the physical side effects of breast cancer treatment. If you can't find a therapist who specializes in breast cancer, look for a general physical therapist in a rehabilitation center or department who has experience taking care of women with breast cancer.

Start Treatment Fast

If you develop sudden-onset lymphedema, seek *immediate* medical attention.

As I mentioned before, infection is your enemy, the prime trigger of edema. If you develop edema, even without obvious signs of infection, I think it makes sense to start antibiotics right away, because infection is one of the only completely reversible causes of arm edema, and it is readily and effectively treated by many available and reasonably priced antibiotics (e.g., penicillin or Keflex). Side effects of a short-term course of antibiotics are usually minimal.

Start antibiotics under the direction of your physician. Call your doctor's office during the day, or page your doctor at night or on the weekend if necessary, to get the prescription. Be sure to let her or him know if you have any allergies to antibiotics. Without prompt treatment, swelling can start and eventually become chronic and progressive.

Cover burns with Silvadene cream and a clean dressing; periodically cleanse, and reapply the cream and bandage. Keep any cuts or abrasions clean: Wash the area two to three times a day with a solution that's half peroxide and half water, and apply antibiotic ointment and bandage.

Ongoing Management

Nonurgent care for edema takes many forms. All therapies for chronic edema require a commitment to a modified lifestyle.

Arm Elevation

If you are experiencing any amount of arm swelling or infection, keep your hand and elbow higher than your shoulder, and higher than your heart. This eases the drainage of lymph fluid from the affected arm back into circulation. Get into the habit of keeping your arm in an elevated position whenever possible. If you rest it on a hard piece of furniture, like the back of a chair, don't put pressure on the armpit area.

Mild Exercise

Exercise is nature's way of moving lymphatic fluid up the arm, against the force of gravity, back into circulation. The contraction of the muscle around the filled lymphatic channels results in a type of "milking" action. Exercise also increases blood flow to the arm, which increases the amount of lymph fluid that needs to be drained. Exercise combined with customized bandaging is a very effective way to pump the lymphatic fluid back into circulation. The force of the contracting muscles against the firm binding of the bandages enhances draining of the lymph. For this approach to work best, the bandage needs to be applied correctly, as described below.

Flexibility exercises are easy to perform and are nonstressful, and they help maintain a wide range of motion. Arm stretches also increase flow in the lymphatic channels. Gradual, strengthening exercises with light (one- or two-pound) weights can be very helpful. Walking and swimming keep the circulation of body fluids at maximal efficiency, and the deep lung action that goes along with vigorous exercise has been said to create a suction effect on the lymph system, promoting lymph flow. Avoid any strenuous activity that involves repetitive, resistance-oriented movement in the at-risk arm. See the Appendix at the end of this book for a description of recommended exercises.

Exercise increases blood flow to the arm, which increases the amount of lymph fluid that needs to be drained. If you have lymphedema, use a compression bandage when you exercise to help drain the extra fluid. And check with your doctor about any new exercise plans you'd like to undertake.

Compression Sleeves and Wrapped Bandages

Compression sleeves are a longstanding therapy device. These elasticized sleeves are customized to your arm. They can be used on their own or in conjunction with manual lymphatic drainage or mechanical drainage (as will be described). All stitching and seams should be parallel to the length of your arm; stitches from the hand up should be small at first, and larger as they near the shoulder. To prevent the sleeve from rolling down—which diminishes its effectiveness—apply a water-soluble adhesive lotion under the top of the sleeve. (Soap and water remove the adhesive.) Buy two sleeves and alternate their use, washing them in lukewarm water every two to three days (dry flat, don't wring); they'll last much longer if you have two and treat them with care.

A roll of specialized elastic material (such as an Ace bandage) is an alternative to the sleeve and is easily modified to your needs. It should be applied first by a trained therapist, who can then train you to apply it yourself.

Weight Loss

Weight gain is common with chemotherapy, hormonal therapy, and the inactivity that tends to accompany treatment, compounding your arm edema problem. Losing weight can really help you reduce edema.

But weight loss is so hard to accomplish. (See Chapter 14.) Restricting your salt and sugar intake will reduce the amount of fluid your body retains, thus helping you control your weight as well as reducing the fluid buildup in your arm. You still must remember to drink lots of water.

Diuretics

Diuretics are a type of medication that removes excess water from your whole body, including your arm. They may be able to ease your discomfort and reduce the asymmetry of your arms, but they do not eliminate these problems, and the relief is temporary. Diuretics remove water from your arm, but the protein remains in the tissues, drawing fluid back to cause the arm to swell up once again. A woman with normal heart, blood vessel, and kidney function, who drinks lots of water, does not have increased fluid buildup. The extra water is simply excreted by the kidneys, and diuretics are unnecessary.

Diuretics require a physician's supervision; regular blood tests must be taken to make sure your blood chemistry is not out of whack. I tell my patients to avoid the use of diuretics unless no other therapy has worked for them, or they have a general underlying medical condition that warrants fluid restriction and the use of diuretics anyway (such as high blood pressure, congestive heart failure, or general edema).

Manual Lymphatic Drainage

Manual lymphatic drainage, known as "complex decongestive physiotherapy," consists of manual stimulation of all soft tissues of the arm. (More traditional massage concentrates mainly on muscle and can be quite vigorous. If it makes you sore, it could potentially worsen lymphedema rather than making it better.)

A professional therapist gently stimulates the affected arm, starting at the hand, using delicate movements of the fingers on the surface of the skin, moving the skin about, slowly, with a pumping motion directed toward the shoulder. The manual lymphatic drainage technique requires specific training and certification.

At the end of every session, the therapist applies a customized bandage or sleeve, which provides light compression of the arm without restricting the flow of lymph, to minimize reaccumulation of fluid.

You'll be prescribed exercises to perform with the bandage in place. Arm elevation is recommended.

Therapy is often one or two sessions a day, five days a week, for from three to nine weeks. Sessions are usually one hour to an hour and a half. The procedure is expensive and usually *not* covered by most medical insurance plans. The success of manual drainage is closely tied to the skill and enthusiasm of the therapist.

Pneumatic (Air-Driven) Pumps

Pneumatic pumps are a component of traditional edema therapy. Your arm is placed into a full-length plastic sleeve that fills with air, compressing your tissues, thereby moving the stagnant fluids out of the swollen arm into channels of normal lymph flow.

An effective pump must have two features. One is *gradient pressure,* meaning the pump exerts stronger pressure on the hand area than it does on the upper arm, to propel fluid in the proper, upward direction. (Less useful pumps exert equal pressure over the whole arm.) The second necessary feature is *sequential pressure*. The pump should exert pressure that moves from the hand up the arm with a sort of "milking" technique.

This treatment requires about a two-hour commitment each day to accomplish transient though significant relief. This therapy is done in your home while you are reading or watching TV, but it must be supervised by a qualified professional. Good pumps are expensive to buy ($5000 to $6000), but they can be rented from a surgical supply store. There has been a sudden surge of medical practices and independent companies promoting the pump; some of these companies lack trained physical therapists to supervise an individual's care. Watch out. Buy or rent a pump only from a rehabilitation center or through the recommendation of your physical therapist. Most medical insurance plans cover part if not all of the cost.

Benzopyrones

Benzopyrones are a class of drugs used in Europe to treat lymphedema, but the Food and Drug Administration (FDA) has not approved their use in this country. Coumarin is the most commonly used benzopyrone. (Don't confuse it with Coumadin, the blood thinner.) Its proponents say it can take weeks, maybe years, to experience its benefits. The manufacturer claims the drug facilitates the confiscation of proteins in stagnant lymphatic fluid; as proteins are "eaten up," the water and edema diminish as well. But the action, efficacy, and safety of these drugs have not been satisfactorily demonstrated by clinical trials or laboratory studies.

I have had no experience with these drugs, either directly or through the breast cancer physical therapists with whom I work. Until the drugs pass the FDA testing process, I would not use them.

Surgery

Surgery has been the last resort for cases of lymphedema that do not respond to the less invasive, less aggressive techniques described above. The principle behind the surgery is to create new avenues through which the fluid backup is permitted to escape the arm.

This surgery is done mostly in Europe. Approach this option with *extreme caution*. This procedure, even in experienced hands, can result in a worsening of your condition. Consequences can be disastrous. I do not recommend it.

Long-term Care

Lymphedema can be a very frustrating condition, limiting your comfort and full range of activities. Women who have this problem deserve careful attention, support, and the best medical care.

A movement is afoot to promote the wearing of a pink bracelet on the at-risk arm, for instant recognition and trauma prevention.

Fortunately, most edema, when it occurs, is mild, and most women are spared the condition. Prevention is the key. Follow the Do and Don't guidelines and take quick action at the first sign of trouble.

11

Other Lingering Side Effects of Treatment

The lingering side effects of treatment that you may continue to experience beyond treatment depend on what treatments you've had: surgery (what procedure was performed), radiation therapy, chemotherapy, or bone marrow transplantation.

Infection can follow any kind of treatment. Be alert for the signs: persistent drainage from the incision, particularly if the fluid is mucuslike, green, or foul-odored; or redness, swelling, and/or warmth at the incision and the surrounding area. See your doctor at the first sign of infection.

Other side effects, such as hair loss, fatigue, edema, and infertility, are such important concerns that I've devoted separate chapters to them.

Side Effects of Surgery Alone

Lumpectomy

After a lumpectomy, you can expect numbness and tenderness in the biopsy area. You may also experience some shooting discomfort in the breast and the underlying chest wall for some time beyond the first month. Tenderness resolves over a few months. Most numbness resolves over six months, but minimal residual numbness usually persists around the incision area well after healing. If the incision was around the nipple, you may experience numbness in this area, which can affect your sexual pleasure. Your skin may also feel thick or leathery.

A few weeks after any kind of surgery, you may notice little suture (i.e., thread) ends rising from the incision; that's your body's attempt to eject them. (It's safe for these suture ends to stay inside you, which they usually do, whether they're absorbable or not.) If there's no pus as these ends emerge, there's no problem and you have nothing to worry about.

When lumpectomy is done for an invasive breast cancer, a lymph node dissection is almost always performed as well. This procedure may result in side effects similar to those described below when lymph node dissection accompanies mastectomy.

Total Mastectomy

Total mastectomy involves removal of the breast. After this procedure, numbness of the skin along the incision site and adjacent area is common. Mild to moderate tenderness and stiffness are also common; you'll feel it more when you reach, stretch, or sleep on your chest (there is less give in the skin, and the breast is no longer there to cushion your chest wall).

Some women have a hypersensitivity to touch within the area of surgery, because the fine nerves to the skin (which lie just beneath the surface) have been cut. This effect can last indefinitely, although most women who experience this hypersensitivity find it improves over time, as the nerves grow back. (This condition can make it very uncomfortable—if not impossible—for these women to wear a prosthesis.) Nerves grow very slowly, however, so it will take a number of months, possibly six, before sensation starts to return to normal. As the nerves regrow, you may get odd sensations in the area—some women say it feels like bugs crawling across their skin—as well as itching and tenderness.

Modified Radical Mastectomy

This procedure is the removal of the breast and the lymph nodes under the arm. In addition to the side effects already mentioned, you can expect some alteration of sensation in the armpit, and sometimes a numb feeling along the inside of the upper arm, usually with some tenderness. You may also experience stiffness, and your range of arm and shoulder motion may be compromised for weeks or sometimes months. Stiffness and reduced range of motion respond nicely to exercise. (See the Appendix for a description of recommended exercises.) There is often swelling of the underarm tissues, because some of the lymph fluid draining vessels were disrupted when the lymph nodes were removed. Fluid that builds up can accumulate diffusely in the armpit, or it may accumulate in smaller areas; it can feel like a golf ball under your arm. This combination of numbness and fullness is common and can be very annoying.

Because you are accustomed to using your arm all the time, after surgery you're frequently aware of the asymmetry and discomfort, which become a persistent reminder of your breast cancer experience. The good news is that both the swelling and numbness improve with time. After six months, you'll probably be able to ignore or adjust to any residual asymmetry or discomfort, especially as you know it will continue to improve.

You may also have some swelling of the breast area from backed-up lymphatics leading from the armpit area; for the same reason, your arm may have some swelling; this swelling tends to be mild. (See Chapter 10.)

Lymph nodes are usually removed along with a pad of fat from under the arm, so another "cushion" is lost: less soft tissue to protect you from bumps and bruises.

Occasionally during lymph node resection, a minor nerve that keeps your shoulder blade in position in your back is damaged. If this has happened, you may notice that your shoulder blade sticks out slightly with certain movements of your arm. This nerve may not re-generate, but the intermittently altered shoulder blade position should not result in any disability of motion or function.

Radical Mastectomy

Radical mastectomy, rarely performed anymore, used to be the *only* kind of breast cancer surgery performed, removing the breast, all lymph nodes, and muscle beneath the breast. Women who have had this procedure have a large concavity of the chest, below the collar-bone between the shoulder and chest. You can easily see the ribs just under the skin, with little tissue left as a cushion. The shoulder is no longer quite as strong as it was, without the muscle, and some arm function may be limited. Arm edema is a considerable risk after radi-cal mastectomy, because all of the lymph nodes are removed from under the arm. There are many women who had this procedure twenty or more years ago still living full lives today, despite its linger-ing side effects.

Mastectomy with Reconstruction

Side effects of reconstruction at the time of your mastectomy, or at some later time, depend on the type of reconstruction. If you had a TRAM flap procedure, your abdomen and chest may hurt for some time. (The incision for the flap goes all the way across your abdomen.) Numbness and tenderness will occur in both places. One month after surgery, most women find the discomfort tolerable with just Tylenol. If you had a tissue expander put in place after mastectomy, the skin overlying the implant will be stretched and under tension. (See Chapter 23.)

Radiation Side Effects

Lingering side effects of radiation therapy to the breast can involve persistent pinkness, redness, and soreness of the skin, and swelling, stiffness, and tenderness of the underlying breast tissue. The skin irritation is usually most prominent in the upper inner corner of the treatment field, in the crease beneath the breast, and along the lower underarm area. Your skin's angry reaction should significantly improve starting one week after treatment, and it will show dramatic improvement by three weeks after treatment.

The most common reason for a *return* of skin redness is infection—requiring your doctor's immediate evaluation and antibiotic treatment (I like good old Keflex)—or a reaction to certain chemotherapies given after radiation is finished. Uncommonly, a woman may experience sudden onset of redness within the entire radiation treatment fields after all treatment—including chemotherapy—is over, which is most likely to be an infection. Occasionally, this same presentation can represent psoriasis, activated by the irritation of radiation, usually in a woman who already has a history of psoriasis. Uncommon is new redness in part or all of the breast years after surgery, which may be due to cancer recurrence.

What takes longer to go away are the textural changes of the breast: the firmness (a combination of healing scar tissue and swelling), color alterations (a pink or tan hue to the breast, or, occasionally, paleness), and tenderness. These changes may resolve relatively quickly or may take years—two to three years is not so uncommon. As the breast area softens up, don't be surprised to feel a new area of prominence where the prior surgery was performed; it's been there the whole time, but it was "buried" within the generalized firmness. This buried area also continues to soften and become less tender with time.

Lingering skin dryness is not uncommon either, and should respond nicely to your favorite moisturizer. Remember that irradiated skin is more sensitive to sunburn, even if your treatment is years past. So protect your skin from the sun with a lotion of SPF 30 or higher, reapplied frequently. A T-shirt alone is inadequate protection, having an SPF of only 8.

The chest wall directly beneath the breast, made up of ribs, muscles between the ribs, and nerves here and there, falls partially within the treatment field. Shooting discomfort may persist here after treatment, brought on by different kinds of movement. The ribs within the treatment field remain slightly more fragile, with one in one hundred women breaking a rib from a fall or injury—but occasionally from only a violent cough. If you have pain in one particular spot on the chest wall, you may have a broken rib. Your doctor may want to get a bone x-ray to confirm the diagnosis. Many doctors, however, base their diagnosis on a physical exam alone (a rib fracture heals on its own). Obtaining rib x-rays does not affect management of a fracture.

Occasionally, scar tissue develops in a small ellipse of lung tissue beneath the chest wall, within the radiation treatment portals, just as it might after an old pneumonia. Symptoms are uncommon (occurring in less than 5 percent of women); they include cough, shortness of breath, and fever, which usually respond to a limited dose of steroids. Changes in the lungs, if they occur, are usually detected coincidentally by routine x-ray for an unrelated reason. (Keep this in mind if, in the future, you're asked by your employer to get an x-ray, or if a new doctor wonders if you ever had pneumonia on the same side as the radiation.)

All these changes can also happen if you had radiation therapy to the chest wall area after mastectomy, with or without reconstruction, to reduce the risk of cancer recurrence in the skin and underlying tissues where the breast used to be. These tissues often get bright red, sometimes peeling like a blister. Radiation is aimed at the skin itself, as well as the tissues lying just below it, so the reaction after treatment can be more intense than general breast radiation (which is aimed further beneath these areas), and it can persist for a longer period of time after treatment is finished. If chemotherapy is given at the same time, the reaction may be even more pronounced.

Radiation side effects to the heart are rare today. If your doctor treats the internal mammary lymph nodes that are located just beneath the chest wall on each side of the breastbone, the risk of heart side effects increases. (This procedure is no longer common because there is no proven long-term benefit from treating these nodes.)

Fatigue after radiation is not uncommon and is discussed in Chapter 8. Blood counts can be slightly depressed after radiation therapy.

Chemotherapy Side Effects
Weight Gain

I hear a lot about weight gain from my patients. It's one of those unanticipated extra insults that follows the diagnosis and treatment of their breast cancer, those ten or twenty extra pounds (or more). There are plenty of reasons for this weight gain. Perhaps it's the result of a sudden arrival of menopause, physical inactivity, or maybe it's a consequence of "relief" eating.

Some of the antinausea medication regimens include steroids, which increase your appetite and alter your metabolism. One of the major reasons for weight gain is that the queasiness, nausea, or hollow feeling that comes with chemotherapy is relieved by eating. If you stopped smoking during or after treatment, eating is a way to distract yourself from the craving for nicotine. And, of course, a lot of people eat when they're feeling stressed. Plenty of stress comes with breast cancer, with diagnosis, treatment, and trying to get back to so-called normal. For more on weight gain, see Chapter 14.

Other Side Effects of Chemotherapy

Nausea is a nasty side effect of chemotherapy, but fortunately it rarely lingers past treatment. Occasionally, a reminder of your treatment will bring back that old feeling with unexpected intensity. "I vomited every time I went to chemotherapy. After a while, just going to the doctor's office, the smell of the place, would set off my nausea."

Chemotherapy can lower blood counts; how low your count goes depends on the kind of chemotherapy you are having and on the dose. If you are having low dose chemotherapy and are in overall good health, your blood count will probably recover relatively quickly, perhaps by a couple of months after treatment. If, however, you had a bone marrow transplant, you will experience a more profound and prolonged drop in your blood count. (See Chapters 15 and 22.)

Other side effects of chemotherapy are related to the type of drugs you get. Cytoxan can cause bladder irritation. Taxol and Taxotere can cause numbness of the hands and feet. You have a 10 percent risk of developing heart muscle weakness, or cardiomyopathy, if you take adriamycin in doses of more than 450 mg per square meter. (Most women receive only about 350 mg with a six-cycle treatment course.) This risk of cardiomyopathy may be reduced with the heart-protecting medication Zincard. Investigators are trying to develop another form of adriamycin without this complication.

There is a tiny risk of developing leukemia from chemotherapy; it happens with certain drugs, such as methotrexate, more than others.

Most treatment side effects improve with time and don't interfere with your ability to lead a normal life. More debilitating side effects and their management are discussed in other chapters.

FOUR

Caring for Your New Self

12

Intimacy, Sex, and Your Love Life

"I'm disfigured. And lopsided, too. I have no hair, and I've gained ten pounds. Admit it! If I think my body is so repulsive, how can you say it doesn't make a difference? I miss my breast so much!" Emily was distraught.

"I miss your breast—but I'd miss you more. It doesn't matter to me. I mean it," her partner insisted. "You're here, and that's all that counts."

Partners Who Care

In spite of what you may imagine or fear, studies show that what partners* of breast cancer patients care about most is that their loved one is alive. They find the loss or alteration of a loved one's breast almost meaningless in contrast. "I don't care what they take from you as long as I can see your face." I talk to and hear from many couples, and what I've learned is that most caring partners see their lovers as having many parts to love, and as more than the sum of those parts.

Nobody is promising there won't be ups and downs; this is a rough deal. While you're worrying about any number of issues, including feeling less attractive, your partner is riddled with worry, anxiety, and maybe even guilt, about you and him/herself: "Could I have been responsible? Could I have been too rough, too amorous? Could I in some way have contributed to this breast disease?" As well as: "Can I be affected by the radiation if I touch her, if I touch her breast? Is her cancer contagious?" Or: "When will I be able to worry about myself for a change? Am I selfish because I want our old life back?" It helps the progress of treatment and recovery, and the maintenance of a

* Partners include men and women.

sound relationship, to have your partner share in the conferences with your managing physician, so that you both get a chance to air and dispel fears when possible, and supplant myths and false information with facts.

Breast cancer is not good for relationships, but good relationships can be made stronger by sharing hardship. It's not easy, and it's only fair to appreciate that your partner can have doubts, and miss and mourn the old you (just as you may be doing). But that doesn't mean he or she is prepared to trade you in. "My husband was there through all my *mishagas*. He stood by while I cried and screamed, and he hugged me when I let him get close enough. Our marriage is better now than it ever was before."

Doubt-Riddled Relationships

Despite assurances, testimonials, and sweet talk, if you see yourself as damaged goods, you assume your partner feels as you do. Emily: "I feel so diminished. How can it not matter to my husband? I just can't believe him when he says he doesn't care." There's a common misconception that "my experience is your experience." It isn't so, but if you are anxious and dejected, it's hard to convince you otherwise.

One consequence of feeling less than lovable is fear of being abandoned—all those stories of women left by their mates even as they go into the operating room. "Right after my diagnosis, he abandoned me emotionally, then spiritually, then physically. He just couldn't handle real life. In the end I was better off without him, though I didn't realize it at the time." Occasionally a man sees his partner's altered body as a personal reflection of his value—and just wants out. But partners leave for innumerable and often inexplicable reasons; some simply come apart under stress. Marriages or relationships that dissolve because of cancer were flawed before they were ever put to a test. A marriage that can just about manage the average stresses that life presents may simply not have the resources to handle the trauma of breast cancer.

It may surprise you to learn that following a diagnosis of cancer, as many women leave their husbands as are left by their husbands. These women decide they don't want to waste their time in an unfulfilling, unrewarding, unhappy marriage.

But, in fact, flawed marriages don't have to come apart, with or without breast cancer. The incidence of divorce does not increase because of a breast cancer experience. Maybe, sometimes, the shock of a cancer diagnosis will push partners within a troubled relationship to consider the source of their problem and seek counseling. Perhaps the excuse of this crisis will give you permission, and courage, to turn to someone who can help you help each other and stay together on new, improved terms. "I'm no longer the same person," says one survivor. "I need to be known in a new way. I don't care if he feels the same way about me. *I* don't feel the same way about me."

When your partner reacts in ways you don't comprehend, misunderstanding tends to escalate and become destructive. "My husband was very resentful toward me for having breast cancer! As though I did it on purpose. He finally came around after he saw I was going to survive, but for a while I thought it was the end of our marriage." Another survivor was stunned when the end of her eleven-month treatment triggered inexplicable nastiness from her husband. It lasted a few painful weeks, then stopped as suddenly as it began. Five years later the marriage is just fine.

You may be the one who responds unpredictably. I had a patient who was supremely independent, but upon diagnosis suddenly became overwhelmed, uncertain, and very dependent. It devastated her. She had a hard time adjusting to this new "frailty," and her marriage went through a rough spell till she finally returned to something of her old self.

Partners tend to help in concrete, significant ways: shopping, preparing meals, allowing you extra time to rest and recuperate—a much appreciated demonstration of love and support. But what may be most important to you is something more personal and intimate: sharing what's on your mind. " 'What do you want to do?' My husband asked me after the doctor recommended mastectomy. 'I want to live.' A breast meant almost nothing by contrast."

Try to figure out your needs and concerns, and tell them to your partner. You don't want to make light of what your partner has already done for you, so phrase your requests as carefully and positively as possible. "You've been working so hard, doing so much—and it's made an enormous difference. But what I really need right now is to be close to you and tell you what's making me nervous and anxious. I need you to listen, and maybe just hold me. Simple reassurance, such as 'you're doing great'—doesn't really help me."

Talking, Telling, Supporting Each Other

It would be nice to have a partner who understands and helps you feel better as you work to get back your old confidence, but that may just be unrealistic. He or she is probably suffering, too, and is less able to express that suffering than you. So each of you has all this emotion buried somewhere inside. Ginny could not understand her husband's silence. "What's the matter with you? Why don't you talk to me about what's happening? I have *cancer*! I could die! Say *something*!" Ginny felt as though she was yelling at a stone wall.

Most people haven't got a clue about how to talk about something as big as cancer. "When I was young, people didn't talk about a breast, let alone cancer!" Start somewhere: Talk about vacation plans or the weather, if that's all you can manage. Once you are talking, try to introduce some conversation about your fears if you can, of how your illness has changed you, of what matters most to you: relationships. You've got to try to discover how your partner really feels, and to let your feelings gradually come out. "My husband said, 'Put it away.' He didn't want to deal with it anymore. But I insisted. I talked and he listened. I think I talked him out of denial. He didn't say much, but he was there after that to help me with everything, including the dusting!"

There's got to be a lot of talking to get comfortable with how things are now. It may be that you have to reassure your partner that it's okay for him or her to feel and express fear, ambivalence, and depression. "She's got the cancer. What right have I got to add my problems to hers?" You may need to give your partner that right, that permission, the reassurance that expressing honest feelings won't destroy you— which is not saying it won't upset you.

If all that talk is simply too hard for you, and seeing a therapist together to help you through this time seems too big a step for one or both of you, get started by sitting down together with this book and let what it says speak for you. Do what Ann Landers always suggests to readers with communication problems: "Show him what I'm telling you in print." Let us do some of the hard work for you. Further along in this chapter, we may be talking about things you've never done, things you've never spoken of to your partner. Remember, then, that pointing to parts of this book can help you and your partner with the uncomfortable stuff. Dr. Leslie Schover, author of *Sexuality and Fertility after Cancer* (Wiley Press), handles the most awkward issues of intimacy, sexuality, and communication with unequaled sensitivity, insight, and information. It's a "must read" for anyone with questions on this subject. Please see Selected Readings for other recommendations.

Changes in Your Sex Life:
What's Real and What's Myth

The most uncomfortable stuff to talk about is probably your sex life and the changes that have taken place with your illness. You may not know what needs fixing or how to fix it, but you do have a measure of what's different. Less sex than you had before your illness, according to many of my patients. One reason is that the breast cancer experience slows your body down. It takes longer to do lots of things, including getting interested in and starting and finishing sexual intercourse. Another powerful reason is that sex may be uncomfortable or even painful for you if you've been thrown into sudden-onset menopause. Sex may be something you just want to get over in a hurry. No surprise that you tend to have less sex, for now.

What you don't need at this time is pressure from popular mythology. Most people have wild ideas about what goes on in other people's bedrooms. Give yourself a break: the carefully researched book *Sex in America* (by Michael, Gagnon, Laumann, and Kolata) tells us that Americans have a lot less sex than the movies, television, and the guys in the locker room would have you believe. Between the ages of thirty and forty, sex averages seven times a month; between forty and fifty, it's six; then five times a month between fifty and sixty. Over sixty, the numbers continue to decline, but now the assumptions that Americans have work the opposite way: that people in their seventies and eighties don't have any sex life. That's just not so. Molly, seventy-eight, described her sex life after breast cancer treatment: "I stopped the action for a while, and then we went back at my request. He was waiting for me to give him the go-ahead." Hilda, an eighty-two-year-old breast cancer survivor, explained that she didn't have a lover "at the moment." Sex goes on even into the nineties for some. Don't let the myths about other people's sex lives get in the way of what's happening in yours.

There are exceptions to every pattern. After Gena's breast cancer surgery, she was suddenly more interested in sex than in food, drink, or television. "I'd tell my husband I want to make love. He'd say, 'Not now, I'm tired.' I'd say, 'Now. It's therapy.' We'd laugh, and we'd make love. It was the only thing that made me feel alive. With the fear of death hanging over me, I needed that sustenance and reassurance."

If your sex life is not working the way you want it to, your doctor or nurse may be able to referee these issues with your partner and you. You can cue your doctor in advance, since she has undoubtedly touched on delicate issues with you already. Maybe she can be the tour guide for the two of you. I discuss the sexual aspects of recovery first with my patients, and again later, with their partners present. One of my patients had told me that her breasts had been a crucial part of her sexual life before the discovery of her disease. She had bilateral lumpectomy, followed by radiation. Her breasts looked great—but her husband was ignoring them completely. I scheduled an appointment that included her husband and was able to reassure him that her breasts would not be harmed by fondling, kissing, or whatever; that he could not catch cancer; and that she was not radioactive. They quickly resumed their former lovemaking habits.

Help from a Pro

Not all physicians and nurses are comfortable discussing sexual issues and practices. Dr. Wendy Schain, a professional sex therapist and twenty-five-year survivor, wishes that doctors who diagnose, dissect, radiate, and reconstruct your body would learn to help you manage the effects of their treatment on your sex life. But many women with a breast cancer experience tell me their doctors don't ask them about their sex life, and don't talk to them about it either, and patients don't usually bring up discussion of their sex life with their doctors. Nobody's talking!

Someone has to break the pattern. Neither partner may want to burden the other with his or her questions or worries. Each one waits for the other to go first; neither can talk about their sex life, or about what's not going right. A trained social worker, sex therapist, psychologist, or psychiatrist can help you open up communication with your partner and finally get around to talking about intimacy and sex issues. A skilled therapist I refer to says not to worry about what you talk about. "Just talk about anything. Any conversation will help you feel better and keep the lines of communication open."

A support group may be more helpful than you might realize. You draw comfort and encouragement from being with other women surviving breast cancer; you also develop a good deal of intimacy with each other. Women in these groups often share advice that extends to the bedroom, ways to increase sexual pleasure that are explicit and specific for women who've had breast cancer.

But maybe real heart-to-heart communication with your partner isn't going to happen. Maybe you just have to live without that level of intimacy. There's a story about the couple soon to celebrate their fiftieth wedding anniversary. She: "You never tell me you love me." He: "I told you I loved you when we got married. If anything changes, I'll let you know."

Meeting Needs in Other Ways

Most marriages have problems that don't get fixed. Marriage is a package deal, and in those marriages that work, the good things outshine the shortcomings. But as a survivor, you may find that breast cancer highlights the deficiencies in your marriage. Can you live with those deficiencies? Can you enjoy your marriage even as you contemplate what's missing? Can you capture the missing pieces in other ways? Give serious thought to your needs and how to meet them.

"I actually sat down and made a list of things I don't get from my marriage—like kisses, conversation during meals, interest in my career—and half an hour later I was still writing! It was great therapy—but there was nothing I could make different or make happen." Jacqueline wasn't writing off her marriage, but she was looking for ways to reduce her frustration. Another survivor told me, "I'm having an affair. My marriage is intact, but after I'd faced death, I decided I needed some passion in my life."

Well, you have to be resourceful, but you can find less drastic ways to keep happy. Fantasy can enrich your life. Countless women read to fill up the vacuum (romance novels are enormously popular). Join a book club, a church or synagogue, or a group that meets to discuss investments, movies, or local politics. Work on friendships; people can be the best medicine of all. Do more with individual friends, like walking, shopping ("retail therapy"), or travel. Strengthen your relationship with family members; make a bigger deal of birthdays and anniversaries. "I never realized how important it is to celebrate simple things with people I love."

Expand your involvement in community or spiritual activities. Get politically active in the breast cancer movement: camaraderie for a cause close to your heart. Linda told an interviewer, "The Living Beyond Breast Cancer$_{SM}$ conferences are like a huge support group for me. I rearrange my life around them—I wouldn't miss that event for the world."

Romance

Are you longing for old-fashioned images that don't work anymore? You may be yearning for a little romance in your relationship, but romance can fade fast in today's daily life. By evening, when partners meet at the end of a stressful day, there's barely enough of you left to get through the basics. "Even when I go out of my way to set up a candlelit dinner, all he wants to do is blow out the candles and get into the sack."

Romance, of course, is not only candles and roses. For one woman it was a vasectomy. "I had to give up the pill, so John just went out and did it. What a gift!"

Another survivor's husband gave up his ritual Sunday fishing to spend the day with her. Each week they have that special time together, and she sets the pace and program. Romance has reentered their lives in real, meaningful terms.

But such attention can also backfire: "When Steve started spending time with me like he never had before, I knew this was it, this was checkout time. Then when he brought me *presents* I was sure my days were numbered, especially because the jewelry was junk. When George Burns gave Gracie an $11,000 mink coat, she was sure she'd get better. Well, Steve is no George Burns, but it's twenty years later, and I'm still around, and so is Steve, and we're doing fine together even though he hasn't paid that much attention to me for a long time." Still, Gena seems pretty happy.

When Debbie, a thirty-five-year-old divorced single mom of a four-year-old son, was diagnosed with breast cancer, she decided to call her old college boyfriend for support. He had never married and was still carrying a torch for her. They got together the very next weekend and fell in love all over again; his family also embraced her. He stayed by her side through chemotherapy, hair loss, early menopause, return of her period (a terrific day, as they desperately wanted children together), and much more. They are about to be married.

Single Women
Finding Your Way

Much of what we've been saying has involved couples, men and women or women and women, but many women recovering from breast cancer are single. Some prefer to remain single, but many want to become part of a relationship, and they worry how breast cancer will affect their prospects. And they worry about how and when to tell those prospective lovers about their condition. Don't allow breast cancer to define who you are. One thing is clear: You don't need to wear a sign that reads "I've had breast cancer," and you don't have to bring it up until you are ready and feel you have some stake in a relationship.

Linda Dackman was thirty-four when she had a mastectomy. She felt terribly angry, more so because she had no way to find help as a single woman looking for a relationship, wanting to know when and how to tell about her mastectomy and her disease. She wrote the book *Up Front: Sex and the Post-Mastectomy Woman,* a personal account of how she coped with these problems. She tells us that each time she met someone new, she had to struggle with when and how to tell, and then how to behave in intimate situations. In the beginning, she would blurt out her history almost immediately, frightening herself and her date. Gradually she got to a point where she was able to wait to the third or fourth meeting, and discuss it without upsetting herself or her companion. And she learned to protect herself during the initial phase of a sexual encounter, by wearing a silky cover-up, gradually working up to full exposure.

Renee had a really positive experience. She told Burt about her cancer history on their first date, including the fact that it was unlikely she could have children. They were married ten months later. "I worked through my fears with him—and they disappeared from my head when we had sex. Sexy lingerie helped me feel confident and attractive."

Breast cancer has become so common that most men have someone close in their life who has suffered the disease. The mother-in-law of one of my patients had had breast cancer, and when my patient was diagnosed, her husband was calm and upbeat—he had been there before. There's no way to predict how any man will respond, but I do know, from patients of mine and others, that more men are supportive and prepared to continue the relationship than you might imagine.

Women may find it easier to talk to one another, and lesbian partners may be particularly sensitive and supportive. It is also true, however, that a woman may feel especially vulnerable and personally threatened if her partner has breast cancer, knowing this disease is one that can affect her as well.

Making the Connection

Finding a suitable and available companion is always a challenge, but there are enough success stories to keep up hope, to take action and make things happen. Your statistic as a breast cancer survivor is irrelevant. You've got to do what any woman out to meet Mr./Ms. Right does, and take your chance, just like anyone else, that you'll be lucky.

There are quality single people out there looking for relationships. They may not fit your ideal fantasy, but maybe it's time to set realistic standards and look for what really counts, like character and responsibility.

Work out a plan. Check out the new-style bookstores, with space for refreshments and socializing. Or upscale grocery stores. The Safeway store in San Francisco's Marina section has a stunning reputation as a scene for meeting new people. Get involved in local politics, join an exercise center, volunteer at your local hospital. Or take up interesting activities that bring out interesting people. Go back to school for computer programming, financial planning, or a carpentry course. Better still, find out what activities your community center, church, or synagogue provides for single members to get together.

You can also take out a personal ad, or answer one. Voice mail is one way to talk to someone new without giving up your cover. E-mail, or electronic computer mail, is another hi-tech route, and a lot of people have fun with it. You scan the possibilities and try out responses, keeping your anonymity until you're ready to jump in. (And then, it's wise to meet in public places at first, until you feel confident that the person you've met in this New Age manner is on the level. There have been reports of women being assaulted by men who had constructed false identities for themselves.) Or you can use a dating service. Or buy an irresistible dog or a quirky irresistible car. I heard about a woman on "Car Talk" (National Public Radio) who advertised a vintage Land Rover for sale. A slew of people came to look at it, but each time she said that, unfortunately, it had been sold and driven away only minutes before each one's arrival. She admitted to the "Car Talk" guys that she had never actually owned such a vehicle, but she did get to meet a lot of intriguing men.

According to *Sex in America*, most couples are introduced to each other by families or friends, co-workers, classmates, or neighbors. So look to the people you know—and tell them you'd really appreciate an introduction to a quality person, a serious date. "A woman at work, someone I hardly know, told me she had a great guy for me. Matchmaking was her passion. She had two marriages to her credit already, she was looking for a lucky third, and she said I fit the bill. He and I hit it off right away. I'm meeting his parents next week."

Don't be shy. Your social network has resources for you to tap, but you've got to let your friends know what you're looking for and talk up your hopes. Keep up your connections and your expectations. You never know which blind date may be The One.

Frayed Connections

This is a tough time, and you've had to do a lot of soul-searching with this disease. Maybe the same soul-searching can help you handle relationships. Breast cancer makes many women angry, a healthy response, but sometimes that anger gets directed at the wrong targets and distorts your perspective. Or maybe other reasons account for why you're having trouble meeting the right person. Maybe you tend to go after the wrong partner, or send the wrong message. If you've had problems with your relationships before breast cancer, those problems are not going to go away. This may be the time in your life for you to look into yourself more closely, perhaps with the help of a therapist.

Accepting the Nude You

If your self-image has been impaired by your breast cancer, you need to work at restoring a positive view of yourself, a noncritical, accepting affection for who you are and how you look. "You've got to make peace with your body. After my mastectomy, I'd dress and undress in the bathroom. Then we took a delayed honeymoon. (We'd had a big fight after our wedding and we never took that first one. I have wedding stories you wouldn't believe!) My husband didn't like my hiding in the bathroom. 'Come on—I love you. Two breasts are better but one is okay.' "

Clothes Cover

Are you going to great lengths not to look at the scars on your chest? (Rosalie would hang a towel on her bathroom mirror so she didn't have to see herself after her shower.) Your reluctance to face the scars is understandable and needs to be respected, but experts on healing suggest it's important to get past this attitude. "For a very long time (six months), I didn't really want to look straight on in the mirror. When I finally did, it wasn't that awful. It was like a patch of white fabric stitched on my chest."

Fancy lingerie or night wear may be the immediate solution to avoiding that initial shock. If you want that protection, that camouflage, go for it. Indulge yourself. Plenty of women keep their clothes on in bed. Beneath clothing, a reconstructed breast or a good prosthesis feels very much like the real thing to your partner; it has the bounce, the weight, and the resilience of a natural breast.

Responding to a discriminating market, small shops have sprung up that offer an excellent variety of prostheses and cleverly adapted prosthesis pockets fitted into underclothing and swim suits. Ask your local American Cancer Society for a list of shops, or look in the Yellow Pages under Lingerie. If you're shy about going into the stores, indulge in catalog shopping (Victoria's Secret can be yours). I think you'll be pleased with what's available. Even for the short term, while you're deciding whether or not to go ahead with reconstruction, a breast prosthesis may allow you to feel more comfortable about your image in clothes and give your self-confidence a welcome boost. So dress up in your favorite nightgown, and maybe you won't feel as though it's hands-off territory.

Easing into Exposure

Frilly lingerie can serve as your first step to getting back into a pattern of relaxed sexual activity, but sooner or later you need to come to terms with your altered appearance. Dr. Leslie Schover suggests "mirror therapy." Use a full-length mirror in a private area of your home, then dress up in your favorite clothes. Study yourself in the mirror for fifteen minutes and pick out three things you really like about yourself. At some other time, study yourself in casual clothes, and find more things you like about how you look. After that, try the exercise in lingerie. Finally, take fifteen minutes to look at yourself in the nude, and again, search out points about yourself that please you. "Focus on the positives."

You need to accept your naked body, even if you never did before, to strike a truce with yourself. And you *need* to let your partner look at you and come to a similar point of view. Take it little by little. Some women I know find it freeing to walk around their room or apartment totally naked. One woman invited close friends over for dinner and when they had finished, she showed off her new reconstructed breasts, to oohs and aahs of approval.

The final step is being totally nude for your partner. This seems to be the last stage in releasing you from the anxiety about your self-image. Cathy, in a new relationship, finally worked up to letting her beau see her naked chest—and he applauded. "You really did something big, letting me see you. But I told you before, it wasn't going to matter to me."

But hold on. Maybe nudity works fine for younger women, but I don't know too many older women, with or without breast cancer, who enjoy parading around naked. You may need to face what you look like, but you don't have to exult in it, or force yourself into behavior that never suited you. Besides, most sex takes place in darkened rooms. When the lights are low and you're getting it on, whether you're totally naked or not may not matter one bit.

Loss of Libido

Perhaps the most frustrating change in your sexual life is the loss of libido. "I just don't have those urges like I did." Apart from the hormonal changes and their consequences, you've lost your hair, your breast is altered or gone, you've put on weight, you have no energy, you're tired, you're nauseated, and you hurt in new places. No wonder you're not feeling sexy.

Your sex life may be altered by vaginal pain resulting from cancer treatment, especially after bone marrow transplantation. Certain chemotherapies can cause ulcers in the body's mucous membranes (mouth, throat, vagina, or rectum). Physical changes may derive from treatment-induced menopause, tamoxifen therapy, or cessation of hormone replacement therapy. Add an assortment of psychological factors, and pleasure from sex may seem like ancient history. Advice from your doctors, or from friends who've been down the same road, may help, but some impairment of sexual function is generally unavoidable. Over time, however, conditions do get better.

"I was so deep-down exhausted, I was beyond desire. I thought 'This is gonna be permanent.' It wasn't. My husband never gave up, thank heaven." Lila was more fortunate than Tess, whose husband was supportive in all ways but one: "We haven't had sex since my diagnosis. I don't know how to get through to him."

Depression and Libido

Depression is a common result of both the diagnosis and the treatment of breast cancer, and it directly affects your interest in sex. If you're depressed, sex may be the last thing you want to deal with. (You may even develop a real aversion to sex.) A sensitive partner picks up on this and holds back. Then, when you recover, your partner may continue to show no interest in sex, and you may assume it's because you're no longer desirable. Back to problems in communication.

If you find you are depressed and unable to turn the corner, you need help. Try to consider the solutions already mentioned: therapists or group support. You've undoubtedly heard of the success of new medications, but you'll have to be cautious. Some therapies for depression may cause loss of libido, including Prozac and Zoloft. Medications must be carefully administered and monitored. Effective dose levels are important and not always appropriately prescribed, and it takes three weeks or more for you to feel the benefit. Depression, however, is too debilitating a condition to ignore, so don't fail to seek help. There are some things that time alone does not heal.

Hormones and Libido

You may find that it has become harder to get aroused, and even harder to experience orgasm. "It takes so long to make it happen," said one woman. Another: "It just doesn't happen for me anymore." This is a consistent complaint, this dullness of response—if you can call it response. You must be explicit with your physician, so that he or she can suggest appropriate medical solutions. Loss of desire and drive may be directly related to your lower estrogen, progesterone, or testosterone levels, induced by treatment.

If you're experiencing problems with sex, you might want to try downplaying the importance of orgasm, at least for a while. While you're recovering, try concentrating on pleasure from touching, kissing, and imagery, rather than penis-in-vagina orgasm. De-emphasizing vaginal orgasm may actually allow it to happen again sooner than you expected.

If your loss of libido continues, and it's a problem (it might not be for some women who've had minimal interest in or opportunity for sex before all this happened), speak to your doctor about the possibility of a hormone evaluation. Women's sex drive is somewhat dependent on the hormone testosterone (the primary hormone in men), produced in the ovaries and the adrenal glands. A little goes a long way. Adjustment of hormone levels may help restore sexual interest, but if your testosterone level is within normal range (20 to 60 nanograms/deciliter), it is unlikely that more testosterone will be of benefit. Too much testosterone can produce acne, irritability, and male characteristics like facial hair or a deepened voice. In addition, it's not known if "testosterone replacement therapy" is safe for women with a personal history of breast cancer.

Pain, Nausea, and Libido

Painful intercourse can demolish your interest in sex faster than anything else. Vaginal ulcers, caused by certain chemotherapies (such as 5-fluorouracil), are a major source of such pain—particularly severe in women who have had bone marrow transplantation. Women with genital herpes can experience an outbreak of the disease brought on by stress and compromised immunity. Steroids and antibiotics can cause yeast infections in the mouth and vagina. Pain medications, narcotics in particular, can also reduce libido.

Menopause, natural or treatment-induced, can cause thinning and shortening of the vaginal walls. Vaginal dryness (lack of natural lubrication) is another menopausal side effect. These conditions can contribute to pain during sex.

Nausea, a side effect of chemotherapy, can kill your interest in anything, particularly sex. Plus some antinausea medications depress libido.

New Conditions, New Solutions
Lubricate

When asked for sex hints for breast cancer survivors, Sue said, "Astroglide, and more Astroglide. The directions say to put it on the penis, but don't forget to smear it in the vagina, too, *lots of it*." "Being slippery is a good thing," says Dr. Margaret Deansley, a physician, breast cancer survivor, and public speaker. You've got to learn to use the "goop," whether it's Neutragena Sesame Oil, Astroglide, Today Personal, Surgilube, Ortho Gyne-Moistrin, Moist Again, Replens, Probe, KY Jelly (a standard surgical lubricant), Women's Health Institute's Lubricating Gel, or Bag Balm (favored by veterinarians). Many women prefer Astroglide, Moist Again, the WHI Lubricating Gel (call 800-537-8658), and Probe over other products, because they spread more easily and last longer. If your partner is using a condom, be sure to use a *water*-based lubricant; petroleum-based lubricants damage condoms.

Some women swear by yogurt (sans fruit)—no embarrassment when you buy it, and *cheap*. "But I don't know how I'd feel putting yogurt in my vagina at night and then having yogurt for breakfast the next morning" was the comment of a surgeon–breast cancer survivor. Hey, whatever works for you.

Learn to use the goop without fuss or ceremony, use it as a matter of course. Begin using it during foreplay, spreading it liberally over the labia and clitoris and into the vagina, as well as on your partner's parts that will enter your vagina; you may need to add more later during intercourse. If you can't get over using your hand (or your partner's) to spread the lubricant inside your vagina, and surgical gloves don't help, choose the product that comes with an applicator. (Our yogurt fans use a turkey baster.) You may also make your choice based on consistency, odor, or taste. Keep a tube in the bedroom, the bathroom, anywhere you're likely to need it. Try using vaginal lubricants the same way you use moisturizing hand cream: frequently and regularly.

Replens is an over-the-counter moisturizer that helps the vaginal wall hold on to water, resulting in thickened tissue that is better able to handle the friction of intercourse. I recommend Replens to any woman suffering from vaginal dryness. Apply it to the vagina three times a week at bedtime, over a period of several weeks. Replens can make intercourse tolerable, comfortable, pleasurable. In one study, 80 percent of women noted a significant improvement in their symptoms with Replens. It may, however, take months to make a difference, and you'll have to keep using it to maintain its special benefits. It's also expensive.

Arousal

Before attempting intercourse, it's important to feel comfortable and relaxed, and then aroused. Some therapists suggest that couples learn to concentrate on comfort and foreplay, and delay having intercourse for some later time, thus establishing a successful pattern of foreplay—particularly genital foreplay—as part of their sexual repertoire. Foreplay is an essential factor for a woman in becoming aroused, particularly for women who find sex painful. The vagina produces natural lubricants, and the vaginal wall relaxes, widens, and lengthens, allowing less painful, more satisfying, penetration. A woman is ready for sex after these changes, just as a man is ready when he has an erection.

If you aren't feeling particularly attractive or sexy, however, your ability to become aroused may be inhibited, or you may want to get sex over with as soon as possible. One way to overcome this problem is to imagine yourself as you would like to be, perhaps as some glamorous movie star or romance-novel heroine. It may be as useful to practice mental turn-ons as it is to practice physical ones.

Arousal can also be started and amplified by movies, erotica, and sex gadgets. I know some pretty straight couples who get positive charging from these sources. Besides the magazines on the hard-to-reach racks, there's the Kama Sutra (an age-old Indian guide to lovemaking), and how-to sex manuals. Very respectable. Lonnie Barbach has a video, "Cabin Fever," especially designed for these needs: romantic, loving, feminine. Her book *Erotic Interlude* has been helpful to many of my patients.

Important: Take a close look at what's happening in your head when you have sex. Are you calling on an erotic fantasy to get you in the mood, or are you worrying about pain or the bills you have to pay? Switch the channels in your head; get off "This Old House" and onto "Passion on the Waves." I tell my patients to keep a journal of their moods through the day. When do you feel the most energized? When do you fade and get prickly? When do you think about sex? Can you detect a pattern, predict when you'd be most likely to consider a little time between the sheets? Now, can you figure out a way to schedule time with your partner that would capitalize on when you feel the sexiest? Can you arrange a lunch break together? A cocktail hour escape? Or an early-morning dalliance? If daylight inhibits you, close the drapes. Let's give this problem as much heat and attention as possible.

Don't count on an exotic vacation to restart your sex life. "I can't think of a faster way to ruin a vacation," says Dr. Leslie Schover. Take the pressure off and take it slow. "Better to think in terms of mini-vacations, short breaks in your normal routine, like closing the bedroom door a couple of hours earlier than usual, with a Do Not Disturb sign hanging from the doorknob."

Understand that a vital reason for fixing problems of arousal is because of their ricochet effect. If you don't feel aroused, your partner is going to feel at least somewhat responsible, and that inevitably is going to affect his or her performance. Partners can be more disturbed by a woman's diminished responsiveness than by the absence or alteration of a breast.

Innovate

Position during intercourse can be crucial. Lying on your side, with your partner entering from behind, is considered the least stressful to the vagina (with the least degree of penetration compared to other positions). It also de-emphasizes the breasts, a plus for some women.

If you want to stay sexually active or you hope to become active, you'll need to keep your vagina lubricated and in condition. That means stretching the vaginal canal, stimulating the membranes to produce natural lubricants, and increasing overall elasticity and resilience. Actual intercourse will then be more comfortable and pleasurable. (It also makes medical pelvic examination more tolerable.) "Use it or lose it." If you don't have a partner to keep your vagina stretched and supple, then it's up to you.

If intercourse continues to be painful, give it up for a while and practice with a dildo, a rubber instrument with the size, shape, and consistency of an erect penis. Don't be surprised at how realistic— veins and all—it may look. (Different sizes, shapes, and colors are available.) It will be more gentle, less emotionally burdensome, and perhaps fun, too. (Be sure to use a lubricant with it.) You can also purchase a box of small, medium, and large hard, straight plastic vaginal dilators, available through special order medical supply companies (ask your doctor or nurse). I find that most women don't like this medical product because it's unnaturally hard, straight, and uncomfortable, and they end up not using it.

I provide my patients with actual prescriptions for dildos for vaginal conditioning. It helps them overcome their embarrassment when they go to sex shops or feminist stores to purchase these items. In fact, many of these stores are aware of the use of dildos for sexual recovery after cancer treatment, and many stores such as Good Vibrations in California, provide mail-order catalogs and ship in a plain brown wrapper. Started by a sex therapist determined to make vibrators more generally accessible and available, Good Vibrations has an 800 telephone number and well-trained representatives who are happy to answer questions in a straightforward, discreet, and helpful fashion. (800-289-8423) Or you can locate a lesbian bookstore somewhere in your area (Giovanni's Room is one in Philadelphia), where you can be sure to get frank, relaxed advice—for all women, not just lesbians.

You don't have to buy any gadgets. You can improvise with a lubricant and an object like a candle or a suitably shaped vegetable, wrapped in a clean plastic bag. But, because I hope you will take this advice seriously and with purpose, the purchase of a commercial device is a step in the right direction. So find a large hat and dark glasses and go shopping!

Beyond Intercourse

Now may be the time to learn more about sexual practices other than vaginal intercourse. *Sex in America* tells us that people do a lot of things besides having sexual intercourse. Sex isn't just penis in vagina; it's all kinds of other activities, too. For example, up to 25 percent of couples between the ages of thirty and sixty engage in oral sex on a regular basis. Maybe oral sex will allow tender parts of you to heal while providing enough gratification to keep you both content. Twenty-five percent is a respectable number, enough to make the practice a normal part of sexuality, enough to give you permission, if that's what you need and want.

There's also the matter of masturbation. For some, just the word itself is enough to induce palpitations. (Just look what it did to Pee Wee Herman and Dr. Joycelyn Elders.) The authors of *Sex in America* tell us something we all know: that it is a practice that few discuss, that's condemned by many, and that makes some of us feel guilty. But, they say, many people, if not most, masturbate. And surprisingly, it's practiced most by people who are otherwise sexually active or married; it stimulates and is stimulated by other sexual behavior. That men are more avid practitioners than women is no surprise. One reason may be how easy and convenient it is for them; they've got their hands on their penis a few times a day urinating anyway, and it's just a stretch of the imagination to get something more going. Women, on the other hand, have to go to greater lengths. You need some place to sit or lie down, you may need some kind of paraphernalia (where do you keep it? what do you do with it afterward?), and you may have to learn technique—and to let go of guilt and inhibition.

You will not harm yourself and nobody will know if you do it or don't. You are in the privacy of your own bedroom and you are entitled to do whatever makes you happy and doesn't hurt anyone else. Masturbation is a legitimate form of sexual activity and release. It provides innocent pleasure and keeps your body healthy.

Massage

Manual stimulation using a lubricant can also provide gratification, a welcome substitute during the period of recovery and readjustment. If your sexual response continues to be sluggish, a head-to-toe massage may play an increasingly important role in your sexual menu. It also allows you to learn more about what pleases you, as well as providing hands-on maneuvering to hot spots, without having to say a word.

Feet are plenty sensual. We abuse them all day long; how nice to give them a little extra attention at night. You'd be amazed at how many women are thrilled by a foot massage. When your lover next wants to do something extra-special for you, ask for a foot rub.

Or a plain old back rub. (In the good old days, any stay in the hospital guaranteed you a nightly back rub; they knew how therapeutic it was.) Massage is a wonderful relaxant and an aphrodisiac. Give it a whirl, music and body oils included.

Your Touching Habits

If your breasts were a crucial part of your sex life before your illness, you'll be experiencing new attitudes and sensations. "Believe me, you can find ways to have great sex without breasts. I was numb—so I figured, why bother?—and we had been very breast oriented before." You may want no touching, more touching, or tentative touching of the breast. Your partner may want no touching, more touching, or tentative touching. The treated breast can be sensitive after healing, or painful, or numb. If your breast has been reconstructed, it will most likely have dulled sensation or none at all.

You may simply not want the area seen, much less touched. You'll have to take hold of the toucher to communicate the touching you do or don't want. You may have to learn to be more assertive than you were before all this. If you can't use words freely, you must use your hand to guide the action, especially if you don't want it going to the breast that is or was. (A few women don't want the healthy breast touched any longer because it reminds them too much of the loss of the other.) Dr. Deansley reminds us that your partner has probably only one hand free for your chest area anyway, so give some thought to how to position yourself, so that the free hand goes to the breast you want fondled.

I suggest that my patients do a little gentle stroking or massaging of the breast area themselves, to try to recapture sensation. If nothing else, it helps you to reacquaint yourself with that part of your body once more.

Endorphins and Exercise

At the same time that you are investigating other solutions to your sexual concerns, try to get back to a regular pattern of exercise, gradually, as you feel up to it. This can help make a difference. Exercise, because it stimulates the production of endorphins (which contribute to your sense of well-being), has been shown to have a positive effect on a person's sex life. Besides, toning and limbering up your muscles will make you feel better about yourself and proud of your self-discipline. A confident you is a sexier you.

Speaking of exercise, you may want to try Kegels, exercises that strengthen the pubococcygeal muscle in the lower vaginal area (also known as the love muscle), the muscle that contracts during orgasm. Tense up, as though you're holding back a bowel movement or stopping the flow of urine, then count to five, release, and repeat. You can practice this exercise anywhere; it's your own private activity. It will help you relax this muscle during intercourse.

It's Up to You

As you learn more about your body and your desires, you'll be encouraged to take some initiative, and even speak up. Be direct and specific: "Please, not now. I'm just not up to sex at this moment." Or "Let's not have intercourse, but please hold me / please caress me / please massage me here / let's try something new / let's try intercourse even if we have to stop." It may be easier to talk about sex when you're not on the verge of starting it; choose a time when you're comfortably settled in together, in a neutral environment.

Talking about sex may be new for you, but change can be exciting. "Be active," Sue advised. She had traveled the distance from posttreatment aversion to sex, to return of interest, and finally, to desire. "Initiate sexual activities, in a lively way. Show that you love it. There's no better turn-on—the sex can be truly terrific."

13

Eating Right for Recovery and Beyond

When my sister and I were kids, my aunt used to push a murky concoction of celery and carrot juice on us, the only guinea pigs within reach to carry out the prescription for good health she was reading about in books by Gaylord Hauser and other fringe publications of the time. She also tried to get us to swallow huge pills of vitamin C and E and B complex. We rejected all her efforts, our jaws clamped shut. We thought she was a little nuts, not realizing she was actually ahead of her time by at least fifty years.

Diet and nutrition: Can you get through a single day without seeing, hearing, or reading something about one or the other? Food, fad, fat, fuss, fraud, fear, fact? What do you do with the information that bombards you, on billboards, in the mail, on the radio and TV, and from well-meaning friends and strangers, each with another version of the Perfect Diet? What can you believe? Because of your breast cancer experience, you want to do whatever you can to enhance your future with the healthiest lifestyle around. Your doctors have told you about treatment—drugs such as tamoxifen, antibiotics for infection, advice on depression—but what should you be eating? Few doctors write a prescription for nutrition. You know the foods you eat and the vitamins and supplements you take may influence your body's ability to fight disease and extend your life. You'd like to make sense of all this information and figure out what's really good for you and what you should do.

But there's even more to weigh in: Your vegetarian friend is working overtime to convince you that eating natural, organically raised food has an inherent value beyond nutrition, that natural foods somehow have inherent purity and goodness, a goodness that has moral overtones, spiritual value, and virtue. Is she right? Another friend wants you to go on a wheat-grass-juice fast "to cleanse the toxins from your body"—and to do it while meditating.

Eating soon becomes an exercise in ethics, and you may be getting the idea that if you really live right, do right, and eat right, you won't get sick again, and that if you do get sick, then it's your own fault. I'm sorry to say that I've counseled many patients who have adopted this viewpoint, which I find disturbing and totally misleading. "I'm sure my breast cancer came back because I couldn't stick to that vegetarian diet and lose weight." *Not true*. No single factor causes or cures cancer. Your lifestyle choices didn't cause your cancer, and simply changing your lifestyle won't make it go away.

Cancer and Diet, What's the Connection?

Scientists have established that at least one third of all cancers can be attributed *in some part* to diet. So, for you and for me, for all women, common sense demands we pay attention to what we eat. When we compare levels of breast cancer in countries all over the world, we find that China and Japan have low rates of breast cancer and the United States and England have high rates. What accounts for these differences? Genetic or racial characteristics might be the immediate assumption, but when women from a low-risk country move to a high-risk country, their cancer rates rise over the years, approaching the higher rates of the new country. The reverse is also true: When women from a high-risk country move to a low-risk area, their cancer levels go down. So it's hardly simple genetics. Can it be the switch from a diet of rice and fish to a high-fat diet of french fries and beef?

Environmental forces of one sort or another—industrial waste, pesticides, automobile exhaust, smog, smoking, and diet, factors often occurring in combination—become suspect. Other factors (family history and genetics, age when menses start, age when women have babies) have a direct relationship to breast cancer risk.

All these factors may contribute to breast cancer risk, and most of them are beyond your control. There's not a lot you personally can do about the pollutants you breathe. You can't change the year you started having periods. You can't decide to have children in your twenties if you're in your thirties. How do you roll back that option? But there is one thing you really can control—what you put into your mouth—tobacco, alcohol, food, and more.

You probably ask next if changing your diet today is likely to make a difference to your health. I'm convinced it will.

Where's the Proof?

When you get diet recommendations from this or that friend, or from well-known personalities or professionals who insist they have absolute, personal proof of how the success of their system promotes their health, you've got to ask yourself, and them, "Where is that proof?"

"That vitamin B_{12} shot was unbelievable! I had my old pep back." Fascinating—but one person's perceived success with a diet plan or remedy may be strictly limited to her experience, and it may not even reflect reality. What helped her may or may not help you, and it could even harm you. Only well-designed, large-scale, randomized studies by a reputable group of scientists, producing results that are verifiable by other investigators, are considered objective, reliable, and acceptable for general recommendation.

Let's say, for example, that a nutritionist tells you that one cup of juiced carrots a day will strengthen your immune system. Sounds interesting, but what is the basis of the claim? Has there been a study comparing carrot juice consumers to non–carrot juice consumers, showing an increase in the experimental group's immune cells and their functions, a lessening of infection, or some other meaningful measure of immune response? Maybe you figure you don't need proof. You like carrot juice, so why not take the recommendation, and if it works—great, and if it doesn't, what have you lost? Probably won't hurt you, though you might take on an orangish hue, and you might be losing some benefits from the carrot roughage you're discarding. Minor drawbacks, you say. But recommendations for other supplements based only on anecdotal reports may not be as innocuous; melatonin, diet pills, and ma huang, for instance, can be dangerous.

Sorting through Nutritional Studies

The Natural Products Division of the National Cancer Institute tests more than 40,000 new natural substances in the laboratory each year for their ability to fight cancer cells. Substances that perform well against these isolated cancer cells are then tested in laboratory animals, and finally in humans.

In clinical studies, investigators can observe a large group of people for many years, reporting on their eating habits, lifestyle, general sense of well-being, type and pattern of illness, and life span. Or studies can compare a specific diet or treatment plan in one group, with a control group whose eating or lifestyle patterns are unchanged. After a designated period of time (years or decades), each group's patterns of eating and lifestyle and the benefits and side effects of their behavior are assessed by gauging the state of their health and their life span. The scientists then formulate conclusions and publish the results, making them available to public scrutiny.

Although even the best-designed studies may have shortcomings, basic standards establish the value of a proper study. First, the reputation of the investigator and the investigator's institution should be upstanding. Second, results should be reproducible by other investigators in the field, a crucial test of any scientific discovery. Then, the study should include people with the same diagnostically established cancer, but selected at random so that the statistical rules of chance apply. The study must factor into analysis the important features of each person, such as pathologic diagnosis and stage of cancer, biological properties of the cancer, therapies received, age, family history, and diet. If the study is about diet, instructions for that diet should be easy to understand, and the participants should be available and supervisable (so if a participant doesn't stick to the diet, the researchers can factor that in). The study should use meaningful endpoints to measure the results, such as weight loss or change in cholesterol level, as well as the participants' sense of well-being, whether other illnesses were contracted, and rate of recurrence and death. Researchers may track results over years so that long-term effects can also be seen. Finally, the conclusions should be analyzed with objective statistical tools that overcome any investigator's bias.

The long process of new drug research and development is often further delayed by the rigors of FDA (the U.S. Food and Drug Administration) safety standards. The FDA holds up the use of promising new drugs until it is fully satisfied that they will not cause harm and that they will produce potential benefits, but waiting for the release of a potential cure is extremely frustrating to anyone who needs a miracle *today*.

Many women, looking for that miracle, turn to dietary supplements, which are no longer regulated for purity and safety by the FDA. Diet supplements' content and safety are in the hands of their manufacturers, and manufacturers have a free hand: Grandiose speculation about possible miraculous benefits sells a lot of supplements without proof of results. Billions of dollars are spent on these compounds yearly.

Approach these products with caution. To protect yourself, read labels carefully and don't take any more than the recommended dose. "Natural" does not necessarily mean safe, nor does fancy packaging, advertising, or space on a shelf in a health food store. Let the furor over ephedrine (the ingredient in ma huang) be a lesson; more than fifteen deaths attributed to ephedrine are warning enough of its threat to health. Buyer beware!

Vegetables: An Important Part of Your Diet

The Benefits of a Vegetarian Diet

I believe the most effective step you can take in your nutritional approach to health and wellness is to become predominantly vegetarian, and to use plants and grains rather than meat, poultry, and dairy foods for much of your protein. The nutritious benefit of soy foods in this context is substantial. They have high protein and low or no fat, and they're versatile, cheap, and easy to get. Many studies of soy's value in people (not rats or petri dishes) show that at least the cholesterol and vaginal cell benefits of soy can be experienced within two weeks of adding it to your diet, even if your diet includes meat and dairy products.

But I want the message to be clear: A nutritional approach to health is a package deal—cut out a lot of the meat, avoid most dairy fats, find a healthful source of protein such as soy, and increase the amount of fruits, vegetables, and grains in your diet. Adding a little tofu here and there between stops to Burger King or Taco Bell won't do the trick.

Soybeans

Early laboratory, clinical, and epidemiologic studies show that soybeans offer many health benefits: high nutritional value, possible anticancer properties, and the ability to reduce hot flashes, lower blood cholesterol, and maybe even keep your bones strong.

Nutritional Value of Soy

Any recommended low-fat diet, particularly a vegetarian low-fat diet, will be rich in soybean foods (see Table 13.1). Soybeans are the most widely used, least expensive, and least caloric way to get large amounts of protein with very little fat and no cholesterol. Weight reduction and control are easier with soy protein because it has fewer calories than chicken, meat, and even fish. For example, a no-fat Boca

TABLE 13.1. Soy Products

Product	Serving size	Calories per serving	Protein (g)	Fat (g)
REAL FOOD				
Nutlettes breakfast cereal	1/2 cup	140	25	1.5
Textured vegetable protein (TVP)	1/2 cup dry	90	15	0–1
Roasted soy nuts	1/2 cup	450	40	21.6
Tempeh	4 oz	182	24	6
Low-fat tofu	4 oz	40	6.6	1.5
Soft tofu	4 oz	85	9	5
Firm regular tofu	4 oz	120	13	6
Silken tofu	4 oz	72	9.6	2.4
Smart Dogs (hot dog)	1 dog	45	9	2.5
Tofu Pups (hot dog)	1 dog	60	8	2.5
Gimme Lean	4 oz	140	18	0
Soy Boy ravioli	1 cup	180	10	3
Roasted soy butter	2 tbsp	170	6	11
Natural Touch Garden Vegetable Patti	one patty	100	10	2.5
Boca burgers, 98% fat free	one patty	84	12	0
Morningstar Farms Fat Free Patties	one patty	70	11	0
INGREDIENTS				
Miso	2 tbsp	70	4	2
Soy flour	1/2 cup	165	24	0.5
Flaxseed	3 tbsp	140	5	10
SOY MILKS				
Regular soy milk	1 cup	140	10	4
Low-fat soy milk	1 cup	100	4	2
Original EdenSoy milk	1 cup	130	10	4

Continued on next page

TABLE 13.1 Soy Products *(continued)*

Product	Serving size	Calories per serving	Protein (g)	Fat (g)
Vanilla EdenSoy milk	1 cup	150	6	3
1% WestSoy Lite	1 cup	90	2	1.5
WestSoy Plus	1 cup	130	6	4
Vanilla Malted	6 oz	240	6	12
EXTRACTS, PILLS, POWDERS				
Vege Fuel	35	120	30	0
Fearn soya powder	1/4 cup	100	10	5
Take Care High Protein Beverage Powder	2 scoops	100–130	20	0.5–1.5
Naturade 100% Soy Protein	2 rounded tbsp	100	25	0
Fearn Soy Protein Granules	1/4 cup	140	22	0

Nutlettes-Dixie Company: Call to order: 800-347-3494.
Take Care Powder: Call 800-445-3350.
United Soybean Board: Call 800-TALKSOY.
Soy Foods Association of America: Write to 540 Maryville Centre Drive, Suite 390, St. Louis, MO 63141

soybean burger contains no fat and fewer than 100 calories; a beef hamburger of comparable size contains about 250 calories and 20 grams of fat (including cholesterol).

Many soy products contain high levels of calcium: Among these are whole soybeans, texturized vegetable protein (TVP), tofu curdled with calcium, and fortified soy milks. Some soy products (primarily the fermented ones, tempeh, miso, and especially soy sauce) also contain very high levels of salt, something you probably want to avoid.

Cancer-Fighting Properties of Soy

Intriguing data suggesting anticancer benefits from a diet of soy have been compiled from laboratory experiments and from studies of the levels of cancer risks among various world populations. Asian women living in Asia have about one fourth the breast cancer rate that American women have. For years, public health researchers pointed to the high-fat diet in the United States versus the low-fat diet in Asia as the explanation. But now we know that fat is only part of the equation. More likely, the reason Asian women have lower risks of breast cancer is that their low-fat, low-calorie lifelong diet is predominantly vegetarian: very little meat, chicken, or even fish, and few or no dairy products. Obesity, a known risk factor for breast cancer, is uncommon in Asia. Asian women smoke and drink far less than other female worldwide populations. In addition, people in Asia are more active physically than most people here in the United States—who tend to jump in a car to go a distance of just a few blocks.

The major source of protein in the Asian diet is soybeans, in the form of tofu, soy milk, and miso. And scientific data are emerging that substantiate the benefits of soy; it seems to help protect breast cells from forming new cancers, and it may inhibit the proliferation of cancer cells already present. The components of soy with potential anti-cancer properties include *protein kinase inhibitors,* which help prevent normal cells from becoming cancerous, suppress activity of cancer-causing genes, inhibit enzymes that help cells break down various types of protein, and are thought to control cell growth; *phytosterols,* which inhibit cholesterol absorption from the bowel; *saponins,* which can also reduce cholesterol levels, enhance immunity, and inhibit DNA synthesis and cancer cell growth; and *phenolic acid* and *phytates,* which act as antioxidants.

Some soy products also contain high levels of *isoflavones* (genistein and daidzein), which are weak estrogen-like substances from plants—phytoestrogens. The amount of isoflavones consumed by women in Asia is 100 times greater than that consumed by women in the United States. Genistein, the most common type of soy isoflavone, can function as a weak estrogen, which in effect acts like an anti-estrogen, much as tamoxifen does, and binds to estrogen receptors (which are present in two thirds of all breast cancers). Estrogen stimulates cell growth and activity by interacting with the estrogen receptors of the cells, so if estrogen can be blocked from the receptors by weaker estrogen-like compounds, then stimulation of breast cell and breast *cancer* cell growth should be diminished.

Genistein is thought to have weaker estrogen-like activity than your body's own estrogens: estradiol or estrone. The estrogen-like activity of genistein is thought to be 1/1000 to 1/10,000 that of estradiol. Two hundred milligrams of isoflavones is estimated to be biologically equivalent to 0.3 milligrams of conjugated estrogen from a pharmacy (Premarin is an example). The ratio is based on how readily isoflavones bind to the receptor relative to estrogen. Think of genistein and estradiol as playing musical chairs, each scrambling to get into the estrogen receptor before the other. If the two molecules are present in equal number, estradiol will get most of the seats. But, if you've got significant levels of genistein in your system from soy, there may be enough to keep most of the estradiol from making it into the receptors, allowing genistein to fill most of the "chairs." Once genistein is bound to the receptor, it may keep the estradiol out, and genistein is believed to deliver a less potent estrogen message to the cell than estradiol.

Also consistent with their role as a quasi-anti-estrogen, the isoflavones in soybeans are thought to do the following:

- Reduce the brain's hormonal stimulation of ovarian estrogen production; increase progesterone relative to estrogen.
- Increase liver production of sex-hormone-binding protein, which binds to estradiol, making it less available to cause trouble.
- Neutralize reactive free radical molecules (as tamoxifen does).
- Inhibit the enzymes that help DNA replicate itself and transmit growth signals to the rest of the cell.
- Prevent or significantly delay the formation of breast cancers in rats.
- Inhibit the formation of new blood vessels that breast cancers need to nourish their growth and sustain their activities. (Extremely high levels of genistein, however, were required to get this effect, beyond the levels that could be sustained by diet alone.)

The soybean-related possibilities for fighting cancer are provocative, and they warrant additional research to determine which are proven most useful and important, how they work together, which soy products contain the necessary components, how much of the soy products must be consumed to achieve the desired effects, and whether there are side effects, including cancer-promoting effects, that need to be weighed against the perceived benefits. Some of these questions are explored in the remainder of this chapter.

Managing Menopausal Symptoms and General Health Concerns with Soy

The weak estrogenic effects of soy seem to result in a reduction of menopausal symptoms. In a recent study, postmenopausal women who consumed 45 grams of soy flour daily experienced about a 40 percent reduction of hot flashes. This response is real, but only moderately better than the 25 to 30 percent response one would expect from taking a placebo, a look-alike pill or substance substituted for the real substance under study. (See a discussion of hot flashes in Chapter 18.)

Soy can also revitalize the cells that line the vagina in postmenopausal women who were given supplemental 45 grams of soy flour or 25 grams of flaxseed while otherwise following their usual diet. These women underwent an analysis of their vaginal cells every two weeks (something like a Pap smear of the vaginal wall). With both the soy and the flaxseed diets, significant vaginal cell maturation occurred, becoming more like those of a premenopausal woman. About two weeks after stopping the soy or flaxseed, the vaginal changes started to revert, and by eight weeks, the vaginal cells had gone back to their baseline menopausal status.

Soy's ability to lower cholesterol levels in men and women was assessed in a combined analysis of twenty-nine studies, reported in *The New England Journal of Medicine*. A daily intake of 47 grams of soy protein was found to lower blood cholesterol levels by 9.3 percent, low-density lipids (LDLs, or "bad" cholesterol) by 12.9 percent, and triglyceride (fat) levels by 10.5 percent; and there was a minimal increase of high-density lipoprotein (HDL, or "good" cholesterol). Another study showed an improvement in cholesterol levels with 25 grams of soy protein per day, and an even greater effect with 45 grams daily.

In a study of people with a hereditary form of high cholesterol, comparisons were made between the cholesterol levels in people consuming a traditional low-cholesterol diet and levels in people whose animal protein diet was replaced by large amounts of texturized vegetable protein (TVP) (70 to 90 gm per day). During the four-week period on high soy intake, a 20.8 percent reduction in total cholesterol and a 25.8 percent reduction of LDLs were observed. No appreciable reduction was noted in the people on the traditional low-cholesterol diet. When they stopped eating the soy, their blood cholesterol profile returned to baseline within six to eight weeks.

Studies have suggested that soybeans are a factor in preventing osteoporosis. An effective osteoporosis drug used in Europe, Ipriflavone, contains daidzein, one of the isoflavones found in soybeans, but the therapeutic value of daidzein is unconfirmed.

Soy foods contain significant levels of calcium: 4 ounces of tofu curdled with calcium has 550 milligrams, whereas 1 cup of cow's milk contains 325 milligrams. One study showed that soy protein was better than milk protein at building and maintaining bone mass in rats. Stay tuned for results in people.

Which Soy to Buy and How Much?

While soy isoflavones (genistein and daidzein) produce the purported menopausal benefits, it is not exactly clear which soy components in what soy foods produce the reported anticancer benefits. I therefore urge you to stick to whole or lightly processed soy products, and to avoid the highly processed derivatives or supplements that may actually have limited levels or none of the valuable elements of soy or they may have too much isoflavone that could have too much estrogen effect. Side effects of these derivatives, if they exist, are not known.

The level of isoflavones in food depends on how the food is processed. Protein is usually measured in grams, isoflavones in milligrams. Dr. Mark Messina, internationally known soy expert, estimates that 1 gram of defatted soybeans contains roughly 2 milligrams of isoflavones. The following products have the most isoflavones: soybeans (½ cup contains 35 mg of isoflavone), soy flour (½ cup has 50 mg), tofu, tempeh, or miso (½ cup of each contains 40 mg), soymilk (1 cup has 40 mg), and Nutlettes (½ cup has 122 mg). The amount of isoflavones in soy-protein-concentrate products, such as TVP or protein powders, can vary tremendously, depending on how they are processed. I've been told that water-processed soy proteins contain the most isoflavone. Any product derived from soy flour should be high in protein and isoflavones. Some products that contain many other ingredients, as soy hot dogs do, may have low amounts of isoflavones.

Some scientists say as little as 25 grams of soy protein a day will make a difference to your health, although 40 grams may result in even greater benefits. *Dr. Susan Love's Hormone Book* and the *Harvard Women's Health Watch* newsletter recommend between 40 and 50 grams of soy protein per day.

Preparing Soy Foods

Whole soybeans require more soaking and cooking to soften them than the average bean. Cook them in a tomato or barbecue sauce (add the tomato sauce toward the end so it doesn't interfere with the softening process), or make them into Boston baked beans. Roast them, serve them as nuts, candy them, or sprout them.

Soy flour can be used just as wheat flour is, to thicken sauces and in baked goods. It is gluten-free, making it a good alternative to wheat flour if you are gluten intolerant. Because yeast breads require some gluten, your bread dough should contain no more than 15 percent soy flour if you want your baked product to rise. In nonyeast breads, you can substitute up to a quarter of the flour with soy flour. Take soy flour baked goods out of the oven a little earlier to keep them from getting too brown and too dry and hard. Buy defatted soy flour to save on calories and get even more protein per serving. (For more information about using soy products, call 800-TALKSOY).

The most concentrated form of soy protein is TVP, an inexpensive, textured vegetable protein, which can be added as a filler to many dishes. TVP has the least amount of fat (none) of any soy product, and a long, convenient shelf life. Soy veggie burgers (I like the Boca brand best), soy cheese, and soy ravioli are other products. The meat substitute made with processed soy protein called Gimme Lean has 18 grams of protein and no fat per serving and can be used like ground beef. Nutlettes, very high in protein and low in fat, are good as a cereal, or sweetened and used as a crunchy topping on sliced baked apples.

Soy milk has been around a long time for use by people who are lactose intolerant, for infants allergic to cow milk, and for people who keep kosher. But some variations end up with too little protein and too many calories to be worth the cost. Read the labels. The low-fat varieties are simply diluted regular soy milk, with less fat but also less protein, and not that much difference in calories. Soy milk may taste a little odd to you at first. You may be able to jazz it up with spices such as cinnamon or nutmeg, or vanilla, coffee, or chocolate syrup. Or use it plain on cereal and in pancake batter.

Tofu is a popular source of soy protein, made from curdled soy milk. Regular tofu has a significant amount of fat in it, but the low-fat and silken varieties have a better protein-to-fat ratio. (Cautionary note: Bulk tofu, sold in barrels of fluid, may have bacterial overgrowth.) You can use the firm variety in soups and main course dishes, or the soft style blended in soup, drinks, salad dressing, and dips, or as a substitute for ricotta cheese in lasagna. If you're not used to eating tofu, it can taste like chalk Jell-O until you learn how to combine it with other ingredients to make it tasty. Nina Shandler, author of *Estrogen, The Natural Way,* dislikes the taste of tofu, but by the time she gets through adding all kinds of herbs and flavorful foods, "It's delicious." My favorite use of tofu and TVP is in hot-and-sour soup, which is easy to make at home, especially if you add ingredients like black tree fungi (also very good for you), dried Chinese and canned straw mushrooms, dried daylilies, and coriander. I also enjoy roasted soy nut butter with a bit of my favorite jam.

There are several fermented soy products that make soy more flavorful, but they usually end up reducing the nutritional value by adding lots of salt and diluting nutrients such as isoflavones. (There may also be a connection between fermented food products and stomach cancer.) Tempeh is a compressed cake of fermented soy beans that can be marinated, sautéed (use spray oil in the pan), or roasted. Natto, made of fermented cooked whole soybeans, has a cheesy consistency that is easier to digest than regular whole soybeans. Used as a condiment with rice, soup, and vegetables, and in marinades, it adds a pleasant, nutty flavor. Miso is a rich salty paste made of ground fermented soybeans and rice (or other grains); it is used as a condiment in all kinds of foods, most commonly in miso soup. Soy sauce is a dark, salty liquid made from fermented soybeans: Shoyu contains soybeans and wheat; tamari, only soybeans; and teriyaki contains soybeans, vinegar, sugar, and spices. Unfortunately, soy sauce has none of the nutritional value of the other soy products. It contains only a small amount of protein and no isoflavones, and it has a very high salt content. Think of it only as a flavoring, and use it sparingly.

Soy oil contains no protein or isoflavones; it is the most frequently consumed oil in the United States, making up nearly 100 percent of what is labeled vegetable oil. Soy oil is high in omega-3 fatty acids, thought to help reduce cholesterol levels and calories.

It's not known if taking soy genistein from powder extracts is as effective as eating genistein in food. As with vitamins, nutrition experts advise eating the whole foods that contain beneficial elements rather than taking capsules, because we don't know what other elements in these foods may be valuable or what form of these elements best serve up the benefits. Asian women living in China or Japan consume soybean curd or tofu with an abundance of vegetables and minimal animal protein and fat; they do not eat powdered soy products cooked in food or dissolved in juice.

Is Soy Really Safe?

You may in fact be concerned that these various plant estrogens may really be acting like the strong estrogens produced by your body once they manage to bind to your estrogen receptors. Understanding estrogen receptors in some detail may ease some of your concerns.

There are various estrogen receptors in your body, each with unique "assignments." Brain receptors control temperature (hot flashes), memory, sleep, and concentration; breast receptors are responsible for breast cell growth; uterine receptors stimulate uterine lining and wall cells; bone receptors determine bone mass and strength; and liver receptors process both sex hormones and cholesterol. How these receptors function differs widely, depending on the following:

- The actual state of the receptor—whether it's been busy working 'round the clock or hasn't worked in days; its condition; its configuration.
- The presence or absence of coactivators—other proteins and complex molecules that interact with the estrogen or the estrogen-like substance and the receptor to determine this effect.
- The various estrogen and estrogen-like substances that are in the

vicinity of the receptor. Receptors in a test tube, undergoing study, are in a highly controlled environment, with exact amounts of other specific substances, but the scene at your body's receptors is more like an orgy. Who and what and how long and which position they are all in is critical to how a receptor responds.

Tamoxifen is probably the best understood of the breast-cancer-fighting compounds that target the estrogen receptor, with both anti-estrogen and estrogenic activity. It is widely prescribed and promoted for its anti-estrogen effect on breast cells. It has added estrogen-like benefits, keeping bones strong and cholesterol down; but it also produces unwanted anti-estrogen side effects at the brain's temperature control center (to produce hot flashes) and as a weak estrogen in the uterus (associated with a slight increased risk of endometrial cancer with long-term use).

Drug companies are busy searching for the perfect molecular compound to *turn on* all the right receptors in cholesterol processing, in bone, and in the brain and to *shut off* the "wrong" receptors in the breast and the uterus. Where will this compound come from and how will it get to you? We're waiting to find out.

Flaxseed

Flaxseed contains a high concentration of lignins, which can act like a very weak estrogen, and therefore as a relative anti-estrogen, in much the same way as genistein. The lignins are concentrated in the hull of the seed. Once the flaxseeds are swallowed, your intestinal bacteria convert the lignins to enterolactone and enterodiol—the active ingredients—which are then absorbed into your bloodstream. Lignins are also found in many vegetables, fruits, and grains.

Flaxseed is also a good source of soluble and insoluble fiber, as well as an excellent source of alpha-linoleic acid, an omega-3 essential fatty acid, which can help reduce the low-density lipoproteins in the blood.

Anticancer Properties
Some early research studies indicate there are anticancer properties in lignans. Lignins kept female rats that were exposed to breast-cancer-causing chemicals from developing malignant changes leading to breast cancer; in rats who already *had* breast cancer, flaxseed slowed the growth of the cancer. But in other laboratory studies, lignins stimulated the growth of breast cancer cells. Laboratory and animal results don't necessarily translate into results for people.

Flaxseed can inhibit the enzyme that your fat cells use to convert androstendione to estrone (a "male" hormone to a "female" hormone). Flaxseed's enterolactone and enterodiol seem to exhibit weak estrogen-like activity similar to that of genistein: decreasing hot flashes, increasing the ratio of progesterone to estradiol, and regulating ovulation.

How to Add Flaxseed to Your Diet

Flaxseed can be ground and added to multigrain breads, cereals, cookies, muffins, and biscuits; or use it in seed form in soups, breads, salads, vegetables, and chopped meats. Try some of Nina Shandler's recipes. (See Selected Readings.) Use ground seeds immediately; whole seeds can last months in the freezer. Regular flaxseed oil is less practical because it can tolerate only moderate heat, it's quite expensive, it contains minimal amounts of lignins once processed, and it becomes rancid rather quickly. (A high-lignin oil adds back the flaxseed fiber particles that contain the lignins.) All flaxseed oils come in dark bottles and are stored in the refrigerator (opened or not) to minimize the chance that the oil will oxidize and spoil. I think Barlean's high-lignin flaxseed oil is the best one to buy, because of its freshness. If you want to use flaxseed oil for salad dressing (I like the nutty taste), be sure it's fresh, and keep it in the refrigerator. I mix flaxseed oil and balsamic vinegar, fifty-fifty, just before serving (it doesn't store well as a salad dressing, even in the refrigerator).

More Vegetables

These familiar vegetables are extremely nutritious, tried-and-true, with recipes in all the best-known cookbooks (unlike soy). They may well be more important than soy, but the disproportionate attention to soy that precedes this section was intended to introduce you to a bean that has only been gaining notoriety and respect in this country within the last few years.

Cruciferous vegetables include broccoli, cauliflower, brussels sprouts, cabbage, kale, and mustard and collard greens. They contain indols and dithiothioles, which are believed to block several cancer-promoting substances. Broccoli seems to be on every list for every crucial protective factor. Steam it; sprinkle it with lemon and maybe salt and pepper. I love it raw or barely steamed, or marinated in a little vinaigrette with half olive oil, half balsamic vinegar. (Cooked broccoli is more digestible for some people.) A friend of mine first sprays the vegetables lightly with olive oil (using a spray gun), then tosses in the balsamic vinegar. By making the vegetables taste better, you're bound to eat more of them. Olive oil is one of the more healthful oils. According to some studies, it may have cancer-fighting properties, but it does count as a fat and it does have lots of calories. Avoid the dips served with raw vegetables at cocktail parties because they're usually full of fat and salt, and the types of fat generally used are not healthy.

Umbelliferous vegetables include carrots, celery, parsley, and parsnips. Besides key vitamins, they contain enzymes that may protect you against some toxic substances, and may also modify prostaglandin levels.

Allium, the onion family, is best represented by garlic. Garlic's main active ingredients are allicin, which some people claim lowers cholesterol levels, and S-allyl cysteine (SAC), which has been shown to lower the incidence of colon tumors in mice. Fresh or enteric-coated preparations are recommended (4 gms of garlic per day), as is the cheapest source: garlic powder. Oil-based products are ineffective. An obvious consequence of garlic consumption is its odor, which not only affects your breath but also may permeate your skin. Unfortunately, there are no conclusive data proving garlic's value for all that's claimed it can do for you, but some of us put garlic—fresh garlic—and onions in every dish we can because we so love its flavor, especially to jazz up the flat taste of soy.

Lycopersicons, tomatoes, contain high levels of a natural carotenoid called lycopene, a powerful antioxidant that is under active study as a promising anticancer agent. (Pink grapefruit, watermelon, and guava also contain lycopene, but in much lower levels.) Countries with diets rich in tomato products (Italy, for instance) appear to have lower levels of cancer of the gastrointestinal tract and prostate gland; studies in Israel are investigating its possible value in protecting against breast cancer.

Tomato sauce in one form or another is popular worldwide. Cooked deep-red tomato products have the greatest lycopene benefits, but the products must be consumed with at least some fat—like olive oil—for the body to absorb the lycopene. Spaghetti with soy-TVP-enriched tomato sauce is an easy, healthful, and popular meal.

Vitamins, Minerals, Supplements

Vitamins A, B, C, D, and E, fiber, aspirin, selenium, ellagic acid, green tea, and cruciferous, umbelliferous, and allium vegetables all have elements that are reported to help prevent cancer. So, should you be popping pills or devouring heads of broccoli?

Many of the vitamins and trace minerals we list are *antioxidants,* substances that neutralize (or buffer) potentially damaging *free radi-*

cals. Free radicals are molecules generated at injured or diseased parts of the body; their job is to attack harmful invaders, but they sometimes turn against the body's own cells, breaking down the cell wall and invading internal structures of the cell—especially the DNA in the nucleus. Because cancer can start with genetic damage (damage to the DNA), controlling potentially dangerous free radicals is a high priority. Your body is constantly neutralizing these radicals with the help of important vitamins and minerals you get from the food you eat. (See Chapter 15.)

So, if a little in the food you eat is good, would more in the form of a pill be better? Results of studies on the value of added vitamins and supplements have been contradictory. Approximately half the studies show a benefit, the other half show no benefit, and a few even suggest possible danger to your health. Megadoses, doses that can be many, many times, even hundreds of times larger than the recommended daily allowance (RDA) of supplements, can be harmful, sometimes even fatal, but there are people who ignore this danger and consume excessive levels of supplements.

Some of the benefits attributed to vitamins may actually be due most directly to other healthy lifestyle choices that vitamin-takers make. People who consume proper levels of vitamins and minerals are generally more likely to avoid smoking and excess alcohol, exercise with some regularity, get regular checkups and pay attention to warning signs of disease. So it's no surprise that, statistically, these people live longer than others.

In an effort to do everything possible to fight breast cancer, many women have been enthusiastic consumers of vitamin and mineral supplements. But the bottom line is that it's much better to get these elements naturally in the foods you eat than in pill or capsule form. There are other factors present in these foods that add to their health-giving benefits. So take moderate amounts of vitamin supplements (with your doctor's okay) if you want to cover all bets, or if you can't find or don't enjoy eating vitamin-rich foods all seasons of the year. And try to keep to a well-rounded diet of real food.

You can get most of the vitamins and trace minerals you need from a diet rich in fresh fruits and vegetables. Cooking does reduce vitamin content in some foods, but for many people cooking makes it easier to swallow and digest larger quantities of vegetables and fruit.

Important vitamins such as niacin are found in animal fats and proteins. If you are limiting your intake of these foods, ask your doctor if you should take supplements in multivitamin form. Some brands of flour, cereals, and breads are fortified with niacin.

Vitamin A and related retinoids and carotenoids (including beta carotene) help reduce the production of prostaglandin and fatty acids, substances that fuel production of free radicals; this in turn is thought to stifle cancer development by forcing cells to "behave" in healthy patterns.

Vitamin A is found naturally in green, orange, and deep yellow vegetables, particularly carrots. Studies have shown that people who eat lots of fruits and vegetables have lower rates of cancer and heart disease than the general public; this same group of people appeared to have high levels of beta carotene in their blood. Scientists made an association between the high levels of beta carotene and the low rate of cancer, and based on these findings, beta carotene supplements became very popular. However, no one knows what other elements in fruits and vegetables may have contributed to the beneficial results from eating these foods.

Well, you can't pop a few vitamin pills and expect miracles. In January 1996, Dr. Charles Hennekens of Boston's Brigham and Women's Hospital, who conducted a major study of the value of the beta carotene dietary supplement, declared, much to his own chagrin, there was no benefit in these supplements. Clinical evidence shattered the expectations of millions, that taking beta carotene supplements would protect them from cancer or heart trouble. Fruits and vegetables still help protect against cancer and heart disease; scientists just haven't yet been able to pinpoint the precise elements in these foods that provide that benefit.

A recent large study indicated that women who take excessive amounts of vitamin A can have babies with serious birth defects, so women who are thinking of getting pregnant should be careful to avoid high doses. Stay within the recommended dose: 4000 I.U.

Vitamin B is actually a family of B vitamins. Vitamin B_3, also known as nicotinamide, blocks the action of enzymes called proteases, which break down or dissolve protein. Proteins are the building blocks of cells, including cells that may help contain cancer (i.e., they keep cancer cells from spreading to other parts of the body). Also, tumor suppressor genes do their job through the proteins they make.

Vitamin B_6 can ease treatment side effects such as nausea, vomiting, and diarrhea. A lot of people report that B_{12} boosts their energy. There are studies that suggest B_{12} may be a tumor inhibitor, but when taken in very high doses (many times over the RDA limits), it can also be a tumor promoter. Some people decide they can self-medicate, and they think if two vitamin pills are good, maybe ten are a whole lot better. "After all," they say, "they're only vitamins. How can they hurt?" Well, too much can.

The B vitamins, found in nuts, seeds, and wheat products, should be consumed in moderation, within recommended limits: 1.6 milligrams for B$_6$, and 2 micrograms for B$_{12}$.

Vitamin C, or ascorbic acid, is believed to boost the immune system by stimulating the production of interferon, which neutralizes free radicals and toxins that can damage normal cell structure and function. Linus Pauling, a Nobel prize winner, believed that vitamin C could fight viruses, such as those that cause the common cold, if taken in high enough doses. Impartial research has not been able to verify his results, but vitamin C may reduce the duration of viral infection and minimize the effects of a cold.

Vitamin C, diminished by cooking, is found in citrus fruits, peppers, cabbage, cranberries, cherries, and many Amazon rain forest fruits. Most of these exotic fruits have yet to reach American markets, but reports of their remarkably high concentration of vitamin C make them very appealing—something to watch for. In addition to vitamin C, citrus fruits contain other important substances, such as carotenoids, flavonoids, limonoids, terpenes, and coumarins, all of which are believed to help neutralize carcinogens. Bioflavonoids are antioxidants, present in many fruits and vegetables: cherries, berries (black, blue, cran, rasp), grapes, radishes, rhubarb, sweet potatoes and herbs. Flavonoids are believed to be the elements in red wine that contribute to red wine's purported protection against heart disease.

If your doctor okays vitamin C supplements in high doses, take timed-release capsules or pills. The recommended dose is between 60 and 200 milligrams once or twice daily, with occasional higher doses if you're trying to beat a cold.

Vitamin D helps regulate calcium levels, important for bone strength and integrity. Women at high risk for breast cancer are participating in a study to test the ability of vitamin D to lower their risk. In trial studies with rats, vitamin D was shown to inhibit the development of breast, colon, bladder, and skin cancers.

Non- or low-fat dairy products are an excellent source of the vitamin, which is metabolized in part by exposure to sunshine. (Muslim women who cover almost all of their skin surfaces can experience low calcium levels.) Excess vitamin D can lead to excessive levels of blood calcium, risking problems such as kidney stones. The recommended dose is 400 IU daily.

Vitamin E is an important antioxidant that neutralizes free radicals and is believed to stimulate the immune system. It has been shown to aid in preventing colon cancer and to inhibit breast cancer formation in laboratory animals—but so far there are no conclusive data for human beings. Vitamin E is also believed to reduce the risk of heart disease. Studies on the significance of vitamin E and cancer are on-going.

Some women find vitamin E (dose: 400 to 1000 IU daily) helpful in reducing the intensity and number of hot flashes.

Vitamin E is found primarily in oils and fat, and in soybeans, corn, sunflower seeds, and lettuce. If you are restricting fats in your diet, it may be important to take vitamin E supplements to maintain a proper balance of this vitamin in your system. The standard recommended dose is 30 IU daily, but for possible additional immune system benefits 200 to 400 IU a day is suggested. While higher doses of vitamin E are believed to have few side effects—compared, for example, with the harmful side effects of high doses of vitamin A—very high doses of vitamin E may do more to interfere with the immune response than to bolster it.

There is strong evidence to support vitamin E's importance to human nutrition. It can also help reduce hot flashes and it may even have anti-cancer properties. But there are breast cancer experts who have expressed concern about the safety of vitamin E consumption in women with breast cancer, pointing to (small) studies that show higher blood levels of vitamin E in some women with advanced breast cancer. The significance of these studies is unclear: it does not mean that vitamin E is causing or stimulating the cancer. One possibility: Vitamin E's presence may result from the body's overactivity or preoccupation with fighting the cancer, cutting back the normal process of breaking down and getting rid of the vitamin E molecules. We don't know—yet. More studies are necessary, and until then vitamin E continues to be recommended to women with breast cancer to reduce hot flashes by renowned medical authorities such as the Mayo Clinic and the National Surgical Adjuvant Breast Project. Foods rich in vitamin E are recommended for their overall health value.

Fiber from whole grain cereals and breads, beans, fruits, and vegetables has been shown to reduce the risk of colon cancer. Because fiber is not absorbed into your body, it stays within your bowel, providing bulk that acts as a natural laxative. Because the contents of your bowels move through your body faster, there is less time and opportunity for your body to absorb toxic waste elements.

Soluble fiber contained in products such as oat bran, peas, barley, beans, Metamucil, Citrosel, and many no-name brands can bind to unhealthful substances and escort them out of your system. Insoluble fiber, which provides bulk, includes fruit, vegetable skins, and some bran.

Another fiber plus: Because you don't absorb either type of fiber into your system, it fills you up without adding calories. People eat large quantities of fiber for this reason alone. The recommended amount of fiber is between 25 and 35 grams per day, not to exceed 35.

Some people reason that clearing or detoxifying one's system faster and more thoroughly (using enemas or high colonics) can be even more beneficial, and there are therapies based on this concept. But there has been no validation of this theory by objective studies, and if practiced with any frequency, such colon manipulation could prove harmful.

Calcium is a crucial element in preventing osteoporosis, the fourth leading killer of women. Staying healthy means paying attention to calcium intake, but new research shows that women should not take more calcium supplements than necessary, or they may deplete their bodies of other vital minerals. Calcium is available in milk (300 mg in 8 ounces of skim milk), cheese, yogurt, ice cream (buy low-fat or no-fat), tofu, and leafy green vegetables. The recommended dose is 800 milligrams daily. If, however, you are undergoing chemotherapy or have metastatic breast cancer, your calcium level may be elevated, so check with your doctor before starting any supplemental calcium.

Aspirin has become a daily supplement for millions, to reduce their risk of heart disease, colon cancer, and, more recently, breast cancer—although aspirin's preventive benefit for breast cancer is still under debate.

Reliable studies have indicated that, over five years, risk levels for heart disease and colon cancer drop by up to 40 percent with regular small doses of aspirin. The effect apparently occurs because of the blood-thinning properties of aspirin (salicylic acid). One baby aspirin a day (81 mg) (or even every other day) is the usual prophylactic dose, but don't take aspirin regularly without checking with your doctor first. Aspirin, like any drug, has side effects and is not for everyone.

Selenium is essential to general good health, but you need it only in tiny amounts. Selenium may reduce free radicals and inhibit the oxidation of unsaturated fats; some believe these effects reduce cancer risk, but there is no conclusive evidence. Selenium is present in minute amounts in vegetables, cereal, seafood, dairy products, red meat, and chicken. Supplements are unnecessary.

Chromium has been promoted as a "fat burner" in health food stores, but research by the U.S. Navy on chromium picolinate has shown no such effect. New tests suggest chromium picolinate may actually promote cancer. A report in the journal of the Federation of American Society of Experimental Biology says that in the absence of adequate testing, chromium supplements cannot be presumed safe for human use.

Ellagic acid, present in red grapes, red wine, raspberries, and other fruit, is believed by some to protect the body by neutralizing reactive chemicals or carcinogens, diminishing prostaglandin synthesis, and protecting DNA. I'm not recommending the health benefits of red wine; the increased risk of breast cancer associated with alcohol is greater than any benefit of ellagic acid. Besides, you would have to drink an enormous quantity to get the benefit.

Green tea is an antioxidant that is consumed in vast quantities in Japan, where many people are heavy smokers, but where there is a much lower rate of lung cancer than in the United States. Green tea contains nicotinic acid, which some believe lowers cholesterol as well as lung and breast cancer in rats. The flavonoid EGCG (epigallo-catechin gallete) is reputed to be the factor that provides the anti-cancer benefits of green tea. No for-profit company is likely to fund research on green tea, because it's already so widely available and so cheap. Decaffeinated green tea does not appear to have quite the same benefits as regular. Black tea also has these properties, but to a lesser degree. Some scientists say you shouldn't use milk in your tea; it may counter potential benefits—one explanation for why the tea-drinking English don't reap tea's reputed anticancer benefits.

Pollutants and Pesticides

To protect your health, it is advisable to avoid foods that contain pesticides, hormones, and antibiotics. The Environmental Protection Agency has indicated that about seventy pesticides currently in use are suspected carcinogens. DDT has been implicated as a possible carcinogen for breast cancer, because its breakdown products act like estrogen and can accumulate in breast tissue for years.

Because animal fats, including dairy fats, accumulate pesticides, hormones, and antibiotics, one way to avoid these substances in food is to restrict the amount of animal fat in your diet. If you have a weakness for fried foods and you indulge in them even though you know better, make sure the food is fried in monounsaturated vegetable oil (preferably olive or canola) rather than in purified animal fats. (A recent National Academy of Science panel report stated that natural and synthetic cancer-causing chemicals in food were much less a concern as factors in human cancer than the high consumption of dietary fat and calories.)

Fish that contain significant amounts of fat tend to concentrate pesticides in their fatty tissue, so limit your consumption of fatty fish from areas suspected of high pesticide use to no more than once a week. Large fish, high on the food chain, such as tuna or swordfish, may contain high levels of mercury or other pollutants. Freshwater fish may contain unsafe levels of PVC (polyvinyl chloride, a chemical used in making plastics). Try not to eat these fish more than once a week, or even once a month, according to some authorities. Cold-water fish, like salmon, haddock, and mackerel, contain omega-3 fats, considered health-promoting.

Imported foods are more likely to contain residual pesticides, because many countries that export fruits and vegetables to this country do not regulate pesticide use, and it's impossible for the FDA to adequately inspect imported foods. (Ironically, this country exports many pesticides whose use is illegal in the United States, which may come back to us on fruits and vegetables we import from countries who buy these chemicals.)

It is worth spending a little extra to buy the following fruits and vegetables grown to organic food standards because they tend to soak up more pesticides than others: strawberries, apples, raisins and grapes, bananas, bell peppers, spinach, cucumbers, and celery.

Hormones and antibiotics used in food production are also suspect compounds. The move toward organically grown foods (foods raised without chemical fertilizers, pesticides, added hormones, or antibiotics, which are common in red meat and poultry) has gained ground each year, and prices are coming down to more attractive levels. Many supermarkets offer certified organic products along with conventional foods, and various supermarket chains (Vestro Natural Foods, Cascadian, Alfalfa's and Wild Oats, Whole Foods, Fresh Fields, and Bread and Circus), as well as some phone order services (Colorado Prime) are devoted to organically raised foods. In addition to supermarket sources, local seasonal products, available at neighborhood stands or farmers' markets, are usually grown with minimal or no pesticides and only natural fertilizers. But there's nothing magic about the word *organic*. You can't assume that just because a food is labeled organic that it's truly free of hormones, pesticides, or antibiotics. Ask your store how they verify their claims that these are safe foods. Federal standards and regulations are now coming into place to ensure the accuracy of the organic label.

To protect yourself from surface pollutants, wash all fruits and vegetables, adding a drop of hand dishwashing detergent to the wash water. Rinse thoroughly. Scrub potatoes if you plan to eat their skins. Peel fruits and vegetables whose skins are waxed (such as apples and cucumbers). Discard the outer leaves of head lettuce and cabbage.

Eat Smart

Researchers are continually investigating the power and value of all kinds of dietary supplements to figure out which new substances will really make a difference to your health. But while all this research is going on, what do you do? What should you take? Our sober advice: Eat smart! A well-balanced diet should supply all the necessary and desirable elements for good health. If you do take supplements, take them in moderation, and don't expect miracles. Restrict the amount of fat you eat, and eat only the healthiest kinds. When possible, buy organic foods.

Substitute soy products for some of the meat and cheese you use in your old-style recipes, or get a good start with an easy-to-follow cookbook, such as Penny Block's *A Banquet of Health* (call 847-942-3040) or Shandler's *Estrogen: The Natural Way*. Don't be scared off by the title of the latter; use it for its practical and inviting recipes, rather than for the benefit of soy's purported estrogen effect.

Enjoy a meal in a vegetarian restaurant, or a vegetarian meal in a regular restaurant, the least expensive way to dine out healthfully.

Food is one of life's great pleasures. And some foods are especially good for you. The trick is to figure out a healthy diet that is also a pleasure to eat. Food that gives you pleasure is not just a bonus, it's an inherent part of eating and nutrition. You should enjoy every bite you put into your mouth. Think of the improvement of your nutrition as an improvement in lifestyle that will ease the effects of growing older and the stressful effects of cancer therapy. And because increasing age is one of the greatest risk factors for breast cancer, easing the aging process on your cells also means decreasing your chance of developing a new cancer.

14

Weight Control

I wasn't doing too bad with my weight until I went on tamoxifen. I put on thirty pounds in no time. I managed to take off ten pounds by watching what I ate and taking the stairs instead of the elevator, but I can't seem to budge the other twenty. I feel good, so I've decided not to torture myself about those extra pounds. I'm not trying to be glamorous anymore. I think I look good enough.

How Pounds Accumulate

A nibble here, a nibble there, and pretty soon another five pounds is sitting on your hips. The metabolism of all women slows as we age—decreasing by as much as 30 percent after menopause—and that means we use fewer calories to get through our day; if we don't cut back what we eat, those unused calories are stored as fat. "I eat just what I always have—but my weight keeps growing and I can't seem to manage to get rid of what I gain. It is so frustrating."

If weight was a problem for you before breast cancer, it's probably a bigger problem now. At least a third of women gain weight during chemotherapy, usually an average of five to ten pounds, and for many, the tendency to gain weight continues even after chemotherapy is finished. For women taking tamoxifen, the tendency to gain weight is a common report. Losing those extra pounds can be an awesome challenge.

Hormonal changes from chemotherapy and tamoxifen or just plain menopause, decreased physical activity, and the food you eat to relieve chemo-related nausea, queasiness, discomfort, and stress, all contribute to the weight gain problem. Certain antinausea medication, such as steroids, can increase your appetite and alter your metabolism. Chemotherapy can cause a hollow feeling in your stomach that is relieved by eating. And women who stop smoking during or after treatment tend to gain weight.

Some research suggests that a taste for high fat and sugar is common among women affected by breast cancer, because these foods create a relaxing effect, stimulating the release of endorphins (opiate-like, feel-good compounds). The pleasure of these very rich foods may have helped ease you through hard times; cutting back to a healthier diet when treatment is finally over can be a real battle.

How Weight Gain Affects You

Maybe if our society were less infatuated with pencil-slim women, it wouldn't be such a big deal if we gained a few pounds, but as it is, few of us can escape the message that "fat is ugly." At least as important, however, are the health issues involved in excess weight.

Most women who gain weight during treatment, or who were already at more than ideal body weight, suffer a constant assault on their self-image and self-esteem. (After breast radiation, one breast may gain weight along with the rest of the body, and the treated breast may not, which can add further stress to self-image issues. (See Chapter 11.) Many women feel unattractive and helpless, and they worry in addition about the harmful impact weight may have on their overall health and risk of breast cancer recurrence.

Excess weight may be a health risk factor for women who have had breast cancer, although the issue has not been fully resolved. Fat cells help make a weak form of estrogen. The more fat cells, the more estrogen there is to stimulate breast cells, including breast cancer cells, if any are present. That's why blocking or eliminating the effects of estrogen is one of the goals of breast cancer therapy.

The location of fat cells may also have an effect on breast cancer risk. Studies suggest that certain female torso shapes are more at risk than others: apple-shaped women have a higher incidence of breast cancer than pear-shaped women. Maybe excess fat on the belly is more likely to produce estrogen than fat located on the hips. It's not known if changing your shape, assuming that were possible, could change your risk.

Fat cells can also be repositories of pesticides and other carcinogens consumed over a lifetime, in food, water, and air.

Excess weight is also a significant risk factor for lymphedema (see Chapter 10), so if you've had lymph node surgery, you have to be especially careful about weight gain. If you have had any lymph nodes removed, you must be cautious about performing exercise that strains the at-risk arm, so exercising for weight control can pose a challenge. Avoid lifting and repetitive-resistance-oriented movement; try walking or swimming to aid fluid circulation and help with weight control.

How to Lose Those Pounds

Is excess weight a problem for you? Are you ready to devote thought and energy to the problem? After all the trauma you've endured with breast cancer, you may not be up to any more challenges. But it needn't be an all-or-nothing proposition. Start out slowly. Your first step will be to select the eating plan that's right for you, from the mass of articles, studies, and media bites that feature one miracle solution after another. Then check out your plan with your doctor—and while you're there, work out a realistic course of exercise that you will enjoy and thus be sure to follow. Exercise, as you know, is a crucial part of any weight control program.

Avoid Crash Diets

Avoid crash diets and attempts at rapid weight loss. If you lose weight too fast, your body goes on starvation alert. Your metabolism starts to slow down to conserve energy, defeating the very purpose of your hard efforts. You shock your system with a diet that's impossible to maintain for long, and you start to lose more muscle than fat.

The all-protein diet is another misguided notion, and is also hard to maintain. It puts an unhealthy strain on your system, especially your kidneys.

Slow and steady wins the battle over the bulge and helps you stay the winner over the long haul. No startling formulas or dazzling diets will do it, although some people do need the boost of rapid weight loss in the beginning to encourage them and give them confidence to move on to a more steady-paced, long-term plan.

Every successful approach to weight loss suggests moderate consumption of nutritious foods from the essential food groups, eight glasses of water a day (not as easy as it might sound), some supplements—and exercise. You won't keep fit and well-shaped without exercise, and it will provide you with a feeling of control, enhance your sense of well-being, and extend your life, whether you lose weight or not.

Boost Your Metabolism

Eat less; move more. (If only it were that simple!) The ideal way to approach weight loss is to slowly decrease the calories you consume and to increase your physical activity and your body's metabolic rate. (Metabolism can be described as your body's furnace.) Your metabolic rate determines how many calories you use to perform your body's essential work. Exercise builds up muscle and raises your basic metabolic rate, thus increasing the number of calories you need just to breathe and stay alive. (A fuller discussion of exercise comes later in this chapter.)

Some people's metabolic rates are more efficient and slower than others': They need fewer calories to do the same work as people with higher metabolic rates. If people with slow metabolic rates eat what most other people do, they end up storing the calories they don't burn as fat. Metabolic rates decline as you age. So if you're eating less than your skinny friends, but you still can't lose weight, it's not because you're lazy, unmotivated, or "pigging out." It may be one more cruel downer of aging.

Limit Your Calories

To lose weight, you need to limit the number of calories you consume. To do that, you need to know the numbers: the number of calories in the foods you eat and the number of calories to aim for. The average woman needs about 1800 to 2000 calories per day, but this count varies depending on age, height, weight, and body type. It is unwise to go below a daily intake of 1200 calories for any extended period of time.

Weigh portions, and keep a calorie-counting book handy, along with a kitchen scale. Use measuring cups and spoons to figure the portion sizes suggested on the Nutrition Facts section of the labels on the packaged foods you buy. Also listed are calories, fat, cholesterol, sugar, salt, fiber, vitamins, and minerals. You can eat a lot of things you like, even high-calorie favorites, as long as you limit the portions and understand how many calories you're actually consuming. You will probably be amazed at the difference between what you consider a reasonable portion and what the label recommends. "Those labels changed my life. I don't eat a thing till I read the fat and calorie content. I'm enjoying meals more than ever, and I've lost ten pounds."

Write out your goals and keep notes on what you eat, so you can plan your calorie intake before you sit down at the table, at least in the beginning. "Think about every bite," says Sherry, a successful dieter, "and enjoy every bite you take." "Count thirty seconds between bites," says Dr. Art Ulene of NBC's Today Show.

Many women find it works best to stick to a strict number of calories for at least two weeks at the start, in order to acquire a true sense of what each food "costs." Keep in mind that all calories are not the same. For example, calories from refined sugar are more readily available to your body than complex sugars that are contained in plant fibers (fruit) that your body only partially digests.

If you don't learn to count the calories in your food, your understanding of how to lose weight will be compromised. That doesn't mean keeping to strict accounting forever. Once you get the drift of how calories add up, you can discard the weighing and the totaling up of exact numbers. You can average out the desired number of calories over a few days, thus allowing for an occasional splurge on one day by cutting back calories the day before or the day after.

Cut the Fat

The tried-and-true standard healthy diet recommendations are to cut total fat, including cholesterol, eat plenty of fruits and vegetables (five to nine servings a day) and high-fiber foods (35 gm of fiber daily), and limit alcohol, salt, and smoked and nitrate-cured foods. It's vital to restrict the amount of fat in your diet. Too much of it, saturated or unsaturated, may increase your chance of developing heart disease or colon and endometrial cancer. The direct connection between dietary fat and breast cancer is controversial. A recent report of combined data from seven studies in four countries, with information from over 300,000 women, showed that dietary fat—whether less than 20 percent of daily caloric intake or over 40 percent—had no effect on breast cancer rates. But other smaller studies do suggest lower breast cancer rates with a low fat diet.

Typical fat intake in this country is close to 40 percent of total calories. For your general medical health, even if it doesn't reduce your risk of breast cancer, it's best to shoot for no more than 20 percent of your daily calories from fat, but that is a hard level for most people to reach, a real challenge to your self-control. Reducing fat levels to between 25 and 30 percent of your daily caloric intake may be a more reasonable goal. (If your recommended caloric intake is 1800 calories a day, you could restrict your fat to 25 percent of your daily caloric intake, or 450 calories. Divide 450 by 9 calories per gram of fat—50 grams of fat is your daily limit.) Zero percent fat intake is also unhealthy: your body needs some dietary fat for normal function.

To get closer to a 25 percent dietary fat level, here's help with low-fat food choices to substitute for more popular selections:

NO, NO	YES, YES
ice cream	sorbet, ices, frozen fruit pops, or fat-free frozen yogurt
butter	unsweetened fruit preserves
cream soups	gazpacho, vegetable soups in broth base
sour cream dip	salsa
potato chips	pretzels
doughnuts, iced cakes	angel food cake
brownies	gingersnaps, fat-free cookies
croissants	bagels
salami, bologna	turkey, lean ham
oil-packed tuna	water-packed tuna
french fries	baked or boiled potatoes
sour cream	yogurt or low-fat cottage cheese
mayonnaise	mustard
corn chips	air-popped popcorn
cheese from whole milk or cream	part-skim mozzarella, ricotta or soy cheese
whole eggs	egg whites, Egg Beaters
ham-and-cheese omelet	vegetable and egg-white omelet
fruit-flavored yogurt	nonfat yogurt with sliced fresh fruit
olives	celery or raw vegetable strips
whole milk	skim milk

Scan your grocery shelves frequently; new nonfat versions of fat-filled favorites appear every day. Single out the foods you like and familiarize yourself with ways to prepare or serve them. Once you're into the swing of the list, menu planning and calorie counting are easier. It's still a challenge to make food tasty when you're keeping fat intake low, but keep with it. Keep in mind that the leading source of fat in a woman's diet is salad dressing, followed by cheese, butter, and ground beef. Your taste will change, and you may lose your "fat tooth." Limit the amount of oil you use (preferably olive or canola), choose beans (canned or dry), grains, pasta, seafood, and skinless chicken or turkey white meat—and serve yourself reasonable portions (four ounces, the size of a deck of cards, is a reasonable serving of meat). Fill up, if you must, with fresh fruits and vegetables. At least fill your refrigerator with plenty of healthful foods to choose from. Libraries and bookstores can supply you with shelves full of stimulating books for the preparation of delicious, healthful meals.

Cholesterol and Oils

Cholesterol doesn't cause breast cancer, nor is it thought to stimulate its growth, but it *is* involved with heart disease. So while you're cutting calories, eliminate the ones that aren't good for you.

Cholesterol is a waxy substance present in many animal food sources that is a necessary biological building block. It is not the same as fat, but cholesterol and fat work together in the structure and function of your body's cells. Unfortunately, cholesterol has a tendency to accumulate in blood vessels and interfere with blood flow. Animal food sources that are high in fat are usually high in cholesterol, and include eggs and dairy products. Vegetable sources of fat contain little or no cholesterol, but even if a food has no cholesterol, it isn't necessarily healthful; oils or foods labeled cholesterol free may still contain large amounts of fat. Limit the amount of cholesterol in your diet to under 300 milligrams per day.

Try to avoid saturated fats such as butter, coconut and palm oils, and hydrogenated vegetable oils; minimize your use of polyunsaturated fats such as safflower, soybean, sunflower, and corn oils. (The soy that's good for you is soy protein, not soy oil.) The best oils to use are monounsaturated: canola (rapeseed) and olive oil.

Olive oil may actually protect you against breast cancer. Studies of women in Greece and Spain, who have a high fat intake—consuming most of that fat as olive oil—have breast cancer rates 50 percent lower than women in the United States. Of course, you can't attribute that reduced rate just to olive oil; many complex factors we don't fully understand are undoubtedly involved in that statistic, but if you're going to consume oil in some form, olive oil is more acceptable than most (or flaxseed oil, which contains high levels of omega-3 fatty acids—considered another healthful choice).

Use cooking techniques that require little or no fat. Microwaving, broiling, and steaming are better than deep-frying and sautéing. Try using applesauce or other fruit purees instead of butter when baking. Use two egg whites (fat- and cholesterol-free) for one egg. Check the bookstores for low-fat and no-fat cookbooks and for inspiration.

Tips on Dining In and Dining Out

When you eat in a restaurant, don't be embarrassed to ask what's in the dish you want to order. Enough people are interested in healthy eating to have made this a commonplace request. Ask to have sauces served separately—butter, sour cream, or salad dressing on the side—and skin taken off the chicken. One thing you can be sure of: Restaurant food has a lot more calories and fat than you or even a trained dietician might imagine or predict. And in restaurants that serve large portions, you may have to leave food on your plate. (Ask your waiter to wrap it up so you can take it home.)

Many menus highlight healthful choices, so ordering can be uncomplicated and streamlined. Even fast-food chains have joined the campaign, with lean specials and take-out literature containing nutrition facts about their popular food items.

Mind Over Mind

All those food facts are very nice to know, but in practical terms they may not make dieting any easier. Plain-spoken rules, discipline, and, especially, mind-over-mind techniques are necessary to stay on track.

Coping with Food Cravings

You may be able to convince yourself that pure vanilla Häagen-Dazs is good for you (proteins for muscle and calcium for your bones), but your intuition about food fats and calories is frequently unreliable, colored by food desires and a mixed self-image. How many calories can there be in a couple of chocolate kisses or in a crisp dry pretzel that looks and tastes like it counts for nothing? Don't trust these presumptions. Most snacks people reach for start off at a hundred calories. It's wildly frustrating, budgeting calories much as you budget money. How do you satisfy your desires with the limited number of calories you can afford?

It's best to try to curb your sweet tooth, or use complex carbohydrates for sweetening—like barley, rice, malt syrups—rather than sugar substitutes like Sweet'n Low or Nutra-Sweet. These chemicals sustain your level of craving or desire for sweets. (Although problems have been reported with each sweetener, they pose no proven health risk.)

If your resolve starts to slip and you think you might be heading toward a binge, try to recapture control; don't let your mind make matters worse. You know the "line" that leads down the road to broken resolve: "I've lost out on today's diet, so to hell with it—I'll forget about today. I'll start off tomorrow, and I'll just finish up the cake now—and that half-empty carton of ice cream." So then you feel guilty and discouraged: "Is it really worth trying to start over again?" Meanwhile, the family wedding, the vacation at the beach, the big birthday party have all come and gone, followed by depression and self-reproach. "Why bother? I never do things right, and who really cares about the way I look? My fashion statement will always be sweat suits."

Don't buy into this negativity. You can fight it off. There's always another vacation or big event to come. Lose one, win the next.

Avoid Temptation

Concentrate on your food shopping. Don't allow high-calorie foods, such as high-fat specialty ice cream or rich entrees, into your house. Select lots of fresh fruits and vegetables (five to nine servings a day), nonfat milk products, grains and pasta, fish, soybean meat substitutes, white-meat poultry, and lean meats, for a full, balanced diet.

Don't shop when you're hungry. Don't drop *anything* that isn't good for you into your shopping cart. When you get that urge to nibble, unwholesome choices won't be available; you'll have to settle for healthful snacks. Keep an ample supply of fruits and vegetables in your refrigerator (and you'll have to eat them just to keep your refrigerator tidy), with plenty of cut-up raw vegetable snacks in water, ready when you are. If you need more flavor to satisfy you, keep the vegetables in a vinaigrette (two-thirds balsamic vinegar to one-third olive oil) instead of water. A whole watermelon goes a long way. Extra-tempting fruit is a smart investment. So are special, tasty low-calorie treats. Dried fruit can be as good as candy—but here, too, the calories can mount up.

Keep the food *in* the kitchen and yourself *out* as much as is possible; it's too easy to taste or pick up a bite of this or that. No more peanuts in the family room and pretzels in the den. Out of sight, out of your mouth. And get out of the house—for exercise, work, or shopping with friends, activities where no food is served or available.

Eat Slowly

Eat only when you are hungry, not when you think it's time to chow down, and eat slowly, in a pleasant setting. It takes a full twenty minutes for your body to figure out that it's had enough and to send that signal to your brain. If you're eating too fast but expecting to stop when you feel full, you're beating out the signal that will help you stop. So slow down and enjoy what you're eating.

Schedule meals far enough apart so that you're hungry when mealtime comes around, but not so far apart that you want to consume everything in sight. Don't eat on the run, because you'll tend to eat more than you think. Pay attention to your food so you really get the most out of every morsel (that means no reading while you eat).

Distract Yourself

Distract yourself with mind-over-mind exercises. Find ways to ignore food cravings. Force yourself to think about everything you've done throughout the day, plan tomorrow's schedule, call a friend, turn on the TV, read a book, work on imagery, play music that is upbeat, inspiring, or soul-satisfying, or take up knitting or handiwork so your fingers are too busy to pick up food.

Make a pact with yourself to stay away from food for the next half hour, or the next ten minutes. If the urge for food won't let up, think about how and why it's got that grip on you. Set your mind against the craving. Remind yourself that *you* are in charge of your life and your weight, not the insidious urge that keeps nagging you. And because we're not machines, allow yourself some rewards through the day or week, but plan them ahead of time so there's less chance of grabbing something you shouldn't, or worse, of bingeing.

Get Peer Support

Peer support is important. Find someone to share your pain and gains, someone you can call when food desires get overpowering, who'll shore up your resolve, who'll talk you past the desperate moments. Control begets more control.

The Weight Watchers program appears to be the most successful program for long-term weight management. It depends on group support and reinforcement, regular meetings, weigh-ins, calorie counting and kitchen-scale measurement of food, and filling yourself with large, healthy, balanced meals. That's one of their lures. You don't suffer food deprivation; you get to eat a lot of real food, not powders or potions. Weight Watchers emphasizes behavior modification by teaching ways to alter bad eating habits, such as snacking, eating on the run, and consuming excessive portions.

Take Charge

Stay in charge. Avoid the martyr role. If you are cooking for a family, especially one with teenagers, you are set up for a real challenge. It can be torture to watch young people wolf down huge numbers of calories, while you try to restrict yourself to an austere menu. What willpower you need! Face the problem. Can you handle it? Can you

get your family to accept a low-fat diet? How much fat can you eliminate from the rest of your family's diet (setting them on a healthy
course for their future)? Should you eat before the others, or at least
eat something that will ease your appetite? Should you prepare separate dishes for yourself?

Chemical Aids to Weight Management

The weight gain–weight loss issue may add up to more than counting
calories and confronting mind-over-mind ploys. Managing your
weight may be beyond your control. Although high-fat diets and
sedentary lifestyles are responsible for most weight gain, more and
more research shows that genes can be the cause of particular weight
problems, such as a low metabolic rate. Genes and chemicals, factors
beyond your control, may be at the root of your struggle. There's an
enormous amount of research going on, especially for weight control
aids; so far, there's nothing totally acceptable for long-term use, but
there are a few tantalizing possibilities.

Some people may just have to live with being overweight, so maybe
it's time to accept your body as it is, resolve not to gain any more
weight, and stop reproaching yourself. But if you're not about to give
up the struggle, and you've explored other routes to weight management, such as organized hospital-based weight control programs or
Weight Watchers, Jenny Craig, or similar plans, diet pills may prove
your last resort to achieve control over your weight gain.

Diet pills are not recommended for women who want to lose five to
twenty pounds; they are considered appropriate only for people 20
percent over their ideal weight with weight-related health problems,
or 30 percent over their ideal weight without weight-related health
problems. All of these "new" diet pills require a doctor's prescription.

The weight-shedding benefit of diet pills lasts only a limited time,
and then decreases in effect. Long-term use (beyond a year) of medication for weight loss is not yet fully approved because it can have
consequences that are worrisome and difficult to determine, yet long-
term use may be required to maintain the weight lost. Proceed with
caution, and only use diet pills under your doctor's supervision.

New Diet Pills

Fenfluramine (pondimin) is dispensed alone or in combination with
another drug, *phentermine* (ionamin), to suppress food cravings. (The

FDA, however, has not officially approved the combination of these two drugs.) Although these two drugs were approved for weight control over twenty years ago, it wasn't until obesity was recognized as a chronic disease that the idea of prescribing these long-term medications became accepted and popular.

Fenfluramine and phentermine increase brain serotonin, a natural substance believed to control compulsive eating. Large numbers of people taking this medication lost up to 15 percent of their starting weight over a period of a year, and then leveled off. Indefinite use of these drugs may be necessary to maintain the weight that is lost, but no study on the safety of long-term use has been completed. The pills don't work for everyone; if you don't lose weight within the first month or so, these medications probably won't help you.

Weight loss is not the only advantage of these medications; they also have a positive effect on cholesterol, blood sugar, and blood pressure.

These drugs can have significant side effects. Mild to moderate side effects include dry mouth, drowsiness, constipation, diarrhea, mild confusion and short-term memory loss, anxiety, bizarre dreams, heart palpitations, and increased blood pressure. These lesser side effects may diminish over time. Serious, even life-threatening side effects are pulmonary hypertension (increased pressure in the arteries that go to the lungs) and heart valve damage. Both are rare but irreversible, possibly progressive, and possibly fatal. Disturbing reports of these terrible side effects in young women are just beginning to surface. Furthermore, long-term studies are not available and may be a long time coming. The complete story on the consequences of taking these drugs is unknown. You must exercise careful judgment and extreme caution, as we've said before.

The new pills are believed to be nonaddictive, whereas amphetamines, popular in the past, were addictive and caused agitation and abnormal heart rhythms.

Dexfenfluramine (Redux) is related to fenfluramine and phentermine, but it is twice as expensive. It has been used in many other countries for years, but the Food and Drug Administration has only recently approved its use. Some consumer health groups have protested the release of the drug because laboratory testing demonstrated that high doses of dexfenfluramine cause brain damage in test animals. They are also concerned about evidence that dexfenfluramine might cause erratic behavior or depression.

Like fenfluramine and phentermine, dexfenfluramine is advised only for people who are more than 20 percent over their ideal weight.

Prozac, otherwise known as *fluoxetine,* also increases brain levels of serotonin; it can lead to weight loss, but after a few months its weight loss benefit appears to diminish. (Prozac is typically used as an anti-depressant.)

Leptin is a protein that has a dramatic effect on the body fat of an unusual strain of obese mice. Leptin practically dissolves their fat away, binding to unique receptors in the brain, suppressing appetite and speeding up metabolism. Remember, though, results for mice (and a special strain of mouse at that) don't necessarily translate into results for people.

Except for what may be a rare genetic abnormality, people who are overweight, in fact, appear to have high levels of leptin in their systems, and recent studies reveal an abnormality in the gene that is in charge of leptin in a significant number of obese people. It's not clear what that leptin is doing. A lot of detective work remains to be done on the role of leptin in human obesity; until human studies are available on the safety and long-term effects of leptin, it will not be available for general use. Amgen Incorporated has spent $20 million to initiate clinical trials of leptin on human subjects. Scientific speculation so far is that large, frequent, long-term doses of leptin would be necessary to have any slimming effect.

Xenical, or orlistat, is a prescription drug that blocks fat absorption, up to a third of what is consumed, but it has all the unpleasant side effects that accompany those "free-from-fat-absorption" potato chips: diarrhea, gas, and problems with malabsorption of nutrients such as vitamins D, E, and beta carotene. (The vitamins slide out of the body along with the fat.) Oily stools may also result in "leakage." Enough said.

But for people with serious weight problems Xenical does offer help with modest weight loss that continues into the second year of use. It also appears to result in slight drops in cholesterol, blood pressure, and blood-sugar levels; all these effects are promising benefits against heart disease.

Exercise for Purpose and Pleasure

No matter how good you are about dieting, it's much harder to lose weight by diet alone than by a combination of diet and exercise. Couch-potato dieters seem to get only so far; they lose weight up to a point, and then the weight loss trails off. People who exercise and diet are able to continue losing weight, and, more important, they are able to continue to maintain their weight loss.

But exercise has importance beyond its role in weight reduction. Exercise can reduce your risk of cancer and heart disease, help prevent or lessen the severity of diabetes and osteoporosis, and enhance your sense of well-being. It reduces fat, increases muscle, strengthens bone, promotes immunity, helps overcome depression, lessens hot flashes, and improves memory, sleep, and sex. That's a whole lot of dividends from something you can get for a moderate degree of effort and little or no money. "I started swimming because I was getting too stiff. After I got into a regular schedule, my arthritis improved and I felt so much better—and younger. I've also made friends with a whole new group of upbeat, energetic young women. I have been told that swimming doesn't do much toward fighting osteoporosis—but I come from a family with strong bones, so I'll keep on swimming."

Frequent exercise appears to reduce the presence of free estrogen in the body. A study of premenopausal women who exercised between one and three hours a week found breast cancer risk was lowered by 20 to 30 percent; exercising four hours a week brought the risk down by 60 percent. Similar findings were demonstrated by yet another, more recent, study.

The important thing is to get started, to overcome your natural inertia. Most people start off tentatively—a fifteen-minute swim once in a while, then once a week, then maybe twice a week, and pretty soon those reinforcing endorphins pop in, and the swim goes to twenty, then thirty minutes three and four times a week. Reinforcement comes from looking good as well as feeling good, and reading and hearing all the media hype on the benefits of exercise. Once you get started, you'll find it fun, or at least habit-forming, because of the release of those endorphins that comes with activity—and your pride in being fit. Endorphins make you feel good; that's why runners get hooked on running, and why people perform the vigorous activities that border on pain.

You don't have to twist yourself out of shape or buy fancy equipment. You don't have to join a fitness club. You don't have to hire a personal trainer. To get started, you just have to take a walk, or swim, climb stairs, wash your windows, or dance. (Find some irresistible tapes of country western, rock, R & B, reggae, klezmer, tango, or jazz, and improvise your own steps.) Anything to get you out of your chair and moving.

To make exercise a regular part of your life, integrate it into your daily routine, and plan it for your convenience at a time and place, no more than ten or fifteen minutes from home or work, that will allow you to keep going, season after season, year after year. Pace the floor when you're talking on the phone. Skip the elevator whenever sensible; get into the habit of climbing stairs. One flight up is worth two flights down. And do more walking; park your car a little farther away from where you're heading. Most people are prepared to walk to any place that's no farther than five minutes away. Give yourself and the car a break; try extending that boundary to ten minutes away.

To begin with, aim for a minimum of fifteen minutes of activity, three or more times a week. Check with your doctor to work out a reasonable plan. Moderate exercise is good; vigorous exercise is better. Two hours a week is good, three hours better, four hours or more best—but any exercise is worthwhile. Thirty minutes a day is ideal, even if you break it into ten-minute segments.

Keep exercise fun, practical, and convenient, so you'll want to keep it up. Do whatever is necessary to make exercise a permanent part of your life. Lack of time is supposedly the biggest obstacle to exercising regularly, and boredom is the spoiler of many a well-intentioned plan. Your head is really what counts in establishing a successful exercise program. (Again: mind over mind.) Liven things up with music or companionship so you won't lose interest. (If you use a radio or tape headset outside, keep the volume down so you don't miss street sounds and jeopardize your safety.) Exercising with a friend makes it a social event and reinforces the pleasure of the experience, making you more inclined to keep going.

Eat properly before you exercise, especially if you engage in a particularly vigorous activity. (You must have a high-carbohydrate component in your diet to provide the fuel you need to burn off body fat.) Dress properly when you exercise. Wear comfortable shoes that give you support, and loose-fitting, layered clothing so you can peel off layers as you heat up.

Some experts recommend exercising only four out of seven days a week, explaining that rest and recovery are an important part of the exercise-to-benefit equation. The body rebuilds and grows stronger in those interim rest periods.

Overdoing exercise is almost as bad as doing no exercise. Don't overexert yourself and don't exercise to the point of pain. Don't follow the advice of anyone who tells you to do anything that causes pain. Pain is a signal that you're at risk, on the edge of injury. Better to exercise longer than harder. Start off slowly; do as much as you can at a level that's comfortable for you.

You can monitor every bite that goes into your mouth, but unless you start some kind of program of regular physical activity, it will be very hard to control your weight. And you'll be losing out on the benefits of agility, tone and shape, vigor, strength, well-being, relief for hot flashes, enhanced self-esteem and libido, better health, better sex, and longer life.

An Ongoing Battle

Anyone out to lose weight has to battle contrary urges every minute of the day. You'll need to use whatever tricks you can find to beat that craving; you need to be alert to any trap that might overwhelm you, any pitfall that might ruin your plans.

At some point, you should weigh yourself. Many women weigh themselves once a day, but once a week is probably better. Then, if you notice an increase of a couple of pounds, you can exercise a little longer or more vigorously, or skip dessert for a while.

After you've made progress and have managed to lose an impressive number of pounds, you may hit a plateau—the pounds stop dropping off. That's how the body works; it has to protect itself from wasting away. It's also possible that as you've lost fat, you've built up heavier muscle, and that balances out the weight loss. Stick to your good habits, and the weight loss should pick up again. If the plateau hangs on too long, try to cut the calories just a bit more and rev up the exercise program, and watch for results. Or simply enjoy the success you've already achieved.

Self-Image and Self-Esteem

It takes a lot of confidence, support, and self-control to eat with restraint and to keep fit and trim. Few of us have such resources. Most of us need help with coping abilities and self-esteem, and we feel like failures when we don't measure up to expectations, when we can't trim down to formidable standards. If you weigh more than you think you should, but you've really worked on weight loss, on your own and with your physician, with limited success, don't punish yourself further. Your self-acceptance and quality of life matter as much as your place in the table of weight statistics.

Self-esteem and self-image depend on more than just weight. If you are not satisfied with your appearance, pay extra attention to what you wear. Clothes can make you feel good about yourself. Wear nice things at home, just for yourself, styles that flatter your figure, colors that suit you and trim you down, not too tight, not too big. Consider how great Roseanne looks on award shows (the 1996 American Comedy Awards, for instance), compared with how unbecoming she looks in those loud, baggy clothes on her own show.

Makeup can be just as important as clothes. Maybe it's not for everyone, but if you like to use makeup, go for it, especially if your skin color is still a little different from normal because of chemotherapy. At least use a dab of lipstick to give yourself that spark of color. And add the final touch—some jazzy jewelry. Wear earrings for fun and a bit of dash and glamour, even if it's only for yourself.

Be Realistic

In this struggle for self-esteem and strength, you need every ally you can get, especially yourself. Treat yourself like your own best friend, not like your own worst enemy. "Accept realistic weight standards and concentrate on the healthful components of your diet," suggests Dr. Kelly Brownell of Yale University. Dr. Brownell studies eating disorders and bizarre approaches to weight control, the downside of dieting. "We have to fight the toxic food environment we live in—the good-tasting, cheap food available at a drive-in window within minutes of home, promoted by sophisticated advertising—that has made for the dangerous rise in obesity in this country. Ease up on the concept of ideal weight," says Brownell. Aim for a reasonable weight, a natural biological weight, one that you can maintain over time.

The battle never ends, and it can be wearing. Smokers who quit tell tales of similar battles: "I haven't had a cigarette for years, but a day doesn't go by that I don't miss that smoke." Hardly a day goes by that I don't miss that late night dish of ice cream. Little by little, your body will adapt to the change in your eating patterns and your exercise program. Your new habits will take hold; you'll lose weight gradually. Your mind and your body will adapt to this new lifestyle—and you'll be so proud of yourself. The challenge then is to keep it off.

15

Boosting Your Immune System

My immune system was hit hard by chemotherapy—but I thought, if it's doing this to me, think of what it's doing to the cancer. I got an awful response to the second bout of chemo: fever, aches, chills, throat ulcers, and I had to go to the hospital. They did a blood count and the doctor came back in a panic. "You have no platelets and as for your white count—there's nothing lower on the scale!" But then my oncologist came in and told me not to worry. "General doctors don't see this reaction, so they get scared. I see it all the time and I know how to handle it, and I know what to do. You're going to be fine, but we need to keep you in the hospital and give you some growth factors." I had a transfusion and I was on IV. After taking time off and taking care of myself, I got back my old strength.

The human body is composed of many organs and systems that are vulnerable to attack not only from outside but also from inside the body: from injury and disease, aging, cell damage, and mutations (genetic changes in gene structure or organization, including those that result in cancer). Vulnerable as it is, the body has amazing strength and security, protected by an immune system that reaches almost every tissue, alert and ready to defend us against danger.

The immune system can distinguish between substances in the body that don't belong, that are foreign (or nonself), and those that are native (or self). It attacks any foreign or abnormal presence in the body, trying to eliminate it, and then stops the attack before the body itself is damaged.

Women dealing with breast cancer inevitably wonder: Can my immune system fight breast cancer? Do the surgery, chemo, and radiation therapy reduce my body's ability to fight breast cancer and infections? Did I get breast cancer because my immune system was weakened by stress, or by the wrong food? How can I fortify my immune system to help me become as healthy as possible? Over the course of this chapter, we'll discuss how your immune system works to protect you, and how scientists are moving to reinforce the immune system's ability to fight cancer—and even to "invent" new immune system defense mechanisms.

The Immune Response

The immune system responds immediately to danger, in an innate, *generalized,* nonspecific reaction, such as inflammation, to fight any threat (for example, a virus or an injury). This response is like an army artillery attack—shells bursting all over, indiscriminately damaging and killing all varieties of bacteria, viruses, and any other microorganisms that happen to be in range, as well as some of the body's own cells. Key cells involved in this innate reaction, macrophages and neutrophils, produce powerful destructive chemicals known as free radicals.

As the immune response continues, it becomes adaptive and more *specific:* The white cells of the blood and immune tissues—lymphocytes—produce proteins called antibodies that selectively kill the invading organisms. Other cells of the body are left undamaged by this specific response. In addition, the adaptive response to this danger is remembered, allowing for a quicker immune response to a similar threat in the future.

Generalized Response

Crudest of your body's defense forces are free radicals, highly reactive and unstable "warrior" molecules, released to take quick action against the enemy or insult. These free radicals are produced by white blood cells that are quickly mobilized by the presence of cancer or the invasion of a dangerous microorganism. Free radicals are nonspecific—they react in the same way to bacteria as they do to a bruise, and even to the cells of normal tissue, if they get beyond their target area or hang around too long. Free radicals and other elements in the generalized defensive response induce swelling, redness, heat, and pain (which together make up inflammation).

After the free radicals have finished their work, they are "turned off," converted into nonreactive, harmless molecules. Antioxidant vitamins are essential to this conversion process, which is why you hear a lot about free radicals (antioxidants) and vitamins A, C, D, and E. (See Chapter 13.) This benefit of vitamins actually produces a dilemma. Because radiation therapy works in part by producing free radicals that attack cancer cells, some scientists wonder if vitamins might reduce this radiation effect and therefore should be avoided during radiation therapy.

After the production of free radicals, white blood cells go on to do more specialized work to fight threats to your health.

Specific Defense

As the response to danger continues, the immune system's distinctive organs, cells, and molecules come into play, employing precise, specific actions that constitute a more specialized means of defense. This defense process is a highly targeted form of combat.

A foreign agent, or *antigen,* enters the body, flows in the blood and lymph, and at some point encounters a matched, or complementary, *antibody,* a specialized fighter protein. Antigen and antibody link, and the immune response progresses, with the generation of huge numbers of antibodies that react with corresponding numbers of matching antigens.

The B lymphocytes, or B cells, the immune cells that produce antibodies, have a long memory for their enemies—those specific antigens. These B cells may remain in the body for years, ready to wage war quickly and powerfully by the explosive production of antibodies whenever that *particular* antigen shows up in the body again. This process is how your body acquires and sustains immunity after vaccination with the specific antigen of a particular infection, such as polio, measles, or the flu. If your B cells have never met up with that particular antigen before, however, there is no antibody response.

There are a number of different ways in which antibodies destroy antigens. Antibodies cause the antigens to clump together, immobilizing them, so that they can be swallowed up by macrophages. Or antigen-covered cells are perforated by antibodies, their insides leak out, and they die. Or, antibodies interlock with the antigen-covered cells, attracting immune cells (macrophages, in particular) like flies to honey, and the harmful cells are gobbled up.

It takes a while for the body to develop and implement the specific immune response. In contrast, the generalized or innate immunity process responds immediately to a threat to your health.

The Immune System's Defense Team

The major organs of the immune system are the thymus, spleen, bone marrow, and lymph nodes. The white cells of the blood are also part of the immune system, and there are five types: Lymphocytes (1)—T and B cells—are central to the immune system because they carry out immune responses against antigens. Macrophages (2) are necessary helper cells derived from white cells (monocytes). They and neutrophils (3), eosinophils (4), and basophils (5) are cells that contribute to inflammation, which is the initial, innate immune response.

The thymus acts like a nursery for the development of T cells. The spleen accumulates macrophages (large cells that engulf and digest microorganisms and other antigens), which it filters from the blood. Lymph nodes filter lymph fluid, removing antigens, bacteria, and cancer cells that get trapped in their weblike structure, where macrophages, antibodies, and T cells can destroy them. You have hundreds of lymph nodes located throughout your body, so the removal of any lymph nodes during breast cancer surgery does not affect your overall lymph node protection.

The bone marrow generates T cells, B cells, and macrophages; these cells travel throughout the body in the blood and tissue fluids. B cells and T cells are long-lived white cells with a memory for specific antigens; they circulate and recirculate through the body until needed. They are the key elements of the immune system, embodying the distinguishing elements of immunity: specificity for a given antigen and memory of that antigen if it reappears in the body. White cells mobilize quickly to destroy the enemy and stop trouble almost anywhere in the body.

How the Immune System Finds and Fights the Enemy

Foreign organisms such as bacteria invade the normal tissues of the body, or cells of an abnormal growth within the body proliferate. The surface of these bacteria or of the abnormal cells of the body bristle with antigens, and it's these antigens that stimulate the immune system.

The antigen-covered cells travel through the body and are swept up into antibody centers such as the spleen and lymph nodes. There they swirl about in a sea of specific fighting proteins, the antibodies, produced by B cells. Antigens and antibodies brush against each other constantly in this huge crowd packed with countless different antibodies. When the antibodies and their specific antigens find each other, they interlock. This locking stimulates the antibody-producing B cells to pump out millions of antibodies that travel through the body, meeting and destroying the specific invading antigens. This is the way your body acquires immunity (lasting protection) to harmful antigens.

Another Corps of Defense: T Cells

There is another powerful means of defense: T lymphocytes, or T cells. T cells react against antigens only after being introduced to them by special escort cells. T cells can be made to work only when presented with two attached structures: the foreign antigens (nonself) attached to receptors on the escort cell (self).

After meeting the antigens, the T cells secrete potent substances that attract fighter cells, such as macrophages and other defense cells, and keep them "pumped up" and fighting until the battle against the antigen-covered microorganisms is won.

Some antigens, such as those of tuberculosis bacteria, may be very hard to destroy. As in real war, some battles end in a draw: The immune system may not be able to kill the antigen outright, but it can encapsulate and immobilize the antigen-covered bacteria in a web of protein strands so they do little or no harm. This is a job for the T cells: to recruit fighting cells that surround, enclose, and immobilize this resilient enemy.

Battling Cancer

Breast cancer cells started out as normal body cells, but they began to grow out of control because of mutation or other damage to the breast cancer prevention genes. The immune system plays a major role in limiting the development of these mutations, often before cancer has a chance to develop beyond a very preliminary stage, so that many cancerous cells are eliminated before they do harm. Occasionally, however, as cells are changing from normal to abnormal, they appear to be normal when really they're not; their surface self-markers stay the same despite other profound changes. They therefore manage to elude attack by the immune system, and they grow and multiply into abnormal cells without triggering an immune response. Eventually, the tumor becomes so altered and threatening that it can no longer hide its malignant character. The immune system is no longer fooled into recognizing these cells as self, and so it launches its attack.

The attack may succeed, or it may be too late: The tumor may be beyond the power of the immune system alone. The immune system may need help: bold measures such as immune growth factors (pharmaceutical agents that stimulate the production of new immune cells) or vaccines that may be able to turn the tide and arrest the disease, or nonimmune-system intervention, such as chemotherapy, radiation, or the surgical removal of the harmful growth.

Scientists believe that there is a continuous process of cell overgrowth and genetic change, followed by growth arrest, destruction, and "mopping up." Damaged, premalignant cells may be a constant presence, but an ever-alert immune system takes them out and protects us from many assaults of cancer that never get beyond the very earliest stage.

Can a Compromised Immune System Protect Me?

You may worry: "What happens if I lose lymph nodes to surgery or my white count drops dramatically because of chemotherapy? Isn't my immune system weakened, and don't I become vulnerable again to cancer and infection?"

Fortunately, your immune system is very resilient and flexible. Various parts can switch roles and fill in for each other, and there is a considerable reserve or surplus of immune cells and tissues. If some lymph nodes are removed, others take up the load, handling the circulation of lymph and the filtering of cancer cells, bacteria, and other unwanted elements. Key cells of the immune system move readily from place to place in the body, traveling through the tissues, and circulating in the blood. Alerted by signals from cancer cells or inflammation, they quickly arrive at the site where they are needed. Because there is such a large reserve of blood cells, so many more than the body requires, cancer treatment can reduce the number of your blood cells without putting you seriously in danger. New lymphocytes and macrophages can be mobilized in a matter of minutes.

Blood counts are used to assess the possible damage to your immune system caused by chemotherapy or radiation; counts of all blood cells can easily be established from a few drops of blood. The amount that the white blood cell count declines depends on the individual, on the treatment given, and on the dose and the interval between dosage cycles, and the accumulated total dose given. Blood counts are most profoundly affected by chemotherapy, because the chemicals travel to all sites of immune cell production. There's a minimal drop with radiation to the breast alone. When the lymph nodes are also irradiated, the decline is somewhat steeper. Radiation to bones for metastatic disease can cause low counts, especially if the vertebrae, pelvic bones, and leg bones are treated, because the marrow of these bones is where most new blood cells are produced.

Counts can be expected to drop for a period of time during chemotherapy or radiation treatment. Really low levels are usually transient, but may be prolonged after very high doses of chemotherapy that precedes bone marrow transplantation. The bone marrow, thymus gland, spleen, and lymph nodes respond by calling on their reserves and revving up the production of more white cells. Growth factors may be administered to improve blood counts from their lowest levels, but even *with* growth factors, there can be some depression of the immune cell counts that persists for weeks, months, or, in an occasional patient, years. White blood cells contributed by donors can reduce the immune deficiency.

When your immune cell counts fall below a critical level, you are more vulnerable to infection and illness, so immune support treatment is initiated. Your chemotherapist will probably delay the next chemotherapy and, if necessary, give you growth factors to speed up your immune cell production. Once your immune cell counts rise above this critical level, between 500 and 1000 "frontline" cells (the neutrophils), your system is sufficiently intact to fight most infections. If you are in the middle of treatment, it can usually resume when the count reaches between 2000 and 2500, and the dose given will depend on what your immune system can tolerate.

Bolstering the Immune System to Eliminate Cancer
Nontraditional Methods

Nutrition, stress reduction, support groups, exercise—there is an intriguing literature evolving that demonstrates the ability of these fundamental but nontraditional interventions to strengthen your immune system. For example, Dr. Fawzy Fawzy, a California psychiatrist, has documented enhanced immune cell function after regular support group meetings for people with melanoma, a malignant skin cancer.

The value of nutrition to immune function is not yet fully defined, but Dr. Keith Block, of the University of Illinois and the Block Medical Center, focuses on nutrition as a means of reducing cancer risk and cancer death and increasing quality of life. His work emphasizes vegetarian diets and fat reduction, coupled with stress reduction and other complementary medicine therapies, all of which he believes combine to strengthen the immune system. (See Chapter 19.)

Proponents of these innovative, nontraditional therapies cite consumption of high levels of dietary cholesterol and other fats (particularly polyunsaturated oils) and excess weight as risk factors for cancer. They claim that fat appears to reduce white cell production, affecting T-cell and macrophage activity, and, further, that it compromises the lymphatic system, making the body more vulnerable to infection and disease. High protein intake, they believe, contributes to these undesirable effects, which is why protein-based foods are strictly limited in these programs.

All experts agree that vitamins and other important dietary compounds are best consumed in whole foods rather than as processed supplements, believing that whole foods may contain many other valuable components that we currently know little about. Fresh fruits and vegetables, grains, mushrooms, herbs, teas, omega-3 fatty acids, complex carbohydrates, yogurt, and seaweed are believed to increase the activity of T cells and their escort cells, and to promote the proliferation of antibodies and fighting cells. But without reproducible results from controlled studies, these claims will continue to be strong beliefs rather than established facts that call for immediate action.

Any process your body performs is crippled by poor nutrition. This is true for healing a wound, building immune cell blood counts, and even managing stress. Attention to good nutrition makes sense whether it specifically benefits the immune system or not. (See Chapter 13.)

Traditional Methods

A more traditional method of building up the immune system is the production of active immunity by a vaccine, in this case a solution made of weakened or dead breast-cancer cells taken from the tumor that caused the disease, the vaccines from which then serve as the antigen that stimulates an antibody response. You could be injected with the vaccine prepared from your own deactivated tumor with the expectation that your immune system would develop a specific response to your cancer antigens, producing antibodies that would circulate throughout your body, primed to attack and destroy cancer cells. If any new cancer cells appear, the circulating antibodies of the "vaccine-educated" immune system should destroy them.

Although this approach is traditional for infectious diseases, it is very much in the experimental stage for cancer, and it is significantly handicapped by the nature of cancer progression. Cancer starts with a few abnormal cells that keep multiplying, generation after generation; each generation produces variations, so that eventually the cancer has countless faces, with a diverse antigen profile. The vaccine, however, results in one or a limited number of different antibodies that were developed against the specific kinds of cancer cells in the vaccine preparation, and therefore they may not be effective against the full range of newly developing cancer cells.

In addition, an effective vaccine must elicit antibodies that target the bad cells and leave normal cells alone. The trick is to catch or tag the cancer cells as they change from normal to abnormal, from self to nonself, and direct a vaccine against the cells just after they have turned into nonself, or become newly malignant. Researchers are investigating ways to unmask the markers that would identify cancer cells at a very early stage, chemicals that would tag the problem cells and alter them enough to make the immune system perceive them as abnormal and attack. It's just a matter of time before scientists find ways to pinpoint and tag these markers and develop antibodies against the identified cancer cells.

Another research approach is to produce antibodies against onco-genes (genes that cause cancer), such as HER-2-*neu,* and the gene for epidermal growth factor receptor (EGFR). By targeting cancer cell genes, the antibody can more precisely identify cancer cells, destroy them, and spare surrounding normal tissue. An elaboration of this approach is to deliver antibodies with attached poisons, such as nitrogen mustard or a radioactive agent, that will help kill the cancer cells. Animal studies have been encouraging, and clinical trials are ongoing.

A serious obstacle to the success of these immune therapies is that the antibodies manufactured in response to the vaccine may not be able to get into the cells. To do their job, antibody molecules must be able to penetrate the cells' outer (and sometimes inner) barriers to truly destroy these cells.

Other research is looking for ways to boost T-cell activity against antigens, to encourage the T cells and other fighting cells to work even harder and longer to find and destroy cancer.

A selective form of cancer therapy, one that is able to distinguish between normal and abnormal, would theoretically be less toxic to the individual than currently available chemo- or radiation therapies.

The goal of current immune system research is to determine the ways to prevent cancer from ever starting, or, if it has started, to track and eliminate any aberrant cells that have escaped removal or destruction by the methods already in use. Various immune therapies are being studied in women diagnosed with breast cancer. The aim is to destroy the cancer and leave normal tissues alone. Let's hope we have some answers soon.

16

Breast and Chest Wall Self-Examination

I find breast self-examination so confusing and scary. I kind of do it, but I can't tell one thing from another—it all feels lumpy. I'd really be terrified if I found anything suspicious.

Breast self-examination has been promoted for years. Many women (or their sex partners) report finding the lump that turns out to be cancer. As hard as you found breast examination to be *prior* to treatment, it can be a bigger challenge *after* treatment.

Comparing the symmetry of your breasts has limited value, because treatment for breast cancer alters how the breast appears and feels. Your breast may have been removed partially or completely, new tissue may have been brought in, an implant may occupy the site, the breast may be tender or sensation may be absent, and the scars and the tissue underneath feel different. These changes resolve slowly after treatment.

Still, breast and chest wall self-examination continues to be important for women who have had breast cancer. By examining yourself regularly, you can best familiarize yourself with the old, the new, the healing, and the "What-the-hell-is-this?"

Fear and Guilt—Obstacles to Self-Examination

Most women find breast self-examination very frustrating. No one likes it; almost all of us would prefer to skip it; few find it reassuring. "It's so hard to figure out what's okay and what's not, particularly after breast cancer treatment." "Everything feels like cancer to me."

Many women confess to avoiding self-examination, hating the procedure with a passion.

I think it's worthwhile to get to know what the geography of your natural or reconstructed breast or chest wall is like, so you can recognize any change. I recommend breast/chest wall self-examination to all my patients—though not necessarily on a rigid monthly schedule. Although some of them are embarrassed to admit they don't examine themselves at all or with any regularity, a few confess they obsess over self-examination, checking themselves repeatedly each day, almost without realizing it. (I've spotted one woman waiting in a grocery line, palpating her armpit and breast area.)

Help Yourself

You probably have breast cancer on your mind whether or not you do breast self-examination. Looking for cancer can be frightening, but try not to be paralyzed by your fear. Doing breast self-examination doesn't mean you're going to find cancer, just as having fire drills doesn't mean you'll have a fire. Better to confront the possibility and dispel it.

If you end up with a diagnosis of breast cancer that you didn't discover by breast self-examination, you'll probably wonder whether you might have found the cancer yourself, sooner, had you done regular breast self-examination. Guilt and recrimination often follow—we all do it to ourselves—even if you'd been convinced that breast self-examination was an empty and frustrating exercise. When a physician with an international reputation was told she had breast cancer, her immediate, spontaneous reaction was "Should I feel guilty that I didn't find this myself?"

Older women tend not to examine themselves. They may not be comfortable manipulating their breasts; they may also feel they have less to worry about. More to the point, their doctors may never have instructed or urged them to do it. Younger women have heard more about breast self-examination and are more likely to find out for themselves how to do it by asking their doctors for help, reading about it, talking about it, or watching instructional videos.

Anxiety can deter you from following early breast cancer detection guidelines. Several studies show that women who are at high risk for breast cancer are *less* likely to follow breast self-examination recommendations. These women are usually younger and tend to overestimate their actual risk, but *even so* they do not come in for their routine mammograms or doctors' checkups.

Until something better comes along, examining your breast and chest area is a valuable procedure and costs no money. I encourage you to do it.

How to Do It

The first step in breast/chest wall self-examination is to take the time to look at yourself carefully and develop an accurate sense of your new contour, size, shape, and color variations. Stand in front of a mirror and compare one side with the other; they may not be alike. You may have had lumpectomy with minimal change, or you may have had a mastectomy, alone or with reconstruction, an implant or a TRAM flap (see Chapter 6). One breast may be bigger, smaller, firmer, pinker, tanner.

After your close inspection, take the next step and feel around your breast or chest area. If you have one or both breasts, you need to feel the whole breast, including the part that extends up toward your collarbone and the part that lies under your arm. Use the hand opposite the breast you are feeling. (Right breast—left hand, and vice versa.) Some women go up and down and others go round and round, starting with the nipple, and going in increasingly larger circles until they finish the periphery. Use the pads of your middle three fingers together to do the feeling, moving them in a small circular motion, first applying minimal pressure, then greater pressure to feel the deeper parts of the breast. Do your breast examination standing up and lying down—in *both* positions.

If your breasts are large, you may find that shifting from your back to your side will help you feel the deeper parts of your breast.

There's a new device called a breast pad that you may find helpful; it's a soft plastic square with a fluid filling; it helps your fingers glide over the breast and it can magnify the internal texture of what you're feeling. Some women find that using baby powder on their skin makes breast self-examination that much easier.

As you examine yourself, ask your fingers what they are feeling.

Remember, the breast is a milk-producing gland, not just a mound of fat. It has different "neighborhoods," each with its own unique collection of little lumpy glands of different sizes and consistencies: hills and valleys, soft and firm; some like a bunch of grapes, other areas like a dense sponge. You need to familiarize yourself with all these many shapes and textures so you know how to distinguish the feel of normal tissue from something that stands out—like a peanut in a lumpy, bumpy bowl of oatmeal—and that might be abnormal.

If you have had radiation therapy, you may find that your whole breast is firmer. In addition, the area where the cancer was, where surgery and boost radiation were focused, can have scar tissue that may be even firmer and difficult to evaluate. Some women, however, can feel the absence of tissue under the scar (corresponding to where tissue was removed).

Your breast will soften over time, often markedly during the first six months. But the healing process can take place over years; three years is not unusual. Firmness and color differences may not resolve until you've finished chemotherapy, as well. After radiation, some subtle color change can persist, with your breast a little tanner, pinker, or, less commonly, paler than the other side. As the firmness gradually resolves, don't be surprised if you're able to feel more of the normal lumps and bumps that have been there all along.

If you have had mastectomy without reconstruction, concentrate your examination on the skin, soft tissues of the chest, and the scar. You need to apply only minimal pressure on the skin and soft tissues. In addition, it's helpful to simply slide your fingers up and down over the whole chest wall area to detect small bumps or irregularities of the skin.

Extra attention to the scar is important. You may feel "suture granulomas": hard, perfectly round bumps beneath the incision that form within weeks of surgery and usually stabilize shortly thereafter, measuring one eighth to one quarter of an inch. These represent scar tissue that forms a bump in reaction to the surgeon's suture material or stitches.

If your breast is removed, your ribs are much closer to the skin surface than they used to be. Ribs can feel just like a breast cancer lump and scare you to death, especially at a point several inches to the right and left of your mid-breastbone where cartilage meets your rib bones, forming a heaped-up junction that can become tender. The good news is that ribs don't move, and you can figure out whether what you're feeling is bone or soft tissue by moving the soft tissue back and forth over the hard, fixed rib. (Also, neighboring ribs can be easily identified.)

Reconstructing a breast after mastectomy usually involves a number of incisions. If skin/muscle was brought in from your back or stomach, it will have a different color, texture, and hair pattern than true chest wall tissues. Hard, irregular lumps can occur with transplanted tissue, usually near its outer perimeter, close to the incision. These lumps are "fat necroses," fat that didn't survive the transfer process, curled into a ball and hardened. They pose no threat but can drive you nuts until you can prove that they are not something worse. Persistent tenderness after any type of treatment is not uncommon.

If you had a silicone or saline implant or tissue expander placed after mastectomy, the implant may be either tight or loose beneath the skin (loose implants may look and feel wrinkled under the skin). Your body may make a scar tissue capsule around the implant that can make it feel hard and unnatural. Expanders that can be kept as a permanent implant once they are filled to the appropriate size have a hard, buttonlike removable port beneath the skin surface.

If you received chemotherapy treatment through a venous port (usually located a few inches beneath the collarbone), this will also feel like a big button under the skin.

Recurrent cancer can occur as a discrete lump, a pale or reddish nodule just below the skin surface, a swelling, a persistent and progressive red rash, or a dimpling of the skin (the lump is beneath the surface pulling the skin down).

Keep in touch with your body—literally—and you'll learn to make sense of the different things you feel.

17

A Child in Your Future? Fertility, Pregnancy, Adoption

I was thirty-two. We had no kids. We were looking to get pregnant when I got cancer instead. After treatment was over, we went to a fertility specialist, and I had a laparoscopy. I couldn't take fertility drugs, so we tried natural techniques—ovulation test, temperature stuff. But my ovaries had shrunk from the chemo, and I had weird periods, maybe signs of early menopause. I suspect we'll probably pursue adoption.

If you are at a point in your life when having a baby is the biggest thing on your mind, and breast cancer is also a fact in your life—how do you decide what's most important to you, what's possible, and what you should do?

You may be thirty-five years old, just diagnosed with breast cancer and about to start chemotherapy, when your doctor says you have a 40 percent chance of going through premature menopause and becoming infertile from the chemotherapy. Yet another blow. Overwhelmed as you may already be by your diagnosis, with trying to find the "right" doctors and trying to choose the "best" treatment, and unsure about what the cancer will mean to your future, you now must worry about whether cancer and its treatment will alter your chance of having a child.

Or perhaps you are past the early shock, finished with your cancer therapy, with only one thing on your mind: waiting to find out if you're fertile, if you can make a baby happen before it's really too late.

How do you protect your own life at the very moment you're

thinking about starting another? Who and what comes first? Do you have a choice? Is it safe for you to become pregnant? Will you live long enough to raise your child? Are there close family members who will help out if you need them? Is it sensible for you to think about adoption? Your mind fills with questions.

I have taken care of many women in their thirties in this predicament, some of them not yet in a committed relationship, some just married but not quite ready to start a family, and some married, with one child (or more), who want very much to have another.

Each woman's dilemma is unique and profound. I firmly believe that cancer considerations should have priority over childbearing issues—but it doesn't have to be an either/or decision. If you do one, you may still have a good shot at the other. But you have to sort out the cancer considerations from your wishes and concerns and those of your husband or partner, and then work out your priorities, remembering to weigh in the best interests of the child as well.

Is your prognosis optimistic enough to allow you to plan your future as a mother? Or perhaps having a child is enough, creating the family that you and your husband or partner want so badly and have decided is most important, knowing that the child will always be loved and nurtured by you and/or your extended family, even if your survival turns out to be limited. Is it essential for you to have a baby to preserve something of yourself for the future? Will pregnancy endanger your life? These decisions are extremely personal. They reflect your relationship with your husband or partner, your value system, your circumstances, your cultural background, and your support systems. Your doctor can help you by providing you with a broad sense of your prognosis, the safety of a pregnancy, and any other information you ask for. But ultimately, the decision to have a child is one only you and your partner can make.

A "must read" for anyone struggling with these incredibly difficult issues is *Sexuality and Fertility after Cancer* by Dr. Leslie Schover (1997). Her expertise and compassion in handling these issues in an insightful, constructive manner will help you set your priorities and come to your decisions. Let me summarize the issues.

Is It Safe to Become Pregnant?

The question most on your mind may be Is it safe to become pregnant?

Pregnancy produces high doses of female hormones, which have a definite effect on the breast. Estrogen stimulates the growth of breast cells, including abnormal or cancer cells. So it is possible that if you are pregnant and have cancer cells in your body, those cells may grow a little faster during the time estrogen levels are elevated, than if you were not pregnant. Growth slows when the pregnancy is over. Whether this transient period of increased growth will actually harm you has not been demonstrated.

The safety of pregnancy can't be studied by a randomized clinical study—the gold standard of research—because you can't have a hundred women diagnosed with breast cancer, split them into two equal groups (correlated by stage, age, number of prior pregnancies, hormone receptors, etc.), and then tell half of them to become pregnant, and the other half not to, so that you can compare outcomes. Second best would be to look at current randomized trials of young women with breast cancer who are already split into equal groups, and to compare the results of women who become pregnant with those who don't. But we don't have this information either, partly because details of pregnancies and fertility status after treatment are not consistently recorded.

The information we do have comes from a number of retrospective studies that looked back over the medical records of premenopausal women with breast cancer at a particular hospital, or in a small country such as Sweden, comparing the outcomes of women who were pregnant with those of women who weren't. The studies show no apparent long-term increased risk of cancer recurrence or death in the women who became pregnant. Pregnancy didn't appear to cause new cancers; neither did it seem to cause more metastases or deaths from breast cancer. These studies also indicated that if you were diagnosed with breast cancer *during* pregnancy, the pregnancy did not affect your long-term prognosis.

Is It Safe to Stay Pregnant and Delay Treatment?

If you are in the first trimester of pregnancy when you find you have to start chemotherapy, most doctors will advise abortion. If you receive chemotherapy in the third trimester, there should be minimal risk to the baby. If, however, you're diagnosed in the second trimester, you and your doctor will have to come to a decision together about chemotherapy and the termination of your pregnancy, depending on how close you are to the third trimester, the nature of your cancer, and your own feelings about the pregnancy. Radiation therapy is absolutely contraindicated during pregnancy because there can be scatter radiation to the fetus.

Chemotherapy and Fertility: Will You Be Able to Have a Child after Treatment?

If you have just been diagnosed with breast cancer and are about to start chemotherapy, you may want to know how it will affect your future fertility. Will chemotherapy make me infertile? Is there something I can do before chemotherapy to preserve my fertility? What do I do? *How soon do I have to do it?* Is one type of chemotherapy more harmful to my ovaries than another? Is ovarian stimulation with fertility drugs safe? How soon after treatment can I try to become pregnant? What about tamoxifen—won't it interfere with my plans? If I can't produce any eggs, do I have any options?

As you think about the therapy your doctor recommends, organize the questions you need to ask your medical oncologist about fertility issues, especially what your risk of infertility might be with the proposed course of chemotherapy.

Whether or not you have ovarian shutdown (or infertility) after chemotherapy for breast cancer has a lot to do with your age. The younger you are, the more likely it is that your ovaries will survive treatment. The closer you are to the average age of menopause (fifty-one), the more likely it is that you will have permanent menopause.

Apart from your age, the risk of infertility depends on which drugs are used in treatment. Although there is not much information available about how chemotherapy drugs affect ovarian function, it *is* known that alkylating drugs such as Cytoxan hit hardest at rapidly dividing cells such as cancer and those that produce hair, sperm, and ova. A six-cycle course of Cytoxan, methotrexate, and fluorouracil (CMF) produces more infertility than a three-cycle course of Cytoxan and adriamycin, with relatively equal anticancer effectiveness, as reported by Dr. Melody Cobleigh, a medical oncologist from Rush-Presbyterian-St. Luke's Medical Center in Chicago. Half of the women taking CMF stop menstruating. The younger the patient, the better the chance she will resume menstruating once chemo is over, as do one half to one quarter of women in their thirties who use the drug. In another report, from M. D. Anderson in Houston, Dr. Gabriel Hortobagyi found that when women are given Cytoxan and adriamycin chemotherapy (plus or minus a few other drugs), none of the patients younger than thirty years of age had a change in their periods. However, 33 percent of women between thirty and thirty-nine stopped menstruating, 96 percent of women between forty and forty-nine stopped menstruating, and the periods of all women fifty and over stopped completely. After chemotherapy, 50 percent of women under forty got their periods back, but only a few of the women over forty got theirs.

Except for Cytoxan, how each chemotherapy drug affects ovarian function is not well studied. Dr. Cobleigh urges every woman who has received chemotherapy to appeal to the drug company involved to assess the effect of these drugs on ovarian function, just as they assess other side effects.

If your periods continue through much of your chemotherapy, your chance of future fertility is good. If your periods stopped but they are "expected" to return, they'll probably come back within the first six months after chemotherapy is completed.

"Isn't there some kind of blood test you can do that will tell me whether my periods will come back?" Measuring blood hormone levels during chemotherapy is not a reliable way to predict your future fertility, but hormone-level tests six months later are relatively accurate. The blood tests used to assess whether your ovaries are beyond menopause measure follicle-stimulating hormone (FSH) and luteinizing hormone (LH), proteins made by the brain that are supposed to stimulate each month's ovulation by the ovaries. Once the ovaries start cranking out estrogen and progesterone and the eggs ripen, the FSH and LH have done their job and the brain stops making these hormones until your next ovulatory cycle. If your ovaries are beyond menopause, they don't respond to the hormone stimulators, but the brain keeps sending them out. FSH and LH levels continue to be high, 13 to 90 milli-international units per milliliter for FSH, 15 to 50 for LH. If your periods do not return after treatment, and both FSH and LH remain elevated six months after your chemotherapy has ended, your ovaries are probably beyond menopause.

Radiation to the breast doesn't cause infertility, but if you are going to proceed with *in vitro* fertilization (fertilization of an egg with sperm in a laboratory setting), postpone radiation therapy if possible, because you don't want the ripe eggs that will be harvested to receive any possible radiation scatter dose. Eggs that are rapidly dividing and ripening for your current ovulation cycle are vulnerable to radiation, but it's unlikely that the same minuscule amount of scatter dose will have any effect on the unripe, dormant eggs still enclosed within your ovaries.

Your *Risk of Infertility*

All this information is interesting and important, but you want to know what *your* specific risk of infertility is likely to be. If your doctor is able to tell you that your risk of becoming infertile after treatment is very low, you can let go of the agonizing worry about your fertility and concentrate solely on cancer therapy issues.

If your risk of infertility after chemotherapy is significant, or an optimistic projection does not reassure you, arrange to see an infertility specialist prior to starting chemotherapy, to gather as much information as possible about your risk and the management of infertility. You'll need some "pull" to get an immediate appointment with this specialist, so ask your doctor to get on the phone and be persistent on your behalf. You're entitled to special consideration because of the pressure to start treatment, but you do have to ask for it. If there is no infertility specialist in your area, your gynecologist may have to suffice. For many infertility problems, that may be fine, but it still makes sense to do a lot of reading or to go to the Web for as much information as you can dig up. (*Dr. Richard Marr's Fertility Book* should prove helpful, although it does not refer to concerns specific to the woman who has had breast cancer.)

You can and should hold off on chemotherapy and radiation until you deal with these issues. Postponing your treatment for a week or so to discuss your questions and obtain necessary information is time well spent. This short delay will not endanger your health.

Finding Your Way Step by Step

When I have a patient who is struggling with the issues of pregnancy and breast cancer prior to treatment, I outline the issues step by step for a clear picture of what must be weighed and assessed. Here are the considerations, broken down into steps, so you can evaluate your options.

Step 1

Talk to your doctor about the seriousness of your cancer condition. Is your prognosis relatively good, enough so that you feel encouraged to become a parent? Or is your cancer prognosis limited enough that you don't want to take added risks?

You don't need exact answers to these questions; you're not going to make any immediate, irrevocable commitments. (We're talking about pregnancy after the whole course of breast cancer treatment is completed.) You're just trying to get a sense of whether having a child remains a reasonable possibility for you. And no one has a precise answer for you, or for anyone. Consider two opposite examples; one woman with non-invasive intraductal breast cancer would have an excellent prognosis. Another woman with, say, over ten lymph nodes involved, or with inflammatory breast cancer, would have what is considered a very aggressive cancer with a very unfavorable prognosis. But I've seen exceptions to every doctor's "rule" of prognosis, so consider these as guidelines, not directives.

When you ask your doctor for a general idea of your chances for living beyond breast cancer, this is the range of figures you may be given:

Five-year survival for invasive breast cancer

Stage I	80–95%	(tumor ≤ 2 cm, no nodes)
Stage II	60–80%	(tumor >2; ≤ 5 cm, with or without nodes involved)
Stage III	40–60%	(tumor > 5 cm, skin involved, with or without nodes involved)
Stage IV	0–20%	(metastatic)

Step 2

Discuss the safety of pregnancy as it relates to your particular kind of cancer. Although there is no definitive evidence that pregnancy alters your prognosis in general, you might have a very unusual condition that suggests an exception to this premise. There may be circumstances that may give your doctor reason to say that pregnancy in your case may be ill-advised; for instance, if your cancer originated as a rapidly enlarging lump diagnosed during a previous pregnancy, if it is strongly estrogen-receptor positive, and if it was present in lymph nodes as well. In such a case, you would need to rethink the safety of any subsequent pregnancy for you. Fortunately, this instance is quite rare.

Step 3

If your doctor says your prognosis is relatively good and there is no particular reason to expect pregnancy to increase your risk for cancer recurrence, then ask an infertility specialist to outline your options for preserving your fertility. (Action may need to be taken before you start treatment.) Can you bank your embryos (fertilized eggs) now, in case you can't produce eggs later? (Current technology can't freeze eggs until they are fertilized with sperm.) Is ovarian stimulation (with subsequent *in vitro* fertilization) the only realistic option to obtaining an adequate number of eggs? Is natural-cycle *in vitro* fertilization a reasonable alternative? How about donated eggs? What is involved with each approach? How long does the process take? Then ask yourself how hard and how long you are willing to work, at this particular time, to keep open the option of having a child.

The standard approach to banking embryos is stimulation of egg production prior to *in vitro* fertilization. You take Lupron to prime your ovaries, then follow up with drugs such as Pergonal, Clomid, or Metrodin to bring a greater than normal number of eggs to maturity, rather than the single one (or occasionally two) produced in a normal cycle. These mature eggs are retrieved with a long suction needle under ultrasound guidance. (Between ten and fifteen eggs are obtained from a woman in her early thirties; a woman over forty will have about five.) (If your ovaries were not fully functioning before the breast cancer diagnosis, fertility drugs may yield only a few eggs, however.) The eggs are fertilized in the laboratory with designated sperm; the resulting embryos are frozen in liquid nitrogen and remain viable for years.

Natural-cycle egg retrieval is the same as the standard *in vitro* technique described above, except that no drugs are used to stimulate the ovary to produce extra eggs. One or occasionally two mature eggs, and perhaps a few immature eggs (normally produced with each month's ovulation) are removed; the mature egg(s) are fertilized and frozen; the immature egg(s) are nourished, and when and if they mature, they, too, are fertilized and frozen. The number of embryos from this procedure is many fewer than when the ovaries are stimulated with fertility drugs.

The advantage to natural-cycle egg retrieval is that you avoid the high levels of estrogen in your body that the fertility drugs produce. During a natural cycle, the estrogen level in your blood peaks at about 150 to 300 picograms per milliliter, whereas estrogen levels can rise to about 2000 pg/mL during the few weeks of drug stimulation of the ovaries.

There is still one other option that can be considered after treatment, when you're ready to start trying to get pregnant: egg donation followed by *in vitro* fertilization. Someone you know, or an anonymous donor, can contribute eggs, which are fertilized with your husband's or designated sperm. The donor's ovaries are stimulated and between ten and twenty eggs are retrieved. The donor eggs are fertilized; the resulting embryos can be used fresh, or they can be frozen and used later on.

After treatment, if you're ready to get pregnant but your periods have not returned, it's time to use your stored embryos or seek out a donated egg. Your uterus is put into action with estrogen and progesterone supplements. The embryos are thawed and checked for viability, and up to four embryos are implanted into your uterus with each attempt. None of the embryos may take, or one of the embryos may successfully implant and proceed to develop. Uncommonly, more than one embryo may implant and develop (resulting in twins, triplets, even quintuplets). The pregnancy is then sustained with supplemental hormones for about the first ten weeks, when the baby's placenta assumes the job of sustaining its home, your uterus.

You have the same chance of getting and staying pregnant as a woman going through *in vitro* fertilization for any other cause of infertility. If you are in your thirties, the chance that the embryos obtained after ovarian stimulation will result in a baby is about 20 percent. If you are over forty, the chance of success is minimal (less than 10 percent). (That's why some centers have an age limit of forty.) If you are in your thirties, the chance that embryos from your natural cycle will result in a baby is less than 20 percent, because fewer embryos are available for implantation. The success rate for donor eggs runs between 25 and 50 percent.

Before initiating the process of *in vitro* fertilization, any woman (with or without breast cancer) and her partner need to consider what will happen to the frozen embryos if you and/or your partner divorce or die. You're into a morass of legal, ethical, and religious issues, with no clear answers. You need to discuss these issues with a lawyer and incorporate your decisions into your will.

Step 4

Next, think about combined cancer and infertility issues: How safe is it for you to postpone your chemotherapy and radiation therapy for at least six weeks for ovulation stimulation and *in vitro* fertilization?

How comfortable your oncologist is with postponing your treatment depends on how favorable or advanced your cancer is. Probably the bigger concern, however, is how safe for you are the effects of the fertility procedures' hormonal manipulations. In general, doctors would be a lot more likely to postpone chemotherapy and/or radiation for infertility management if they felt more comfortable with the safety of the increased level of hormones flooding your body. Which leads us to Step 5.

Step 5

Are the hormones that will be used to stimulate ovulation safe for you? Or might the high estrogen levels be dangerous? Fertility drugs are usually contraindicated for women who have had breast cancer, because no one understands the full impact of fertility drugs such as

Pergonal and Metrodin on breast cancer cell activity. There are no studies that address the issue of whether it is safe for a woman with breast cancer to take fertility drugs.

If you're thinking of using fertility drugs for just one cycle, you and your doctor will have to evaluate the aggressive character of your tumor and determine how risky it might be for you to proceed with the drugs.

Although tamoxifen is used mainly as an anticancer drug, paradoxically it can also be used as a fertility drug, at high doses, taken intermittently. When tamoxifen is used to enhance fertility, it provokes the same concern about estrogenic stimulation of breast cancer cells as do Pergonal, Clomid, and Metrodin.

There has been some suggestion that fertility drugs taken for more than one year may increase a woman's risk for ovarian cancer, but other risk factors may independently contribute. Women who have an abnormal breast cancer gene (whether or not they've had breast cancer) are at higher risk for developing ovarian cancer, and women with ovulation problems also may have a higher risk for developing ovarian cancer.

Step 6

Once you've gone through the first five steps, proceed to the basic fertility questions in the following steps: Eggs need sperm for fertilization, so where are they going to come from? If you're already married, you have the answer, but you still need to know if both you and your husband are highly motivated to have children. If you're not married, is there someone in your life that you are not only committed to but would want to have children with? Is this expectation mutual? Are you single or in a lesbian relationship and willing to pursue sperm donation?

If you are married, before you pursue aggressive fertility procedures, make sure your husband's sperm are tested so you know they are strong swimmers, present in sufficient numbers, and banging on the door. (Why go through a difficult and costly procedure if the other half of the equation isn't there?) In many fertility centers, low sperm counts can be compensated for by combining several sperm specimens or directly inserting sperm into an egg to achieve fertilization.

If there are no viable sperm—or no husband or male partner—in the picture, you have to consider where the sperm will come from. Sperm banks offer a wide choice of donors' physical characteristics and medical, religious, and professional backgrounds. A no-strings-attached sperm bank donor works, but most *in vitro* fertilization centers won't accept a designated sperm donation from a boyfriend who's not in a committed relationship with you, because of the legal and ethical issues about the rights of and to the embryos.

Step 7

Are you open to the idea of having a child born from someone else's egg? Are other options, such as a surrogate mother or adoption, acceptable to you? These answers need to come from *you*.

Answers to questions relating to donor eggs can wait until after treatment, when the status of your fertility is known and you've had more time to consider these options. Any questions that involve your eggs must be considered before treatment.

Step 8

How much will the fertility procedures cost? Do you have the money to pay for them? Are you able and prepared to pay for this out-of-pocket expense if your health plan won't pay? Most don't, but a few states mandate payment for fertility treatment, and maybe you can negotiate ways to get a portion of your expenses covered. (See Chapter 26.)

The cost of each ovarian stimulation combined with *in vitro* fertilization is approximately $8000 to $12,000, plus a few hundred dollars a year to maintain the embryos in the freezer. The cost for natural-cycle *in vitro* fertilization is about $5000 (you save the cost of fertility drugs). The cost of the donor egg process is $20,000 if you're using a paid donor, or about $8000 to $12,000 if the eggs are donated at no charge. Rent on the freezer is the same.

Now Take a Step Back

After you have considered all the issues and sorted out all the answers to your questions, what you will come down to is this: If your prognosis allows you a realistic expectation for having a family, *and* if you are at significant risk of becoming infertile if you proceed with the recommended treatment, *and* if you have figured out where the sperm will come from, *and* if this source meets legal specifications, *and* if you have the resources to cover the cost of the procedures—*then* ask yourself: Is the 20 percent or lower chance of having a child through *in vitro* fertilization with your eggs worth (1) postponing your chemotherapy and radiation treatment to do the procedures, and (2) accepting the risk of transient high estrogen levels that accompany ovarian stimulation? You'll need a team—medical oncologist, radiation oncologist, family doctor, and infertility doctor—to help you with your decision.

Virtually all of my patients in this quandary decide not to pursue *in vitro* fertilization prior to their cancer therapy, praying that their periods will return. Some patients pursue ways to maximize their chance of preserving their fertility throughout their chemotherapy. They may work with their doctor to choose an effective chemotherapy regimen with a lower risk of infertility, or they may decide to take a drug such as Zoladex during chemotherapy, to suppress ovarian function, which may protect unripe eggs from chemotherapy damage. (It works in female rats, but it hasn't been studied yet in women.)

Someday in the future, you may be able to freeze a section of your ovary containing a large number of immature eggs, and then later on have those eggs ripened artificially, fertilized, and implanted in your own (or a surrogate's) uterus, go through pregnancy, and have a baby. (Portions of sheep ovaries have been experimentally removed, frozen, and stored for future fertilization, but this research is years away from any link to human reproduction.)

When or If Your Periods Return

After treatment is over, most women in their thirties get their periods back after a pause in their menstrual cycles, or they never lose their periods, and most of them have been able to become pregnant and deliver a healthy child, although the size of their family may be smaller than they had hoped. For women close to forty or older, however, the breast cancer treatment can put an end to lingering hopes of having their own biological child. Bobby was just married for the first time, at forty-four, to a wonderful man with children from a previous marriage when she was diagnosed with breast cancer. Any chance of having a child herself was over: "That closed the book altogether for me. But my life is full and rich and I'm blessed with all the other things I do have."

I have also taken care of women who never lost their period from chemotherapy but had trouble becoming pregnant later on because of non–cancer-related infertility problems. I've even taken care of women who thought they were infertile, never pursued any fertility treatment, never used birth control, and ended up with a big surprise: a baby.

If you are infertile after your chemotherapy is completed, and if you didn't or couldn't freeze your own embryos, or your implanted embryos did not result in a successful pregnancy, you can still consider becoming pregnant through egg donation. And for any woman, adoption can be a plausible alternative. Remember, if you spend $20,000 for *in vitro* and it doesn't work, you have nothing, but if you spend it for adoption, you have a baby.

If you are ready to have a child but you are no longer ovulating and your periods have not returned, you will have to go back to the infertility specialist. If you didn't bank embryos prior to treatment, you can ask your infertility doctor about ovarian stimulation close to the time you want to become pregnant, to try to reawaken the ovaries and return them to working order, at least for a few cycles. But the safety issue of infertility drugs still prevails, and the success rate for ovarian stimulation after menopause is low.

Your remaining options are egg donation and adoption.

RESOLVE is an organization devoted to providing education and support to individuals with fertility problems. RESOLVE is headquartered in Somerville, Massachusetts (617-623-1156—no 800 number); there may be a local chapter in a city near you.

"How Long Do I Wait Before I Start Trying?"

Many doctors recommend a wait of two years to get you past the time when the risk of cancer recurrence is highest, but it's unclear when to start that countdown—whether from the time of diagnosis or from when treatment ends. (These two points can differ by as much as a year.) Again, your risk of cancer recurrence depends on your unique situation. Also implicit in the recommended two-year waiting period is a value judgment about when you should or shouldn't become a parent. Two years is a long time to wait, if having a baby is a high priority for you, and you are already in your mid-thirties or older. If your periods have returned, you may be assured of normal expectations for becoming pregnant, but you may not be able to count on your cycles continuing as long as if you had not had cancer therapy.

After much discussion and dialogue with my patient, I try to help her make the best decision for herself: no wait, six months, or two years.

"Will Tamoxifen Screw Up My Plans?"

You've just finished chemotherapy and your eggs are jumping up and down and ready to boogie—and then your doctor tells you he or she wants you to start tamoxifen. Taking a medication that may further mess with your hormones is probably the *last* thing you want to think about at this point. "I had a miscarriage six months prior to diagnosis.

I'm thirty-eight years old now, and my periods returned five weeks ago. I'm a perfect candidate for tamoxifen, but what about babies?"

Tamoxifen will not induce early menopause unless you're already on the brink, but it does induce menopausal symptoms while you're taking it. After you stop taking tamoxifen, your body should revert to where it was before.

The first question, then, to ask your doctor is "How important is it for me to take tamoxifen?"

If the bottom line is that you would benefit from taking tamoxifen, then I suggest you take it, for at least the period of time that you are urged to, and have agreed to, wait to become pregnant: two years (from diagnosis or end of treatment). Two years of tamoxifen is better than none, and yes, five years is supposed to be better than two. But if all is going well for you, and you are in your mid-thirties, your time to have children is now. It's a compromise and a calculated risk, but one maybe worth taking. Take tamoxifen for two years; stop the tamoxifen; then try to get pregnant. Or, after careful consultation with your physician, together you may decide that tamoxifen offers you only marginal benefit—and you decide to forgo it.

You may decide for yourself that you want to take tamoxifen the recommended five years. Ann and her husband had been married for four years, had one child, and were about to try for another when Ann was diagnosed with breast cancer. "My husband wanted me to go the distance with the tamoxifen," Ann explained. " 'I don't want you to give away any chances, even as much as we want that child,' he told me."

Liz started tamoxifen and was married in the same month. "My husband would love kids, but my doctor says to stay on tamoxifen for two years; then I can come off and take about six months to a year trying to become pregnant. If it doesn't happen within that time, he says he wants me to go back on tamoxifen for the full five years."

Waiting those five years may put you past forty, reducing the possibility of your having your own biological child. Instead of forgoing these five good years of parenthood, adoption may be worth serious consideration. Later, if you recover your periods, you can have a go at having your own biological child as well.

While you're taking tamoxifen and waiting until you can try to get pregnant, studies *may* be published that show that chemotherapy alone is enough for a premenopausal woman, and that adding tamoxifen may not provide additional anticancer benefits. There are studies now under way to address this issue.

Is Breastfeeding Safe?

The questions don't stop once you've successfully conceived and given birth. Here's one of the first ones you'll ask: Is it safe to breastfeed my baby? The answer is yes. If you still have a breast, breastfeeding is possible after breast cancer.

If you become pregnant after treatment with lumpectomy and radiation, your untreated breast will probably get significantly bigger during the pregnancy than your treated breast. If you had radiation to one breast, it is not likely to produce very much milk, if any. Your untreated breast can usually make enough milk to feed a baby. (There won't be any harmful elements present in the milk.) Under these circumstances, the milk-producing breast can get very big, and some of this asymmetry is likely to persist even after breastfeeding is ended. (You'll need some special fittings to find the right bras to keep you comfortable.) If you are nursing your infant and you are advised to start chemotherapy, you should stop before you start the chemo. (The treatment drugs are likely to appear in your breast milk.)

If you are unable to breastfeed but want to capture the experience, you can try using a breastfeeding simulator—a milk reservoir that empties through a small tube positioned on your nipple. The baby sucks the tube end and your nipple, both at the same time.

Adoption
Starting the Process

Because adoption is a complex, anguishing, and sometimes confusing process, I'd advise you to seek out an adoption counselor who knows the ropes, one who can guide you to a lawyer, an agency, or an independent pathway to a child (domestic or international), take you through the home study process, and help you understand the special psychological aspects of adoption.

Successful adoption may depend on successful management of these psychological issues, including the normal sadness that comes with giving up the idea of having your own biological child. The same holds true for the birth mother and birth family. Counseling for the special problems they face in giving up a child is crucial and can determine the stability of the adoption you are in the process of negotiating.

"The adoption counselor will consider your special needs and find you an agency open to working with all different kinds of people for all different kinds of children," says Abby Rudet, a counselor in the Philadelphia area. "We have never had a problem finding a child for a woman who had cancer in her past and is now considered disease free."

Kathy and her husband found an exceptional adoption counselor who gave them a wealth of information and support: how to find the right agency, where to go inside and outside the United States, what to expect with a new child in their life, and what special legal, ethical, and psychological issues the future may hold.

An experienced and caring counselor can make an enormous difference in how adoption turns out for you. Interviews with an adoption counselor are relatively inexpensive (several hundred dollars), compared with the total costs of adoption—up to $50,000. Costs for domestic adoptions average around $8000 to $12,000; international adoptions range from $15,000 to $25,000. As you have had to do in finding other specialists, ask for personal recommendations from friends and physicians, then ask for credentials and references.

Starting in 1997, you can receive a $5000 federal tax credit (against the federal tax you owe) when you adopt a child. Given the expenses of your cancer treatment and the typical costs of a conventional adoption, this money saved is a welcome break. You may need to work harder at finding alternative and less expensive ways to adopt a child.

I tell women who are thinking of adopting to talk to people who have taken that road. You'll get a lot of personal insights, useful hints, and a sense of the day-by-day details that can be so helpful. Also, some people need that "reality check" to be able to trust what they're told by the professionals in the field.

Meeting Requirements

Of primary importance for you, as a woman who has had breast cancer, is to get a strong letter from your doctor, affirming your health, stating that you are free of cancer and have been for X number of years, and predicting a long and healthy future for you.

You will then go through a home study, where your background is checked (for any criminal records), you are interviewed, and your home is visited to be sure it's a child-friendly place (there is no white glove standard). "I don't think anybody fails the study unless maybe you have a history as a child abuser." The home study can take up to two months; the search for a child can run up to a year or more.

The traditional route to adoption is an agency. The advantage of going through an agency is that the screening, the counseling, and the standards that are included in the process are for your protection as well as the child's. But it can mean a wait of up to a year (or three, or more), depending on the child you are looking for. Of course, adoption is not a matter to be rushed, but a long waiting list may be unacceptable to many women who have been through the experience of breast cancer, who come at last to the decision to adopt, and who want that child as soon as possible. "When we finally figured I was infertile and also shouldn't come off tamoxifen, and we decided that we really wanted to go for adoption, we wanted it *now*. I'd been through so much, I wanted something good, fast."

So what are the alternatives to an adoption agency? Some people choose independent adoption, through an adoption lawyer. A few people—and birth mothers—advertise on their own. And more and more people are choosing international adoption, especially if the adopting couple is older or of the same sex, or if the adoptive parent is single.

Independent adoption can be riskier than an agency adoption, however, unless all technical details are covered. Expect to do a lot more work on your own, starting with learning the details of state law that pertains to the adoption you are contemplating. (Call the state agency that handles adoption and speak with the state adoption supervisor for the information you need.)

Probably the least costly way to adopt a baby is through networking: letting the word out to all your friends and relatives, even to the nurses, social workers, and technicians you met during treatment, that you want to adopt a baby. (Include the word in your Christmas letter, and in your church bulletin or newsletter.) Just be sure you go through all the right steps and get a well-qualified lawyer. (Costs may run about $2000, mostly for legal fees.)

One reason adoptive parents have trouble making their adoption secure is that the natural father may never have agreed to give up his rights, and his signature was not on the release. Not every lawyer is competent, and some birth mothers withhold the truth about who or where the father is, or they simply don't know. You must make absolutely certain that you follow the letter of the law, that every detail of the adoption process is observed. If you can't get every signature (including the father's), you may be able to do a legal search. "But if you get a bad feeling about the way the adoption is going, walk away."

Adoption laws vary by state. Some states allow for final adoption settlement within forty-eight hours; other states require months, almost a year, before an adoption is considered final. Pay attention to pending legislation: A lot is happening politically with adoption. New laws are being introduced and debated that may benefit you or limit your options.

With open adoption, you can meet the birth mother and get to know what she's like, get to know her background and her history. And someday, when your child wants to know all there is to know about his or her birth mother, you'll be able to talk about her as a real person. Some adopting parents welcome this opportunity; others feel threatened by the connection and want to know nothing about the birth mother: "I just want to pretend she doesn't exist."

Jane and Tom wanted to adopt a child as a newborn, rather than a child several months old. "We were anxious to get a baby from the moment he was born. That's not important to everyone, but it was to us. We decided we wouldn't compromise on the baby we wanted, not at the beginning at least. And we did it, our way. But you really need to be your own advocate. I spent a lot of time in the library, reading everything I could find on adoption."

Some people have been discouraged from domestic adoptions because they tend to take longer. They're also motivated by the terrible fear of being forced to return an adopted child if the birth parents change their minds and the legal issues are entangled, a fear hyped by the media in cases such as Baby Jessica and Baby Richard. (Not that this can alleviate your pain and suffering, but there is such a thing as adoption insurance, which reimburses you for your expenses if the birth mother changes her mind.)

Ruth adopted two little girls (both at the same time) from Russia, where adoption is a relatively speedy process; her forebears had come from that area many generations before, and she wanted her children to blend in with her family. Kathy and her husband had been intensely involved in Chinese therapy ever since Kathy's breast cancer diagnosis, and she was spiritually drawn to a Chinese child.

Kathy stayed clear of a few agencies known for having narrow restrictions on whom they would serve. She and her husband arranged the adoption with their lawyer and took off to China for a seven-month-old baby girl. "It turned out to be our version of labor pains. It was hot and humid when we arrived and we were up for another twenty-four hours straight: We had to take two small planes and an overnight train to get to the orphanage that had our baby. But it was worth it. She's opened up a whole world for us and brought in so much love."

China and Russia are currently popular countries to adopt from because of fewer restrictions on who can adopt, but restrictions can change overnight. Nationalistic attitudes shift; governments may decide it doesn't look good to have so many of their babies leaving the country. "Don't be drawn into the designer option of the moment," says an adoption counselor.

You must be cautious with any adoption, particularly regarding the health of the child and of the birth mother. The birth mother should agree to an HIV test before you get caught up in negotiations for adoption of her baby; in fact, you should have access to all her medical records, so you know as much as it's possible to know about the medical history of the child that you hope to raise. There has been mounting concern about babies who have been exposed to alcohol and drugs *in utero,* or who have suffered malnutrition, or who are developmentally delayed, conditions that for many people can add up to too much of a challenging start to parenthood. If you're prepared to consider a high risk child, educate yourself about the demands you may be expected to address, and make a fully informed choice.

Adoptive Families of America (800-372-3300) is an organization devoted to helping anyone interested in the adoption process. One phone call, and a warm and informed organization member can set you on your way.

When you finally make your decision, stick to it—"otherwise you can go crazy." And get going, because the process is "hurry up and wait."

Caring for a Child

The whole issue of fertility forces you to face your mortality. An occasion for expectation and joy can include anxiety and fear. You may find you are more ambivalent than you expected. "When I was first diagnosed, a baby was in our future, a very real desire for us. Now, we're not sure. We try to talk, but not very successfully. As hard as it is to say, I know my husband is afraid of being left alone with a child. Not that he wouldn't love that baby, and take wonderful care—he's just afraid. We're still working on this one. I think I've accepted that we'll skip having kids. We're older anyway, we like our freedom, I can pursue my career—but I don't know."

Or you may be absolutely sure of what you want to do. "Even though my husband knew my prognosis was uncertain, he wanted a child as much as I did. And he vowed he would care for the child on his own if it came to that. 'If I can't have you forever, I want you living on in our child. I want us to share all we can—including a new life.' So far, we've shared day care, carpooling, and chicken pox."

18

Menopause and Growing Older

Everyone wants to live forever—but no one wants to grow old. When I was in my forties, I scorned "old" women who tried to look younger. Now that I'm near seventy, I understand. The face in the mirror may look seventy, but the spirit inside isn't yet fifty. Why is *old* a dirty word? "How old would you be if you didn't know how old you was?" asked Satchel Paige.

I had a lumpectomy, radiation, and then a hysterectomy. The hardest part was I couldn't produce estrogen and I couldn't take it. It was devastating to my sex life. But I started on alternatives, Catapres and an occasional Bellergal, and I began to use Astroglide, and they ALL have helped. And oddly—my husband and I have never been closer and my life has never been better.

"No one likes growing old—but aging is a gift, and it sure beats the alternative," says menopause expert Michelle Battastini. Our culture pushes youthfulness beyond reason—who needs pubescent models setting the standard for what mature women should look like? We need to stir in a little more of Asian culture and its appreciation of the aged.

The aim of this chapter is to help you grow older in the best physical and emotional health possible, before, during, and after menopause. Running, walking, eventually inching down that path to old age is a welcome goal for any woman, particularly if you've had breast cancer. I hope this book can help you become as healthy as possible as you make the trip.

What follows is information that illuminates these special issues of aging and how they pertain to you, including practical solutions that will help you maintain and improve your health and your quality of life. "That we age is inevitable, but we do have some control over *how* we age," says Dr. Battastini.

At some point in every woman's life, her hormone production drops below the level sufficient to sustain menses, the menses stop, menopause occurs, and the ability to reproduce ends. (Hormones are proteins produced by special glands; they travel to other parts of the body and deliver a specific "message.") It's a change in your body that is a natural part of your progress through life, and for many women it's not a particularly outstanding event: You've reached your late forties or fifties, your family is on its way to independence, you're looking ahead instead of back, and you're not sad to see the end of monthly blood flow and emotional ups and downs. If you're one of the women for whom the transition is not particularly eventful, you may not understand all the fuss that goes with The Change, and you may even think all that carrying on is really just an exaggeration of symptoms.

Hardly. For many of you, menopause can affect your sex life, trigger mood swings, cause debilitating hot flashes and high tension, and push you down the road to bone and heart problems. Your body and mind may respond in dramatic ways to the change in your hormonal status—especially if you have gone into sudden menopause because of treatment for breast cancer and you're catapulted into middle-age symptoms years before your contemporaries. "Like, isn't breast cancer enough? I need this insult, too?" An abrupt menopause that leads to hot flashes, loss of libido, weight gain, and even dashed hopes of having a baby can feel like a disease, worse even than breast cancer. It's these menopausal changes, not the breast cancer or the immediate effects of treatment, that may interfere most with your day-to-day quality of life.

Three major factors influence how you age: *lifestyle*—diet, exercise, weight, smoking, environment, personal relationships; *hormones*—estrogen, progesterone, and others; and *genetic makeup*—the genes that come from your parents, the blueprint of your constitution and perhaps your future health, all have a major influence on how you experience aging. The complexity of these factors can occupy volumes, but the point is that no single factor determines your progress through life.

Understanding How Women Age

Lifestyle: Wear and Tear

Your hormones are playing the notes, but your age is the keyboard—probably the most important factor in how you respond to what life is throwing at you at the moment. The age of your heart and your bones is more significant than the hormones that tune them up. If you are a seventy-year-old woman, you are past menopause and your body has weathered seventy years of wear and tear. If you are thirty-five and caught in a medical menopause, your ovaries may be in menopause but the rest of your body is still that of a thirty-five-year-old woman. If you're actually much younger than your menopausal symptoms suggest, and if your hormones are not what they used to be and you can't juice them up with hormone supplements because of your breast cancer history, you are not without options for keeping toned up and healthy.

Human beings have a life span of around seventy-five years. Starting at about thirty to thirty-five, however, the body begins to experience a slow decline in function and activity. It is not as resistant to stress and injury as it once was, and it responds more slowly and less effectively. Reducing stress and injury, therefore, is more important as you age than it was when you were younger. It's not only not too late to give your body a break, but now may actually be better than earlier to make these changes: You're more mature and more likely to follow your resolutions for better health, like eating better and stopping smoking.

Your Genetic Makeup

Every cell comes with a central control panel, a nucleus that contains your chromosomes, on which are carried your genes—the ultimate blueprints to your body's functions. Genes inherited from your mother and your father are largely responsible for how your body and much of your mind behave.

If your relatives are arriving at family get-togethers into their nineties, you've probably got a good shot at the same route. (Tina's mother got breast cancer at eighty and lived to be ninety-four.) If, on the other hand, most of your relatives died before seventy from heart attacks and strokes, you may share their risk for heart and vascular disease. But even with long-life genes, you have to do your part to ensure healthy aging.

Other illnesses strongly affected by your genetic makeup include breast and ovarian cancer, and osteoporosis. Even how you experience emotional stress, anger, or depression may be influenced by your genes.

Hormonal Transitions

The hormonal transitions of your life may be the longest roller coaster ride you've ever been on. During *adolescence,* your ovaries start responding to signals from your brain, producing the hormones estrogen, progesterone, and testosterone. Soon after, monthly ovulation begins, followed by your menstrual periods if the eggs you produce are not fertilized. For about twenty-five years, from age thirteen to forty, you are most fertile. After that, for ten to fifteen years, there's a gradual decline in ovarian function and the amount of hormones you produce. This time of declining ovarian function is called the *climacteric*. Eventually, the amount of estrogen and progesterone your ovaries produce is no longer sufficient to initiate ovulation and perpetuate your monthly periods. The result: Your periods become irregular; you may experience hot flashes; you may feel moody, disconsolate. This one- to three-year period of hormonal flux before your periods stop completely is called *perimenopause*. How mild or severe your menopausal symptoms are depends on how fast your transition to menopause occurs, how much time your body has to acclimate to its changing hormonal milieu, and how much estrogen your body has from other sources, such as adrenal gland androgens (which are converted to estrogens by fat cells—the more fat you have, the higher the level of non-ovarian-produced estrogen). The most commonly reported symptom during this phase is hot flashes.

You might go through *natural menopause* and barely perceive the transition because it is long, smooth, and gentle. Perhaps you have an excess of fat that is making an alternate supply of estrogen, or you started menopausal hormone therapy as soon as you experienced any menstrual irregularity. Either of these factors might have eased your transition through menopause.

But a fair number of you reading this chapter have experienced menopause in an "unnatural" manner because of your breast cancer diagnosis and treatment. Your treatment may have profoundly affected your hormonal status, bringing on the cessation of menstrual periods much earlier than you expected. Certain chemotherapies can force the ovaries into retirement within a few months of treatment; this is *medical menopause*. Fifty percent of women younger than thirty-five who had CMF (Cytoxan, Methotrexate, fluorouracil) chemotherapy go into menopause, as do about 80 percent of women thirty-five to forty-four, and nearly 100 percent of women over forty-five. With adriamycin chemotherapy, the risk of permanent menopause is somewhat less for women under forty, but it is similar to that of CMF for women over forty. Occasionally, chemotherapy-induced menopause is only transient. Tamoxifen added to a cancer regimen produces severe hot flashes in some women, as can other anti-estrogen therapies; although these drugs don't cause menopause, they can mimic some of the symptoms, which may then continue for some time. You might go into menopause literally overnight if your ovaries are surgically removed; this is *surgical menopause*. Both treatments derail the gradual process of lowering hormone levels that normally eases you into the next stage of your life. Dr. Melody Cobleigh, medical oncologist at Rush-Presbyterian-St. Luke's Medical Center in Chicago, describes natural menopause as a fender bender, whereas medical or surgical menopause is like hitting a brick wall at sixty miles an hour.

Perhaps you were on menopausal hormone therapy and you had to stop the moment you were diagnosed with breast cancer. I call this a hybrid of natural and medical menopause—*cold turkey menopause*—characterized by a dramatic drop in estrogen. I took care of an eighty-four-year-old woman who had just been diagnosed with early breast cancer; more important to her, however, her surgeon had just taken her off estrogen hormone treatment, which she had been taking for forty years. "Menopause at eighty-four stinks," she announced. A woman in her fifties said, "Stopping hormone therapy made me feel ugly, unworthy, unwomanly."

You may not know whether you have gone into menopause. You could be in the midst of chemotherapy and miss a few periods. Or you may have had a hysterectomy (so your periods have stopped), but you still have your ovaries intact (and you are not sure if you are continuing to ovulate).

Blood tests can assess whether your ovaries are beyond menopause or not. These blood tests measure follicle-stimulating hormone (FSH) and luteinizing hormone (LH), proteins made by the brain that are supposed to stimulate each month's ovulation by the ovaries. If your ovaries are beyond menopause, they cease to respond to FSH and LH, and your brain reacts by sending out even more of these hormones. Persistent elevated levels of FSH (13 to 90 milli-international units per milliliter) and LH (15 to 50 mIU/mL) are consistent with a postmenopausal state. Normal levels of estrogen before menopause peak at 150 to 300 picograms per milliliter each month (depending on where you are in your menstrual cycle), falling to less than 20 pg/mL after ovarian function declines.

Defining the Hormones of Treatment and Replacement

Terms used to describe treatment for menopause need clarification. The term *hormone replacement therapy* is commonly used to describe the use of estrogen and progesterone pills to reestablish estrogen in the blood to a level between the usual premenopausal and postmenopausal values, about 80 to 100 pg/mL, to ease the signs and symptoms of menopause and reduce the risks of osteoporosis and heart disease.

The term *replacement,* however, implies that something is missing, but it's normal for women who go through natural menopause to have lower estrogen levels. There is no disease, nothing missing that requires replacement. Dr. Susan Love suggests the use of the term *menopausal hormone therapy* (MHT), as more appropriate for women who have gone through natural menopause. But for women who have undergone a medical or surgical menopause while in their thirties or forties, the concept of hormone *replacement* therapy remains appropriate. However, using two different terms for the same treatment can be confusing, so I'll use only the term *MHT* in this chapter.

Estrogen does not disappear from your body after menopause. There are different kinds of estrogens. Some diminish to inconsequential amounts; some are made from other areas of hormone production; and some are the products of conversion from similar molecules. Estradiol is an estrogen hormone made by the ovaries; it decreases after menopause. Estrone is an estrogen formed when fat and muscle cells convert DHEA to androstenedione, a testosterone-like hormone produced by the adrenal glands; this form of estrogen persists after menopause. The degree to which it persists depends on the amount of fat and muscle in your body. The more fat and muscle, the more estrone. Estrone may be further converted to estriol, which may be a safer form of estrogen—particularly for a woman concerned about breast cancer.

All of these hormones are built from the basic material cholesterol by your ovaries and adrenal glands. (In men, the testes and the adrenals build these hormones.) Small modifications in structure create the range of different hormones, and the difference in their function. And many of these hormones can convert from one type to another, like DHEA to estrogen, depending on what your body needs. You can see how much versatility your body and your hormones are capable of providing.

Life Changes and Lifestyle Issues

What do menopause and growing older mean to you? The end of monthly blues, of PMS? That's good. The end of fertility? The end of youthfulness? Maybe not so good—if true. But youthfulness can be a state of mind, so let's work on that and on the condition of your body.

Your lifestyle affects how you age and how you experience growing older. Is your life too filled with stress—are you trying to do too much—or have you learned to roll with the punches? Are you a couch potato or a dedicated walker? Are you attentive to what you eat? Is it steak and potatoes—with ketchup as your other vegetable— or are you a confirmed vegetarian with heavy emphasis on beans and broccoli, and only an occasional lapse for an ice-cream binge?

Exercise, in whatever form you choose to take it, eases the stress and strains of aging; keeping your body in condition helps you stay steady and limber, and feeling good. A healthful diet keeps your body functioning the way it should and helps you live longer. And stress-reducing efforts, including meditation, relaxation, hobbies, or distraction, will ensure that you get more pleasure from each day.

Too much can be blamed on hormones when what's really knocking you out are the plain facts of your life. If your breast cancer occurred close to menopause, and you've experienced the loss of a breast, and a large block of your time is spent getting treatment, the vision of yourself as a healthy woman with a long life before you has been threatened, if not shattered. You've got a lot of pieces to put back together.

And as you move on through middle age, there are tougher challenges. "Growing old is not for sissies." Empty nest, divorce, widowhood, the dependency of sick parents, the death of a mother, or kids in trouble: "You're only as happy as your least happy child." Or maybe you have a dead-end job, or no job at all. And then there's society's view of older women as decrepit and unattractive. It's normal to feel stress, isolation, depression—quite apart from the hormonal changes that relate to menopause.

As you approach menopause (or you're propelled into it) the immediate issues are usually the "in-your-face" symptoms: hot flashes, weight gain, dry vagina, mood swings, loss of energy, skin and hair changes. Long-range issues are osteoporosis, heart and vascular disease, and how to live a full and reasonably happy life.

If you're looking for more reading material on menopause, check the Resources section at the back of this book. I especially recommend *Dr. Susan Love's Hormone Book,* containing the most information for women who have had breast cancer. Also, Janine O'Leary-Cobb publishes a newsletter, *A Friend Indeed,* dedicated to the issues of menopause, with an emphasis on alternative therapies (call 514-843-5730).

Short-term Signs and Symptoms of Menopause

You may have only a few menopausal symptoms, or you may have every one in the book. Under normal circumstances, you should not feel rushed to make decisions to cope with these symptoms, but if they began because of a medical, surgical, or cold turkey menopause, and if a particular symptom is especially debilitating for you, you may be anxious to get help.

In the treatment recommendations that follow, you will notice a range of suggestions covering lifestyle choices, complementary therapy, and medications from conventional medicine. Most effective therapies have some side effects, but the potential benefits should clearly outweigh them. Start with the simplest, mildest remedy with the broadest benefit and the least number of side effects. Careful exercise is an ideal example: it strengthens your bones and heart, controls weight, lessens hot flashes, improves your sleep, boosts your energy, revs up your sex drive, and makes your skin glow—with no side effects to speak of. Then gradually move on to stronger forms or amounts of treatment.

At the potent end of the treatment spectrum is estrogen therapy, recommended almost automatically by many physicians for most significant menopausal symptoms in women without breast cancer. But if you have had breast cancer, you may be just as automatically told you *cannot* have estrogen therapy, as a matter of inflexible policy, without regard to your individual case. Keep an open mind and an eye to creative solutions as well as a full range of therapies that might serve your particular needs.

Hot Flashes

Here it comes: that sudden, intense, hot feeling on your face and upper body, perhaps preceded and accompanied by a rapid heartbeat and sweating, and sometimes accompanied by nausea, dizziness, anxiety, headache, weakness, or a feeling of suffocation. "It's not like being hot, it's like being on fire!" Some women have an "aura," an uneasy feeling just before the hot flash, that lets them know what's coming. The flash is followed by a flush, leaving you reddened and perspiring. You can have a soaker or merely a moist upper lip. A chill can lead off the episode or be the finale.

How They Happen

Hot flashes are primarily caused by the hormonal changes of peri-menopause and menopause, but can also be affected by lifestyle and medications. A diminished level of estrogen has a direct effect on the hypothalamus, the part of the brain responsible for controlling your appetite, sleep cycles, sex hormones, and body temperature. Somehow (we don't know how), the drop in estrogen confuses the brain's ther-mostat (the hypothalamus) and makes it read "too hot." The brain re-sponds to this wildcat report by broadcasting an all-out alert to the heart, blood vessels, and nervous system: "Get rid of the heat!" The message is transmitted by the nervous system's chemical messenger, epinephrine, and related compounds: norepinephrine, prostaglandin, serotonin. The message is delivered instantly. Your heart pumps faster, the blood vessels in your skin dilate to circulate more blood to radiate off the heat, and your sweat glands release sweat to cool you off even more. (Skin temperature can rise six degrees centigrade dur-ing a hot flash.) This heat-releasing mechanism is how your body keeps you from overheating in the summer, but when the process is triggered instead by a flux, or drop, in estrogen, your brain's confused response can make you very uncomfortable. Your body cools down when it shouldn't, and you are miserable: soaking wet in the middle of a board meeting or in the middle of a good night's sleep.

Who Heats Up

Eighty-five percent of the women in the United States experience hot flashes of some kind as they approach menopause and for the first year or two after their periods stop. Twenty to 50 percent of women con-tinue to have them for many more years. As time goes on, the inten-sity decreases. For women who have had breast cancer, hot flashes can follow the same pattern as for women in general, or they can be more intense and last longer, particularly if menopause was premature, or if you are taking tamoxifen and your body hasn't adjusted to it.

There is considerable variation in time of onset, duration, fre-quency, and the nature of hot flashes, whether you've had breast can-cer or not. An episode can last a few seconds or a few minutes, occasionally even an hour, but it can take another half hour for you to feel yourself again. The most common time of onset is between six and eight in the morning, and six to ten at night.

How Hot Is Hot?

Most women have mild to moderate hot flashes, but about ten to fif-teen percent of women experience severe hot flashes for which they seek medical attention. For women who have had breast cancer, the

TABLE 18.1. "Safe" remedies for hot flashes resulting from menopause and chemo/hormonal cancer therapy

To do or take	Active ingredient	Amount/dose	How it works	Side effects (most common)
LIFESTYLE CHANGES				
Keep a hot flash journal	You	Keep a daily record of when you're hot, when you're not; triggers and squashers	Listen to your body; design your own solutions to make yourself comfortable	May be tedious and boring—but when it helps you feel better, your enthusiasm may grow
Exercise, exercise, exercise	You	30 min/day	Endorphins; cardiovascular conditioning	Aches and pains (and, rarely, heart problems), depending on your current health and exercise tolerance and the type and amount of exercise
Layer clothing; stick to natural fibers; use cotton sheets	You			

To do or take	Active ingredient	Amount/dose	How it works	Side effects (most common)
Climate control: fan/air conditioning	You			
Avoid caffeine, spicy foods, alcohol; drink ice water	You			
Stop smoking	You			
Reduce stress—avoid triggers; use relaxation techniques	You			
SUPPLEMENTS Vitamin E	Vitamin	800 I.U. daily (range 400–1000)	Unknown	None at this dose
Vitamin B$_6$	Vitamin	200–250 mg daily	Unknown	None at this dose
Peridin-C (hesperidin and vitamin C)	Bioflavonoid and vitamin	2 tablets three times daily	Enhances small blood vessel tone	Perspiration may have an unpleasant odor

To do or take	Active ingredient	Amount/dose	How it works	Side effects (most common)
Black cohash, wild yams, dong quai, ginseng, licorice root, evening primrose oil	Herb remedies that contain plant estrogen	Doses and potency of many extracts are very variable (see reference books in Resources section)	"Weak estrogen," alters your body's balance of various "female" hormones.	Unknown; likely to share some side effects of estrogen
MEDICATIONS				
Isoflavones (in soybeans)	Plant estrogens	30–60 mg daily suggested, but "correct" dose still undefined	"Weak estrogen"	Unknown, but may share some side effects of estrogen (see Nutrition chapter)
Lignans (in vegetables, flaxseed)	Plant estrogens	1 tbsp flaxseed daily	"Weak estrogen"	Unknown, but may share some side effects of estrogen
Wild yams	Plant DHEA (dehydro-epiandrosterone)	Very variable	Converted to estrogen	Unknown, but likely to share side effects of estrogen
Megace	Megestrol acetate, hormone	40 mg/day for 1 month, then adjust (max. 80 mg/day)	Stabilizes brain's temperature-regulatory center	Weight gain, fluid retention, vaginal dryness, elevated calcium
Catapres-TTS (clonidine)	Nervous system; alpha-adrenergic agent	0.1-mg patch, change once weekly	Stabilizes blood vessels and brain's temperature-regulatory center	Low blood pressure, dizziness, fatigue

To do or take	Active ingredient	Amount/dose	How it works	Side effects (most common)
Aldomet (methydopa)	Nervous system; inhibits alpha-adrenergic nerve receptors and decarboxylase enzyme	250 mg twice a day	Same as clonidine	Dry mouth, fatigue, headache
Betapace (sotalol)	inhibits beta-adrenergic nerve pathways	120–160 mg twice a day	Slows the rapid heartbeats in response to the brain's hot flash alert	Slow or irregular heartbeat, fatigue, dizziness, shortness of breath
Bellergal-S	Nervous system stabilizer	One tablet at night, but may need to increase to twice a day	Inhibits nervous system signals	Dry mouth, dizziness, drowsiness, addictive potential. Do not use with alcohol
Tylenol (acetaminophen)	Prostaglandin inhibitor	325 mg, take 1–2 every 4 hours	Reduces inflammation, reduces hot feeling	Liver damage if taken in excessive doses or if person has underlying liver disease or drinks large amounts of alcohol

number who suffer debilitating hot flashes is probably much higher. Realistic numbers aren't well defined—any study of hot flashes selects women who are having them, making the statistics seem more compelling. Randomized studies provide the most objective data; for example, in a study randomizing women with breast cancer to tamoxifen or placebo, 13 percent of women on tamoxifen for a year experienced severe hot flashes, compared with 3 percent of women taking a placebo.

The faster you go through the transition from regular periods to no periods—the perimenopause or climacteric—the more significant your hot flashes will be. Hot flashes are severe after surgical menopause, and they can also be quite difficult after a chemotherapy-induced medical menopause. If you haven't been warned about hot flashes, a sudden severe episode can be frightening; you might even confuse the flash with a heart attack.

The intensity of hot flashes accompanying treatment with tamoxifen eventually improves for most women (but not all) after the first three to six months. Because of the conversion of androstenedione from the adrenal glands into estrone by fat and muscle cells, heavy or muscular women experience less severe hot flashes than thin women. Smokers, whose blood vessels can't expand as well to increased blood flow that allows heat to escape, may have prolonged hot flashes because it takes more time to radiate the heat.

Beating the Heat with Lifestyle Changes

The best way to beat a hot flash is to treat the underlying problem. Hot flashes have a lot to do with the low levels of estrogen in your body, but there are other factors that cause your temperature control to go out of whack. Instead of estrogen therapy, look at less drastic, nonpharmaceutical measures first, partly because estrogen therapy is not known to be safe for women with a history of breast cancer, but also because your first approach should be the least invasive or aggressive.

Avoid Triggers, Use Squashers

If you can establish some pattern or identify the trigger to your hot flashes, you've made the first step in getting the upper hand. Keep a record of when they occur and what you were eating or doing, or how you were feeling, at the time. Many women find that stress tops the charts as a trigger. Was that hot flash in the boardroom a random hit, or were you feeling under pressure at the time? Solution: Give yourself more time to plan your work, to rehearse your presentation, to deliver your assignments, to arrive where you're going. Plan your schedule so you avoid meetings or decision making when you're most likely to be in a sweat.

Other triggers: anxiety, alcohol, caffeine, diet pills, spicy food, hot food, hot tubs, saunas, hot showers, hot beds, hot rooms, hot weather. Caffeine can precipitate a hot flash by transiently increasing your blood pressure and heart rate. Alcohol can throw off your internal thermometer by dilating your blood vessels and affecting how your liver processes your hormones.

Quit smoking! There is *nothing* you can do for yourself that is more important than this for a full range of health benefits. Plus you need to stop so that your blood vessels will be as healthy and elastic as possible (releasing heat faster and shortening the hot flash).

Hot flash squashers: Dress in layers, so you can peel off one after another as you get warmer. Don't wear wool, don't wear synthetics, and be wary of silk. That leaves cotton, linen, rayon, and more cotton. (Look at the bright side: You'll save on cleaning and you can stop worrying about moths.) Avoid turtlenecks; stick to open-neck shirts.

Keep ice water at hand that you can sip to cool down your insides. Where possible, lower the house or room or workplace thermostat. Maybe it's time for a decent air conditioner or a ceiling fan. Or maybe you'd prefer one of those little hand-held battery-operated fans (in gadget or stationery stores). I prefer the foldable kind you flutter in front of your face. You can find perfectly adequate paper fans for about a dollar, but you can move up the scale to elegant and costly. Try a shop that imports Chinese or Japanese knickknacks. Or call 800-528-5599 for battery-operated mini-fans ($7.20 a dozen) or a variety of hand fans (starting at $1.50 per dozen).

A good night's sleep may be fundamental for fighting hot flashes, but you'll probably have to plan carefully. Wear cotton pajamas or a nightgown—if you perspire a lot at night, your nightclothes are easier to change than the sheets. Use cotton sheets only, not synthetics. Get a bigger bed if you and your partner are on different heat planets but you still want to stay in close orbit. A cool nighttime shower may also help, as might a mild medication like Tylenol. (A step beyond would be Bellergal, prescribed by your doctor.)

Lonnie Barbach's *The Pause* offers several additional creative solutions. "Arrive at meetings early so that you can get the coolest seat. Use your freezer liberally. A number of women talked about opening the freezer at home (or in the market) and sticking their head in when a hot flash hits."

Exercise, Exercise, Exercise

Increasing your level of activity and integrating exercise into your life (e.g., taking the stairs instead of the elevator) can reduce hot flashes and have a positive impact on just about every other symptom attributed to menopause and growing older: insomnia, mood swings, eroded self-image, loss of libido, fatigue, elevated cholesterol, and concerns about the health of your heart, blood vessels, muscles, and bones. Exercise increases endorphin levels (thus increasing your threshold for pain) and may also increase the conversion of androstenedione to estrone. Chapter 14 discusses exercise in greater detail.

Relaxation and Stress Reduction

Additional lifestyle changes include stress reduction and more relaxation. If you can't manage to let trouble roll over you, if stress is inescapable for the moment, you probably need help relaxing. Use relaxation exercises, breathing exercises, meditation, visualization, massage, hypnosis, yoga, or biofeedback techniques to avoid stress, lessen its severity, or shorten the episode. (See Chapter 19.)

Change Your Diet

Dietary modifications can help; some were already mentioned above. Over time, a low-fat diet helps some women with hot flashes. Losing excess weight helps, but losing too much weight, being too thin, can worsen them. As you consider other food changes, keep in mind that natural doesn't mean harmless, an important reality discussed in Chapter 19. Herbal remedies may work because of their plant estrogens, but you can't assume that just because an estrogen comes from a plant it's okay.

Read Chapter 13, on eating right, for information about the plant estrogen in soy foods and about lignin (another estrogen-mimicking substance) in flaxseed.

Chinese Medicine

Chinese medicine has a long tradition of treating hot flashes, but there are all kinds of hot flashes, and the Chinese have descriptions for all of them. Before treating you, a Chinese-medicine doctor takes a full history and performs a complete physical, with particular attention to your tongue and pulse. He or she determines whether you're suffering from a "hot" menopause or a "cold" menopause. If you have gone through a surgical or medical menopause, Chinese herbs are usually not considered strong enough to eliminate your menopausal hot flashes, but they can help. Treatment usually involves a combination of acupuncture and Chinese herbology. Many different herbs are cooked together to make a tea (the recipe is customized to your particular symptoms). Neither the acupuncture nor the herbal tea is likely to have unwanted side effects. If any do develop, treatment is altered to eliminate them.

Acupuncture moves your Xi (your inner wind, energy, or spirit). Maybe you're skeptical, but it helps a lot of women who are troubled by hot flashes.

Common to all Chinese herbal mixes is dong quai, thought to be a plant estrogen. More plant estrogens that women have found effective in treating hot flashes over the centuries can be found in ginseng, evening primrose oil, licorice root, red raspberry leaves, sarsaparilla, spearmint, damiana, motherwort, chasteberry (a.k.a. Vitex), black cohosh, and wild yams. These herbal remedies, Chinese and other, may be effective at reducing hot flashes but, again, their relative safety in women who have had breast cancer is not known. I think avoidance, or cautious use, is best, and never try any of them without telling your doctor.

Mary Ellen Scheckenbach, a Chinese-medicine practitioner with whom I have worked, tells women not to self-treat with Chinese herbs. But if you have no practitioner near you or none on whom you can rely, read the books available on herbal medicine before you start stirring up potions. Scheckenbach recommends *Between Heaven and Earth* as a reference on Chinese medicine (see Selected Readings). "It's really very, very important to get it right," she emphasizes.

Medications

If you have tried these lifestyle, nutritional, and alternative medicine recommendations, and they have not helped, you may feel impelled to go on to stronger remedies, available only through your physician (refer to Table 18.1).

One way to forestall a hot flash is to intercept the messenger: epinephrine, the chemical signal that broadcasts the faulty temperature message. Blood pressure–lowering medications such as clonidine (Catapres-TTS, 0.1-mg patch applied once weekly) and Aldomet (250 mg twice daily) can lessen the severity and frequency of the flushing symptoms. In a randomized study, a group of women were put on clonidine for a period of time, then switched to a placebo; another group were given the placebo first and then clonidine. When the women were taking the placebo, they experienced a 20 to 25 percent reduction in their hot flashes; when they were taking clonidine, they had an *additional* 15 to 20 percent reduction. However, the side effects of dry mouth, constipation, and drowsiness were significant, and most of the women expressed no preference for clonidine or the placebo. Low blood pressure is also a side effect. Betapace (sotalol) which controls how fast your heart beats in response to stress, can help reduce the heat waves in about two thirds of the women who try it. Veralipride works on a chemical related to epinephrine, serotonin—a nerve chemical that works in the brain. However, this drug should probably be avoided by women who have breast cancer, because it may cause breast glandular stimulation as a side effect.

Megace (megesterol acetate) can reduce hot flashes in approximately 80 percent of women who take it, and it is also considered a treatment for breast cancer when taken in high doses continuously. Megace is usually started at 40 milligrams daily, and it may take a few weeks to work. After a month the dose is adjusted up or down. The maximum dose is 80 milligrams per day. Those who reap its benefits and can tolerate its side effects (fluid retention and bloating) may do well on this medication.

If you are having severe hot flashes while on tamoxifen, discuss options with your doctor. You can rethink tamoxifen's potential benefits and your decision to take the drug. If you and your doctor decide that it's important to continue tamoxifen, you could try the approach of Dr. John Eden of the Royal Hospital for Women in Paddington, Australia: Temporarily discontinue tamoxifen and if hot flashes still continue, try Megace for six months. If the hot flashes do not go away, stop the Megace and start going slowly back onto the tamoxifen. Begin with 5 milligrams per day of tamoxifen, and work your way back up to 20 milligrams per day. Most physicians would not recommend estrogen therapy to remedy severe tamoxifen-related hot flashes because estrogen is not known to be safe for women who have had breast cancer, because estrogen may reduce tamoxifen's efficacy, and because of the potential synergistic side effects of the combined drugs, such as blood clots forming and traveling to the lung. There is a study, however, on simultaneous estrogen replacement therapy and tamoxifen in women beyond menopause that showed no short-term problem from combined side effects. Also, ECOG (the Eastern Cooperative Oncology Group) has an ongoing study which combines the two drugs. Share this information with your doctor, and decide together what you want to do.

Vitamin E, 800 I.U. (range 400 to 1000) daily, helps some women, though only a little more than a placebo alone would do (i.e., about a 30 percent response), and is recommended by the Mayo Clinic. The NSABP's tamoxifen prevention trial also recommends vitamin E, or one of the following: Vitamin B_6, 200 to 250 milligrams daily, and Peridin-C (containing antioxidants), two tablets taken three times daily. Bellergal-S, one tablet at bedtime (and up to twice daily, morning and night), can be quite effective and safe when used occasionally, and not in conjunction with alcohol consumption. (It contains belladonna, phenobarbital, and an ergotamine.) Phenobarbital can cause drowsiness and, if you use it regularly, you can develop a dependency for it. The antidepressants Zoloft or Prozac may be helpful in reducing hot flashes and in helping you cope with them.

MHT, or estrogen therapy, is probably the most effective way to treat hot flashes, but its use is highly controversial in women who have had breast cancer. However, if your hot flashes are severe and you have not had adequate relief from lifestyle modifications or nonhormone remedies and medications, your doctor may suggest a limited course of low-dose MHT to ease your transition into menopause, for six months to one year, depending on the degree of your symptoms, tapering off over the last few months. I'll address the controversy over MHT later in this chapter.

Sadness and Depression

Your treatment for breast cancer may leave you feeling sad, bad, or depressed. These feelings are complex conditions, resulting from and affected by so many factors: your cancer diagnosis and treatment, aging, hormonal changes, your life experiences, your genetic constitution.

Sadness is a natural part of your breast cancer experience, something you need to express, and move through. If you don't allow yourself to feel sad and grieve, the unresolved grief gets in the way of feeling better and getting better, and getting past it. Read Chapter 2, on support groups, and find people to talk to.

Depression is more than a feeling of sadness. It's an inability to cope, an overwhelming feeling of helplessness and hopelessness, inertia, inability to concentrate, memory problems, panic attacks, loss of pleasure in what used to make you happy, lack of interest in sex or food, sleep problems. All these are signs of clinical depression. "Someone looks at me cross-eyed and I burst into tears." If you have been thrust into an abrupt menopause perhaps ten years earlier than you deserve to be, with a rapid decline in hormone levels, you may be thrown into a depression not unlike postpartum depression. (Natural menopause is not associated with a greater risk of depression.)

Fatigue, the most common side effect of cancer treatment, may have hit you hard, especially if hot flashes are stealing your rest. If your workday is also interrupted, you are likely to find yourself debilitated and overstressed. The shock of diagnosis, the fear and anger that were pushed out of sight while you kept busy with treatment and then scrambled to restart your life at work or with your family to make your life *normal* again, and the adjustments of menopause—all this accumulated abuse affects your well-being, and there you are, in the middle of a genuine depression.

Depression is more than a side effect of treatment, or even a response to a serious disease. For mild depression, alternative therapies and behavioral therapies may be enough. Estrogen therapy may help the women without breast cancer who take it. But if you have serious depression, MHT may not help—it may even make things worse. You should get help. You must talk to an accredited psychotherapist who can help you get better. Although another round of medication may worry you, antidepressants can be an important and a sound approach to alleviating depression. But it's also important to obtain help by expressing what's bothering you and getting people-support for your problems. Medication can take up to six weeks to begin to make a difference; in the meantime, continue to talk with the psychotherapist who is prescribing your medication. A support group is not sufficient at this point, although, later, it can help keep you on an even keel.

A note about medication: Go to a specialist in antidepressant medications to get the best recommendation from the most highly skilled professional. Your oncologist is trained in cancer treatment, not depression medication. Seek help early to forestall serious trouble and long-term treatment. Sometimes a onetime visit to a psychotherapist can make a huge difference. And make sure you get approval from your health care insurer; insist on your rights for further mental health assistance if you need it. (See Chapter 26.)

Memory Problems

Memory and learning are heavily dependent on aging, the level of your mental conditioning, hormonal changes, medical and psychological health, and your genetic characteristics. A study by the National Institute on Aging concluded that older people cannot commit information to memory as effectively as younger people, but both groups retrieve information from memory equally well.

Fatigue, anxiety, and depression have a potent effect on memory: They interfere with it. Chemotherapy (without tamoxifen) can affect memory. (One of my patients in treatment made three separate commitments for Christmas dinner.) Many women claim that tamoxifen has reduced their memory capacity. (See Chapter 7, on tamoxifen.) Radiation to the breast area has no effect on short-term memory, but radiation to the whole brain for metastatic disease can have a profound effect.

Women entering menopause sometimes report feeling "fuzzy," or losing their mental sharpness. It's not clear to what extent menopause affects memory, or whether this is a consequence of normal aging.

Estrogen does have a significant effect on memory. Studies show that estrogen therapy can improve short-term and verbal memory by sustaining nerve cells, particularly in the brain's main memory center, the hippocampus, but estrogen appears to do little for your sense of organization and spatial memory.

Although most of us couldn't care less about a rat's menopause, that trusty laboratory animal is teaching us a few things about estrogen and the brain that may apply to women. When premenopausal levels of estrogen are present in a rat's brain, (1) its nerve cells grow and are well sustained, (2) the number of connections between nerve cells increases and allows for ever better communication, and (3) the protein that helps prepare the signals sent between cells increases in production.

Early clinical data have begun to suggest that estrogen therapy may lessen the devastation of Alzheimer's disease. Women on estrogen therapy tend to get the disease at a later age, less severely, and with slowed progression of the disease. It's not yet known whether you can wait to start estrogen therapy at the time Alzheimer's is diagnosed and still obtain any significant benefit.

We can use the information we have about estrogen to *speculate* that when your estrogen levels are low, or if you are taking a drug that blocks the effects of estrogen (e.g., tamoxifen), your brain cells' ability to receive, communicate, and store information may be reduced, resulting in decreased memory.

Memory is also very dependent on mental conditioning—how often and how long you use your memory and other brain functions. The more rigorously and regularly you "exercise" your brain, the better it will function. So keep your brain busy; keep learning new things all the time, and stir up your memory by testing yourself on what you'd like to remember—telephone numbers or family birthdays.

For more on memory, see Chapter 8, on fatigue.

Weight Gain

After menopause, many women begin a slow but steady gain in weight. As people age, their metabolic rate slows, so they need fewer calories to maintain their normal weight. If they're less physically active as they age, but consume the same number of calories, the result is weight gain. "Do I need to send my body to college, to give it a new education? How else do I relearn a lifetime's eating habits? I feel like a thin woman trapped in this fat woman's body—it just snuck up on me in the last five years or so, while I was minding my own business, eating the same as always."

Weight gain is a big issue for women who have had breast cancer. Some studies have found a correlation between obesity and breast cancer, and others have refuted the connection. (See Chapter 14.)

Vaginal Dryness

With the significant drop in estrogen after menopause, the membranes of the vagina thin, lose elasticity, and decrease the production of lubricating fluids. Sexual intercourse may be uncomfortable or painful. Pain with intercourse may be largely a result of vulvar soreness, which may benefit from avoidance of any soaps on the vulva, and from the use of a barrier cream like Eucerin or Bag Balm.

For vaginal dryness, try Replens or other lubricants first. Replens is designed to moisturize the walls of the vagina, but it may not in fact be the best lubricant. Many women don't like Replens because it tends to drip out of the vagina. If you need a lubricant, use a lubricant. Chapter 12, on intimacy, addresses the management of vaginal dryness, and lists various lubricants.

Only after you've had no improvement and you're having significant vaginal pain, is it appropriate to talk to your doctor about using a vaginal estrogen cream. A vaginal estrogen cream can help thicken and lubricate the walls of the vagina, but absorption of estrogen through the vagina can be just as complete as absorption through the stomach, so don't assume that vaginal estrogens will remain confined to the vagina. Estradiol is readily absorbed, estrone is less readily absorbed, and estriol is thought to be minimally absorbed. Some studies suggest that estriol may actually protect against breast cancer, or at least that it has less potent effects on breast tissue than estradiol. (See further discussion of estrogen therapy later in this chapter.)

If you and your doctor decide it's okay for you to use a vaginal estrogen cream for vaginal dryness and pain, after you have had no real relief from Replens or the other lubricants that have been suggested, then an estriol cream may be the type of estrogen cream to use. You may need only a very small amount. Dr. Susan Love recommends starting with a dose as low as 0.1 milligram of estrogen per day, applying just a small dab inside the vagina, for up to three to four weeks, and then cutting back to once or twice a week. "If you apply it daily for more than four to six weeks, it becomes less effective," says Dr. Love.

Estriol cream is available in Europe and in some parts of California. Mail order pharmacies that offer estriol vaginal creams in the United States include Bajamar Women's Healthcare Pharmacy (800-255-

8025), Belmar Pharmacy (800-525-9473), Women's Health America Group (800-222-4767), and Women's International Pharmacy (800-279-5708). (Telephone numbers were provided by the Women's Health Advocate May 1996 *Newsletter.*) Your doctor's prescription is required for any of these products.

Troubling vaginal discharge can also occur with menopause. Of the women taking tamoxifen, 80 percent will have no change in vaginal symptoms, 10 percent will have vaginal dryness, 10 percent will have vaginal discharge. Describing your symptoms clearly and accurately to your gynecologist will make it a lot easier for you to get help. The woman who says straight out, "My crotch itches so much I can't leave the house, I have a vaginal discharge that looks like cottage cheese, and I'm convinced that everyone on line with me at the supermarket is disgusted by the odor," is more likely to make her doctor listen and understand what the symptoms mean to her and is more likely to get effective treatment than the woman who mumbles something under her breath about "a weird discharge that makes me a bit uncomfortable."

Wrinkles and Sun Damage

"I prayed to the God I don't believe in: I'll never complain about wrinkles, sagging skin, gray hair, or liver spots if I survive this breast cancer. And I'm here, I'm alive—and I'm not complaining." Okay, so it's not much of an issue compared with breast cancer, but it still may mean something to you and it does to many other women—why else would all those cosmetic companies rake in billions for Retin-A and moisturizing creams if it didn't? Here are a few secrets about how to manage this problem, and then we'll go on to the serious stuff—bones and the heart.

Wrinkles are attributed to menopause, but they are more properly attributed to aging and lifestyle factors. The hormonal fluxes of menopause contribute relatively little to the development of wrinkles. Natural menopause comes at a time when cumulative effects of sun exposure, smoking, aging, gravity, and genetic predisposition produce wrinkles—especially wrinkles on the face. There is no evidence that chemotherapy or tamoxifen causes wrinkles, and little is known about how the lower estrogen levels of menopause affect the skin. It's believed that aged skin has less collagen supportive tissue beneath it, so it loses some of its fullness; add in ever-present gravity and sun exposure and you've got sags and bags as well as wrinkles.

Your genetic makeup also contributes to how resilient your skin is: If your mother went wrinkle-free into her seventies, you can probably skip the skin care creams; if your mother had weathered creases and lines by her sixties without heavy sun exposure or smoking to blame for the effects, expect similar evidence of aging, and save up for sun screen and Retin-A. Although exposure to the sun is probably the most significant lifestyle cause of wrinkles, smoking runs a close second. Smoking constricts the little blood vessels that nourish the skin and results in three times as many wrinkles as for a woman who doesn't smoke.

It's never too late to protect your skin against additional wear and tear. Basic prescription: Stop smoking and avoid the sun. If you're not prepared to give up sunbathing, at least protect your skin from the sun. *Especially protect yourself during 5-FU chemotherapy and protect all areas where you have had radiation therapy.* (This is a precaution you must observe for the rest of your life.) In spring, summer, and fall, when you spend more time outside, it's a good idea to wear a moisturizer or makeup base with a sun protection factor (SPF) of at least 15. If you are outside a lot, go for a waterproof lotion with an SPF of at least 30. Reapply if you go in the water or are at the beach more than a few hours.

If you hate to apply and wear sunscreen lotion (or even moisturizing lotion), as I do, you can purchase special protective clothing with an SPF of 30, or find a long-sleeved, tightly-woven cotton coverall. A T-shirt alone will not protect you—it has an SPF of only 8. You'll also need a tightly woven hat with a brim of four inches or more. When I go to the beach, I have to be particularly careful because I have a bunch of atypical moles (funky cancer-prone spots). I go no earlier than 3:30 P.M. and I wear a Solumbra-brand pants-and-jacket set that is light, cool, roomy—and boring: I look as if I've come straight out of a uniform catalog (phone Solumbra, 800-882-7860). You can wear tightly woven fabrics, such as pima cotton, and get similar protection without sacrificing comfort, as long as the fabric covers you thoroughly. If you can take the time to shop around, you may be able to find something stylish and cheap.

If you have wrinkles and you are unhappy with them, you do have options. Fine wrinkles can be smoothed in a number of ways that provide short-term results: Renova cream, containing the vitamin A derivative tretinoin, increases skin cell growth and turnover, increases collagen production, and reduces keratoses (those raised, scaly, brown-black spots that tend to appear as we age). A 25 percent alphahydroxy lotion and Retin-A are also effective and work the same way. All three require doctors' prescriptions.

Less effective but still worth trying for fine wrinkles are potions from nature's medicine cupboard: fruit and milk acids that cause a mild skin reaction resulting in increased firmness of the skin. These acids include glycolic (from sugar cane), citric (from citrus fruits), lactic (from soured milk), malic (from apples), tartaric (from grapes), and tannic (from wine). For moderate to more pronounced wrinkles, there are options such as chemical peels, collagen injections, laser therapy, and face snips or lifts.

Whether you enjoy, accept, or resent your wrinkles, it's a good idea to keep your skin moist and supple with a moisturizer of your choice. The only thing that truly moisturizes your skin is grease, although it may be cut with water or alcohol to make it more spreadable and appealing. Don't dry out your skin with alcohol-based creams (any ingredient that ends with *ol* means it's a form of alcohol) or harsh soaps such as Ivory and Noxema (no matter how much they advertise otherwise).

If you want to look tan, it's safe to use self-tanning lotions like dihydroxy-acetone, which affect only the uppermost layer of your skin. Tanning parlors are dangerous; I'd avoid them altogether.

Long-term Health Concerns

One out of eight or nine women gets breast cancer, and one out of two or three gets heart disease, but more women fear breast cancer than they do heart disease. Thirty percent of all women die of heart disease (average age, seventy-five to eighty), 3 percent die from complications of osteoporosis (average age, eighty), and 3 percent die of breast cancer. Heart disease is the leading cause of death in women over sixty-five, but one third of all cardiovascular deaths occur in women less than sixty-five years old.

Women who have had breast cancer have a greater chance of dying of breast cancer than women who have never had it, but they are at risk of heart disease just like other women. Death caused by breast cancer occurs over a much greater age range, because women start getting breast cancer at much earlier ages than they do heart disease and osteoporosis: beginning in their twenties and on to over 100.

Bone Strength or Osteoporosis

Bones in Flux

Bones are always in a continuous process of growth and resorption: Old bone is absorbed and removed by osteoclasts, and new bone is rebuilt by osteoblasts. Osteoblasts apply a kind of spackle, collagen fortified with calcium and phosphorus, to the walls of the bony cavities in a process called mineralization. It's rather like having a huge old house that you want to keep in tip-top shape: You're fighting weather and day-to-day abuse, forever scraping and redoing the walls and woodwork. Prior to menopause, particularly before age thirty-five, the rate of resorption is equal to the rate of rebuilding, and the strength of your bones is stable. (You've got enough money in the bank to keep the old house in good shape.)

What Is Osteoporosis?

After age thirty-five, and particularly after menopause, bone resorption gradually begins to outstrip bone formation, resulting in a slow loss of bone mass. Over time, usually many years, bone mass reaches the low end of the normal range; the term *osteopenia* is used to describe this condition. If loss of bone mass continues long enough, osteoporosis is the result. Osteoporosis may be moderate, associated with an increased risk of fracture, or it can be severe, associated with actual fractures.

Loss of bone mass is an inherent part of the aging process of men and women, although it tends to affect women more. Our bone mass is less dense than men's to begin with, and we tend to live longer, allowing more time for bone aging. Bone mass is greatest in your twenties and thirties; it stabilizes between thirty and forty, and above forty there is slow loss of bone strength. After menopause, there is a five- to seven-year period of accelerated bone loss; then the rate slows and returns to an age-related rate.

The aging process has a greater effect on bone loss than the presence or absence of estrogen. Smoking, prolonged bed rest or inactivity, being underweight, and certain medications can increase bone loss. Weight-bearing exercise increases bone mass. Tamoxifen tends to stabilize bone strength, but for the first year of taking it, premenopausal women may experience bone *loss*; postmenopausal women may have some bone fortification.

Osteoporosis can lead to loss of height and small fractures of the vertebral and wrist bones; you're also more vulnerable to larger fractures of the hip. Such fractures can have a significant effect on your quality of life, limiting the comfort of any activity you contemplate. If an elderly woman fractures a hip, forcing her to stay in bed, she is at significant risk for developing complications from the fracture or from the inactivity. Fewer than 20 percent of these older women return to their prior lifestyle. And death can occur in up to 30 percent of women over seventy-five who develop a hip fracture, because of complications from extended bed rest; like a pulmonary embolus (a blood clot from the thigh or pelvic area where the fracture was that breaks off and travels to the lung). These types of scary problems usually occur in women over seventy-five.

Measuring Osteoporosis

At one time, treatment for critical bone loss began only *after* a fracture led to the diagnosis of osteoporosis. Now it is possible to diagnose osteopenia and osteoporosis and predict risk *prior* to fracture, using single- and/or dual-energy x-ray absorptiometry (DEXA) tests. This x-ray scan measures the bone density of your lumbar spine, because the spine is usually the first area to experience loss of bone mass. (A DEXA scan is different from a bone scan, which you may have had to check the health of your bones and to make sure there was no evidence of metastasis to the bone.)

You probably don't need a special scan to identify bone loss if you have lost height each year (a sign of significant osteoporosis). But if you have just recently experienced any type of menopause, you may not have lost significant height so far, and good medical practice suggests stepping in before you lose ground.

Preventing osteoporosis is particularly important when you have just experienced premature medical or surgical menopause. If you are trying to figure out what you should do, if anything, two DEXA scans taken six months apart can tell you the rate at which you are losing bone mass. If you learn that the rate of your bone loss is minimal, you may decide to do nothing. (It's still important to keep your bones strong—see below—and to periodically reassess how your bones are doing.) If, on the other hand, you find that your rate of bone loss is significant, you may be motivated to do more to actively prevent osteoporosis.

For more information about the DEXA scan technique and the location of a scanner near you, and for general information on osteoporosis and the various medications used to treat it, call the National Osteoporosis Foundation's general information line, at 800-464-6700. The cost for a DEXA scan is $125 to $350, but you may have small hope of getting your insurance company to cover the expense. A strong letter from your doctor may do it. The advocacy office of the National Osteoporosis Foundation, however, may be able to help you present your case and fight for what you need. Their phone number is 202-223-2226. (No toll-free number as yet.)

Keep Your Bones Strong

The most effective way to maintain the strength of your bones requires lifestyle changes and medical measures. Lifestyle changes consist primarily of stopping smoking, doing weight-bearing exercise, practicing good nutrition with minimal amounts of animal protein and sufficient calcium intake, and preventing falls. (Most hip and wrist fractures are preceded by falls.) Non-weight-bearing exercise, such as swimming, can also be helpful, as long as the muscle puts repetitive, balanced tension on the bone. Weight-bearing exercise is most effective and should ideally be performed thirty minutes a day, three or more days a week.

Calcium supplements are recommended to most women: 1000 to 1500 milligrams per day (but check with your doctor first to be sure your calcium level is not too high to begin with). Vitamin D supplements (not to exceed 400 I.U. daily) may be recommended if dietary intake is inadequate. Fosamax (alendronate sodium), Miacalcin (nasal calcitonin), or Slow Fluoride (a slow-release sodium fluoride) taken in combination with Citracal (calcium citrate) represent three choices if osteoporosis is present. Consult your doctor about these options.

Fosamax is one of a new class of medications called bisphosphonates that halt the rapid bone loss you may experience beyond menopause and that may even help restore some of the bone mass you have already lost. With a dose of 10 milligrams daily, Fosamax stabilizes bone mass and reduces the number and severity of bone fractures. It is not a hormone and it has no apparent effect on breast cancer. In one study comparing Fosamax to MHT, they were equally effective in halting bone loss. There is evidence that Fosamax can actually increase bone density, not just restore an equal balance of bone resorption and formation.

Fosamax requires your doctor's prescription. It can affect your kidneys if they are not functioning well or exacerbate a problem with your esophagus. Side effects include irritation of the esophagus; gastrointestinal symptoms such as nausea, constipation, heartburn, and diarrhea; and muscle or bony discomfort—all usually mild and transient. The biggest problems with the drug—apart from cost—are that you cannot lie down for at least thirty minutes after you have taken it, to avoid irritation of the esophagus, and that the drug is absorbed well only if taken on an empty stomach. (And you have to wait at least thirty minutes before you can eat or take other medications.)

The hormone calcitonin also reduces the rate of bone resorption, but it is probably not as effective as Fosamax. It comes in two forms, Calcimar and Miacalcin. Slow Fluoride taken with Citracal stimulates bone formation, increasing bone density and preventing new spinal fractures.

Estrogen prevents further bone loss by inhibiting bone resorption, and over time it helps reduce compression fractures of the spine, wrist, and hip, but it does not appear to help rebuild bone or increase bone mass. If you have had breast cancer and cannot take MHT, these other therapies are effective alternatives. Each of these treatments costs about fifty dollars a month.

Aggressive medical management is called for if you have osteoporosis or progressive bone loss with a significant spinal deformity, such as kyphosis (prominent back hump) or scoliosis (side-to-side curvature of the spine) or other severe postural problems. Adopting lifestyle changes—and sticking to them—is essential for you. You and your doctor should consider a medication such as Fosamax to prevent further loss of bone integrity. A new medication, Raloxifene, which protects the bones and heart, is currently being studied. MHT, until proven safe and more effective than alternatives, should be avoided. (MHT will be discussed further in this chapter.)

Heart Health

The aging process creates the most significant effect on the heart; heart disease goes up at a regular rate as you age, for about five to ten years after menopause the rate increases, and then it assumes the previous age-related rate (that is the same pattern seen with osteoporosis). If you take MHT, you avoid the period of accelerated increase in heart disease. Other risk factors in your life also have a major effect on heart disease: high blood pressure, high cholesterol, diabetes, and a family history of early heart disease. Smoking, a sedentary lifestyle, and your diet are also very important factors.

One woman, a two-pack-a-day smoker, was crushed when she was told to stop MHT upon diagnosis of breast cancer. "But I have such a strong family history of heart disease!" That history was not enough, however, for her to stop smoking, which would have had a much greater impact on her risk of heart disease than the MHT.

The best way to keep your heart and blood vessels happy and healthy is through a combination of lifestyle modifications: Control blood pressure, stop smoking, exercise, use relaxation techniques, and change diet to reduce the "bad" cholesterol (low-density lipoproteins) and increase the "good" cholesterol (high-density lipoproteins), consider soybean foods. Loss of excess weight can help with blood pressure, cholesterol levels, and your sense of self and well-being. A baby aspirin per day (if your doctor recommends it) may also be beneficial for your blood vessels. There is a full spectrum of medications to control blood pressure, used singly or in combination, with convenient once-a-day timed-release preparations. Check with your doctor about an exercise program, cholesterol and blood pressure levels and medications, and use of aspirin.

Promising, but very preliminary, results for heart and vascular health have recently been demonstrated with the use of *Ginkgo biloba* extract. The extract seems to reduce cholesterol plaque buildup in the blood vessels of laboratory animals, and to lessen the severity and length of heart attacks. Stay tuned for more studies.

It is estimated that MHT can reduce the risk of heart disease by 50 percent. This indication for MHT is not firmly established; it is not even listed as an indication for the medication in the *Physician's Desk Reference* (the PDR). Tamoxifen's weak estrogenic effects can also reduce blood cholesterol levels and the number of heart attacks, but it is not as effective as "full octane" estrogen at reducing cardiovascular disease; it has not consistently reduced the risk of dying from heart disease in the large randomized studies that have examined the issue.

It is critical to keep in mind that lifestyle changes alone can have a profound effect on heart disease risk, reducing heart disease by up to 50 percent. Effective blood pressure control further decreases heart disease. Dr. Battastini says, "It's just tunnel vision to focus on MHT as *the* answer to cardiovascular risk protection. But if MHT is not part of your care, it becomes that much more important to adhere to a healthy lifestyle and control cholesterol, blood pressure, weight, diabetes."

Menopausal Hormone Therapy

In this chapter, I've tried to build an understanding of how women grow older: the aging process, the effects of hormonal changes and cancer treatment, and your genetic makeup. I mentioned that MHT with estrogen might significantly help you with some health concerns; I also introduced the controversy behind its use, but I have tried to stay away from the question of whether *you* should take MHT, until now.

Menopausal hormone therapy with estrogen is only one kind of menopausal treatment, but it is one of the most effective because it works to relieve many of the immediate symptoms and long-term concerns of menopausal women. Most doctors go by the book, however, and adhere to the 1997 PDR recommendation: "Since estrogens increase the risk of certain cancers, you should not take estrogens if you have ever had cancer of the breast or uterus." Reading this may make you feel angry. Another blow. Only 20 to 30 percent of women in the general public use MHT, but if you are suffering from menopausal symptoms, you may not find this statistic in any way comforting.

It's certainly much easier to take a pill than it is to reorder your priorities or modify lifelong personal and cultural habits about food, weight, and illness. You may find these changes very difficult to accept, and even more difficult to integrate into your family's way of life.

If you have *seriously tried* to make these lifestyle changes and you have worked closely with your doctor, taking nonhormonal medications and nutritional and mind-body therapies—all to little avail—and if your symptoms are sufficiently bothersome, and if they are symptoms that are likely to respond to MHT, it may be time for you and your doctor to assess the role of MHT in your care.

Before I present you with the arguments for and against MHT, ask yourself about your expectations from hormone therapy: What benefits do you expect from MHT? Do you know its potential side effects? What controversies about taking MHT worry you most? Have you made up your mind one way or the other? Or is this issue a constant struggle for you? What does your doctor suggest about estrogen therapy for you? The decision to take any drug depends on balancing all these issues: Is it harmless and helpful, or harmful and helpful? (Or harmful and not helpful?)

Arguments for Estrogen Therapy

1. *MHT improves the immediate symptoms and signs of menopause.* Natural menopause may be a normal part of aging, but medical, surgical, or "cold turkey" menopause can feel very much like a disease— a disease with symptoms that demand treatment to achieve more than can be effected by lifestyle changes and nonhormonal medications alone—*ergo*, estrogen therapy. Hot flashes, low energy levels, vaginal dryness, urinary tract symptoms, aches, memory, concentration, the ability to sleep at night—are all improved with MHT.

2. *MHT improves the long-term health of your bones and your cardiovascular system, maybe even your brain and colon.* Many women with early-stage breast cancer have an excellent long-term survival prognosis, so their long-range risk of developing, having complications from, and dying from non-cancer problems increases. Their risk of death from a heart attack may be equal to or higher than their risk of dying from recurrent breast cancer. Estrogen also helps preserve bone mass, reducing the risk of fractures and associated complications. And recent studies report a reduction in colon cancer and Alzheimer's disease in women taking MHT.

3. *Estrogen is not necessarily dangerous to women with breast cancer.*
- Pregnancy, a time of high levels of estrogen, does not have an impact on the prognosis of breast cancer.

- Long-term use of MHT only mildly increases the risk of breast cancer in women in the general population. In particular, there is no additional increased risk of breast cancer in women without a personal history of breast cancer taking MHT who have either a prior history of benign breast disease or a family history of breast cancer in a first-degree relative (mother or sister). (There are no data yet available that consider this issue in families with an abnormal breast cancer gene.) Breast cancers diagnosed during MHT usually have a more favorable prognosis than breast cancers diagnosed in women not taking MHT.
- High dose continuous estrogen in the form of diethylstilbestrol (DES) is an effective treatment against advanced breast cancer.
- Premenopausal women diagnosed with breast cancer who are taking tamoxifen as an anticancer treatment can have significantly elevated estrogen levels, and so far these higher estrogen levels have not caused any known danger.
- Estrogen levels in the breast are usually always higher than estrogen levels in the blood, and that differential can remain significant even beyond menopause, making some clinical scientists believe that the breast sequesters a higher level of estrogen, or that the breast itself produces estrogen. The result: The breast will see to it that it has the estrogen it needs even if the ovaries and adrenal glands are making only minimal amounts and you are not on MHT.
- In oncology practice today, making sure a woman becomes postmenopausal is not considered a necessary therapeutic objective of breast cancer treatment. For example, it's not proven that women with the same kinds of cancer who get chemotherapy do better if their chemotherapy throws them into menopause; also tamoxifen—which does not produce complete menopause—is probably just as effective as removal of both ovaries, which does produce complete menopause.

4. *The survival benefit* of chemotherapy and its elimination of estrogen production may be outweighed by the potential long-term survival benefits of MHT. There is no question that chemotherapy can improve the survival of women with breast cancer, particularly premenopausal women—but chemotherapy usually produces a permanent early menopause. If your prognosis is very good or even excellent, then you will probably live long enough to encounter the higher risk of heart disease and osteoporosis. When do the risks balance each other? When does one risk overshadow the other?

5. Breast cancer survivors with severe menopausal symptoms who are given MHT *do not show an increased risk of recurrence* in any of the

retrospective or case-control studies performed to date. There are numerous retrospective studies done on small numbers of women diagnosed with breast cancer who were given MHT for significant menopausal symptoms; the observed risk of recurrence was no higher than would be expected given the stage and characteristics of the cancers and the treatment that these women had.

The study I find best on this issue (so far) is a case-control study conducted by Dr. John Eden and his associates in the Royal Hospital in Australia. Of the 1472 women with breast cancer treated within a particular interval, 167 women used MHT after treatment for breast cancer to help relieve their severe menopausal symptoms; they were given equivalent doses of Premarin or Ogen (0.625 mg and 1.25 mg, respectively), as well as 50 milligrams of daily continuous medroxy progesterone acetate. (In this country, Provera is the most common preparation of this drug; it's also related to Megace.) Most of these women had tried at least one month of Megace prior to using MHT. The women who took MHT were younger, closer to the time of menopause, than the women who did not take MHT. The outcomes for these women were compared with those of women of the same ages and with similar-stage breast cancer who did not take MHT. After several years, the results showed that the women who took MHT had nearly *half* the risk of recurrence as the women who did not take MHT: 16 of the 167 women on MHT had recurrences, compared with 31 of the controls. Some of the women taking MHT were taking tamoxifen as well, which was not associated with excess estrogen-like side effects such as blood clots.

6. *Estrogen is only part of the picture*; other hormones may influence breast cancer risk. They include progesterone, dehydroepiandrosterone (DHEA), androstenedione, testosterone, estrone, and estriol. Most of these hormones can convert from one to another.

Arguments Against Estrogen Therapy

1. *MHT may increase the risk of prior breast cancer recurrence and new breast cancer development.*

- MHT may increase the risk for a recurrence of your breast cancer. This big concern, of course, forms the basis of the controversy about the safety of MHT in women with a history of breast cancer. There are no data available that show this, and it has not been studied properly by randomized clinical trials.

- Breast cancer is a hormone-responsive disease. Both laboratory and clinical data clearly show that estrogen makes breast cells—

normal or cancerous—grow. And breast cancer cells are more likely to grow in response to MHT if the cancer has estrogen and progesterone receptors.

- Some of the most effective treatments against breast cancer work by blocking the effect of estrogen on breast cancer cells (e.g., tamoxifen) or by lowering the circulating estrogen in the body available to affect the breast (e.g., ovary removal, Arimidex, aminoglutethimide, Zoladex). Given the power of these anti-estrogen treatments, it's hard to imagine that giving estrogen-based MHT could be safe (but this intuition is not yet proven or refuted).

- MHT may promote the development of a new breast cancer. Long-term use (more than five years) of MHT increases the risk of breast cancer by 10 to 30 percent in women within the general public; but it's unknown if MHT causes a greater increase of risk in women who have already had breast cancer. Unfortunately, there are no long-term data to address this important issue.

2. *A low estrogen level may predict a more favorable outcome.* Breast cancer survivors in the Australia study who had severe menopausal symptoms and were treated with MHT had a lower risk of breast cancer recurrence than women not taking MHT. Presumably, women with severe hot flashes have a particularly low level of estrogen, and perhaps this low level is the reason why these women did better. Taking this premise a step further, it is also possible that treatment with MHT in fact increased their risk of recurrence, approaching, but not quite reaching, the level of risk of women with a higher level of hormones who had less severe symptoms. (To investigate this possibility further, women with severe hot flashes who didn't use MHT would have to be compared with women with severe hot flashes who did take MHT.)

Conversely, women with a high natural endogenous estrogen level, such as those who are significantly over ideal body weight, who often experience few menopausal symptoms, and who have strong bones, are thought to be at increased risk of developing breast cancer. Perhaps both the absence of symptoms and the higher recurrence rate can be attributed to greater conversion of androstenedione to estrogen (in the form of estrone, which is then converted to estradiol or estriol), but the gain may also be caused by reduced exercise and activity, a high-fat diet, and insufficient consumption of fresh vegetables and fruit. In some women, MHT may increase weight gain, thereby increasing their body's own production of estrogen.

3. *There are reasonable, effective alternatives to MHT.* Lifestyle changes, complementary medicine, and nonestrogen medications can

be quite effective at relieving immediate concerns of hot flashes, mood changes, insomnia, vaginal changes, and skin changes. Exercise; cessation of smoking; sustained control of weight, blood pressure, and cholesterol; and good nutrition can produce a major reduction of heart disease. Similarly, exercise, cessation of smoking, good nutrition, sufficient calcium, and, if needed, Fosamax or Miacalcin can help reduce the risk of osteoporosis. Tamoxifen can also be used to address some of the long-term health issues for which MHT is prescribed (i.e., heart disease and osteoporosis), even though it's not as effective as MHT at dealing with these issues.

4. *MHT can make mammograms harder to interpret.* MHT increases the density of breast gland tissue, which can cause a general increase in breast density on mammography in roughly one third of women. The denser the breast tissue, the greater the likelihood of missing a cancer concealed by the gland tissue (the clinical "false negative" rate increases), and the more likely it is to find a change that turns out *not* to be a cancer (the false positive rate increases). This doesn't mean that mammograms are impossible to read; it means they may be just a little harder to interpret.

So, estrogen therapy may be the easiest and the most effective *single* way to ease your symptoms and address future health concerns, but it is also very controversial and potentially dangerous.

Ultimately, It's Up to You: What Do You Want to Do?

I do not feel comfortable prescribing MHT for women who have had breast cancer, because I do not know that it is safe and because I believe that there are effective alternatives to pharmaceutical estrogen. While alternatives like Megace, exercise, and soy foods require a lot more effort and are probably not as effective as MHT, they usually do provide significant relief of symptoms and help with long-term health concerns, representing a reasonable compromise.

Clinical Trials of MHT Safety

There may be a safe and effective role for MHT, but the only way to know whether MHT is safe is with clinical trials. I share the view of Dr. Jeffrey Perlman, of the National Cancer Institute's Division of Cancer Prevention and Control: "It's time to study ERT (estrogen replacement therapy); it's not time to use it."

There are two ongoing studies of estrogen usage in women with breast cancer: ECOG's study by Dr. Cobleigh (ECOG stands for Eastern Cooperative Oncology Group) and the M. D. Anderson study by Rena Vassilopoulou-Sellin.

The M. D. Anderson study offers women MHT if they are not taking tamoxifen and if they have been free of breast cancer for at least two years, if they had hormone-receptor negative tumors, or are at least ten years beyond treatment for a hormone-receptor-positive or receptor-unknown cancer. You can join this study even if you do not live in Houston. The ECOG study does include women who are taking tamoxifen. Off study, some breast cancer survivors do take MHT for a few months up to a year or two, to ease their way through menopause with more tolerable symptoms. This is followed by slow weaning before a complete stop. If you are depending on MHT to keep your bones strong and your blood cholesterol in check, then you would have to continue on MHT indefinitely, at least until a better medication, a more targeted estrogen, comes along that can achieve the same goals without the potential side effects on breast cancer growth.

Is Tamoxifen the Answer?

Some women count on tamoxifen's weak estrogenic effects to reduce their risk of osteoporosis and heart disease. Although estrogen therapy is better able to keep your bones strong, tamoxifen represents a good compromise. Some women with a personal history of breast cancer with only borderline indications for tamoxifen may choose to take tamoxifen because of these added benefits.

DHEA Is Not the Answer

Dehydroepiandrosterone (DHEA) is a hormone that is made by your adrenal glands (which are located on top of each of your kidneys). As discussed earlier in this chapter, DHEA is converted to androstenedione, then to estrone (a type of estrogen) by fat and muscle cells. (Androstenedione can also be converted to testosterone.) Estrone can be modified further to become estriol and estradiol, two forms of estrogen. Thus, DHEA is considered a source of estrogen. DHEA has become very popular and is now widely available in health food stores, but it's an unproven form of treatment.

DHEA levels rise through adolescence and then slowly diminish. By age sixty, DHEA levels are about two thirds of their early peak levels. Levels can drop transiently during times of illness, such as cancer. These lower levels suggest that DHEA may have a role in the aging process and your ability to fight disease—but are they the cause or the effect? We don't know if an increase or a decrease helps fight a particular illness; most supporters of using DHEA as a supplement believe that the lower DHEA levels during illness makes it harder to fight the illness, so they take DHEA to beef up their resistance—but proof is nonexistent.

Most studies of DHEA are limited by procedural flaws. In laboratory animals, DHEA has been shown to improve immune function, prevent the formation of breast cancer, and extend the survival of mice with breast cancer, as well as lower their cholesterol and improve their energy levels and their ability to lose weight. Sounds like really good stuff in a mouse, but how about in people? The many studies so far have not been able to demonstrate any benefit. One study showed that DHEA stimulated the growth of human breast cancer cells in laboratory dishes. Another observed an increase in natural-killer immune cell activity in people taking the drug, and still another noted a significant elevation of blood estrogen levels to above-normal levels for a premenopausal woman.

DHEA is available in health food stores under many brand names, either synthesized, or extracted from food, such as the Mexican wild yam, dioscorea. The most common source of DHEA is food, so it is considered a food supplement and is unregulated by the U.S. Food and Drug Administration (FDA); but the most common available form of estrogen is pharmaceutical, and therefore it is regulated by the FDA. This distinction is arbitrary. That DHEA is natural doesn't mean it is any safer (or more dangerous) than estrogen therapy. In fact, the law governing the use of supplements led the FDA to ban DHEA in the mid 1980s, because it had no proven efficacy or safety. Its return to the health food store shelves doesn't mean that its efficacy or safety have been established, but simply that the FDA no longer regulates vitamin and food supplements.

DHEA should be considered a form of estrogen therapy. Its safety for women who have had breast cancer is unknown. It deserves further study, but research is expensive and there are no patentable rights to be owned by the company who might do the research, therefore no financial incentives. Until its efficacy against cancer and its side effects have been determined, I recommend that you avoid DHEA.

Testosterone: Not for Men Only

Testosterone, a hormone we associate primarily with men, is also present in women. Made in the ovaries and also derived from adrenal gland hormones, most of it is converted into estrogen; it helps sustain our muscles and keeps our skin oiled, our memory intact, our energy up, and our sex drive alive.

Normal levels of testosterone are 20 to 60 nanograms per deciliter. A little too much testosterone can cause acne, facial hair, aggressive behavior and excessive anger, a deep voice, male-pattern hair loss, and depression. Lower than normal levels can make you feel tired and diminish your libido. The difference between too much, too little, and the right level for you is pretty tricky. If normal testosterone levels do not improve low libido, extra testosterone probably won't—another reason for the low or absent libido should be looked for. If you are suffering from memory loss, low energy, and low libido, ask your doctor about testosterone—but do look at the bigger picture, too (see Chapter 8, on fatigue, and Chapter 12, on sexuality.)

As we grow older and pass through natural menopause, our testosterone levels decrease, but not as much as our levels of estrogen and progesterone. With a premature medical or surgical menopause, however, you may experience an abrupt drop of testosterone. A cold turkey menopause, resulting from stopping MHT upon your diagnosis of breast cancer, should have no additional effect on your testosterone, unless your MHT included testosterone in the hormone therapy cocktail.

Whether it's safe to replace the testosterone missing after a medical or surgical menopause, or to supplement testosterone after natural menopause, is unknown. The effects of testosterone on breast cancer are unclear, as frustrating as it may be to hear that said once again. It is true that testosterone in the form of Halotestin, in high and continuous doses, can be used to fight breast cancer; there is some evidence that testosterone at lower doses can increase breast cancer risk.

For the women who have an abnormal breast cancer gene 1 and who don't yet have a personal history of breast and ovarian cancer, and who elect to have prophylactic ovary removal (to reduce their high risk of developing ovarian cancer), the decision to take hormones is a difficult one. If a woman in this situation decides to restore her natural hormonal milieu, then testosterone should probably be part of the cocktail.

Choices

There is often a conflict between what may improve your quality of life and what may threaten your survival. I don't think you should take chances until the risks are better understood. If I am too conservative for you, you should seek information from other sources, and figure out a plan of action right for you.

There are many risk-free lifestyle changes that you can make to improve your future health. Test-drive the various suggestions in this chapter and try to modify the stress and demands in your life, to enhance the quality of your life and help you live as long as possible. Whenever you can, find a practical way to implement these lifestyle changes.

This approach is going to take much more energy and willpower (and cooperation from you and the people in your life) than is required to take a pill. But, *no pain, no gain.* You can't just sit back and hope that you will stay well. This is your life, and you've got to work on it.

Menopause is a wake-up call to a new phase of your life, and so is breast cancer. Two wake-up calls can be more than most people can handle, but what's the choice? You sure can't go back to sleep. So get up and decide what you're doing today—and the years ahead.

19

Alternative and Complementary Therapies

I've visualized, meditated, and joined support groups. I've done Tai Chi, yoga, and animal imagery. I've read everything ever written for the lay person about breast cancer. I've walked around with headphones attached to my ears feeding me positive affirmations. I've changed my diet, exercised, reduced my working hours, and reshuffled my priorities. And you know what? Everything I did made a difference! I never felt so focused, so happy, in my life.

Fifty years ago, American medicine was swept up in science and new discoveries: penicillin, streptomycin, and technological wonders. America's newfound postwar preeminence in medicine focused treatment on scientific method and technology. Alternative medicine was akin to voodoo.

The scene today has shifted, and alternative healing solutions are finding a respected place in the catalog of therapies. These last fifty years have seen a gradual acknowledgment by the conventional scientific medical community of the value of herbal therapies, from rauwolfia and digitalis to treat blood pressure and heart problems, to vinca alkaloids and Taxol to treat breast cancer. Much of alternative medicine is slowly moving from the shadow of quackery toward the arena of accredited, funded research and treatment. One out of three Americans are reported to make use of nontraditional therapies. The Office of Alternative Medicine is now part of the National Institutes of Health, and its intention is to develop new discoveries in alternative medications. I prefer the term *complementary medicine* because I wish to emphasize that women should consider these approaches in *addition* to conventional treatment, not *instead* of it. Confusion and controversy cloud the available therapies, so how do you figure out what's relevant to your needs?

Nature's Bounty

More than 25 percent of drugs in your neighborhood drugstore have natural sources, some discovered by accident, some after methodical searching of a promising ecosystem, some translated from folk medicine to high-tech, extended-release capsule form. The biggest recent splash in nature-based compounds was Taxol, first extracted from Pacific yew tree bark, to fight ovarian cancer and metastatic breast cancer. It took twenty years to learn how to get it properly absorbed by the body; now, it has been partially synthesized, is part of mainstream treatment, and has a strong competitor, Taxotere. It stands as an inspiring example of how nature provides wonder substances to fight disease. Another plant derivative, vinorelbine, is being used in random clinical trials, after more than ten years of studies in Europe and the United States, to establish its precise role as an antimetastatic breast cancer drug in combination with other known anticancer compounds. This semisynthetic alkaloid derived from a vinca plant is one more of nature's promising miracle compounds.

Our government supports research into these compounds ("searching Mother Nature's cupboard") through the Natural Products Division of the National Cancer Institute (NCI). This division collects and tests compounds from forests and oceans and elsewhere all over the world, including deep sea expeditions at the South Pole. Each year, more than 40,000 samples are tested against a full range of cancers. "If we find a specimen that is fat and colorful and *not eaten,* we want it," said Dr. David Newman of the NCI ("it" being a specimen with some unique form of self-defense). The NCI wants compounds that defy attack or that destroy disease-causing organisms, that can eventually be bottled for medicinal purposes. "But we must be careful: We've found poisons that make strychnine look as benign as the sugar on your breakfast cereal."

What Is Complementary Therapy?

How does complementary therapy differ from the conventional medical therapy most of us are used to? Conventional medical practice aims to treat a specific problem, a specific complaint, or a definable disease, to make an accurate diagnosis and cure the patient, or at least to send the disease into remission, by a combination of comprehensively tested and approved medications, surgical procedures, radiation, or chemotherapies. In complementary therapy, the body is typically seen as a force unto itself, holistic, as in Chinese medicine, where Xi (chi) is the body force or energy, and the whole is more than the sum of the body's many parts.

Preventive health care is an important, relatively new emphasis of conventional medical care, whereas it is the primary emphasis of many alternative therapies: Illness indicates a problem within the whole spirit and system of the body. The problem is analyzed by pulse, tongue patterns, touch, patterns of tension and stress, state of fitness, and careful, close attention to the patient's description of her symptoms. Therapy is designed to help the body correct itself, by directing the body's energy to maintain balance and health. Health or wellness is promoted with herbs, potions, purges, acupuncture, massage, biofeedback, hypnosis, visualization, laying on of hands, prayer, meditation, music, movement, and a predominantly vegetarian diet.

Most alternative or complementary care has not been reimbursed by health insurance providers, but this is changing. A few insurers are starting to include massage therapy, chiropractic, and nutrition and diet counseling, but, generally, participants are not allowed to *replace* conventional medical practitioners with alternative medical caregivers.

Few people with cancer seek alternative medicine to the exclusion of conventional medical therapy. Again, I view alternative medicine as *complementary* to conventional breast cancer treatment, *not* as a substitute for conventional therapy. I believe that many but not all complementary therapies can significantly improve your quality of life, which is likely to improve how well you live, and maybe even how long you live. Complementary therapies have helped many of my patients reduce or relieve their stress and unwanted symptoms, as well as the side effects from chemotherapy or other anticancer therapies, such as nausea, pain, edema, hot flashes, and sleep problems. They also promote vigor, appetite, and mood, for an overall sense of well-being.

You may feel impelled to try complementing therapy as an alternative to conventional therapy when all conventional medical options are exhausted—and this may provide you with hope and relief. But be cautious. When you feel hopeless and desperate for anything that might work, stay away from grandiose claims with an all-or-nothing approach and a high price tag.

Relatively little is known about how complementary therapies work, how effective they truly are—and how *safe*. Clinical trials, the key to determining benefits in conventional medicine, have not been widely used for confirmation of results in alternative therapy. There are no large randomized studies, no broad-scale laboratory or clinical testing by a nonbiased outside party with findings that can then be reproduced by still another group of investigators, such as normally are employed to evaluate new conventional medical therapies. Most results from alternative therapies have been collected as anecdotal reports ("I took this, and now I feel terrific."), which represent a particular individual's experience or an individual therapist's experience in practice, but these experiences are not necessarily applicable to anyone else.

To help assess the large and confusing range of treatments, Living Beyond Breast Cancer$_{SM}$ held a conference on complementary therapy titled "Complementary Therapy: From Harmless to Helpful to Harmful." These three H's are the crucial criteria you must weigh for any treatment you investigate.

This chapter is not meant to be a comprehensive guide to complementary therapies; a full discussion of their benefits and drawbacks lies beyond the scope of this book. The material provided here is designed to provide an introduction, a thoughtful perspective, to these intriguing forms of therapy. There is a considerable collection of literature available on the subject to amplify and satisfy your own particular interest. Books by Andrew Weil are among the most popular; Michael Lerner covers the field in *Choices in Healing*; and *Choices* by Morra and Potts focuses on healing after cancer. See the Selected Readings section of this book for more reading choices.

Is Complementary Therapy for You?

How you feel about complementary therapy depends on your cultural, religious, ethnic, and personal background, and on what you have heard or read.

Most people are attracted to complementary therapy because it *seems* more natural, life-supportive, and intuitive; less toxic and intrusive compared to conventional medicine. The rising frustration many women feel about dealing with health insurance coverage—rigid policies and bureaucratic complications—makes alternative medicine seem more attractive with its unencumbered accessibility. (Although most costs are likely to come out of your pocket, some HMOs [such as the Oxford Health Plan] are now reimbursing members for approved alternative therapies.)

Are you getting ready to look into other routes to continuing therapy, to make other choices beyond the scope of conventional medicine? Have you completed conventional medical treatment? Does your physician take care of all your health needs? Do you still have unanswered questions, healing work you want done? Are you intrigued by herbal remedies? Acupuncture? Meditation? Massage? Prayer? What are you comfortable with? What are you willing to try?

Proceed with Caution

You want your medical doctor to listen with an open mind to your quest for complementary care and to respect your autonomy, and to watch for what might be harmless, helpful, or harmful to you. But your physician can't know everything about all therapies; most physicians don't have the background to make a judgment about complementary therapies. When a patient asks me, "What more can I do to keep cancer away?" I ask her in turn, "What do you have in mind?" And then I listen.

If she wants to pursue nutritional therapies, I feel comfortable if she limits her fat to as little as 15 to 20 percent of her caloric intake; derives most of her protein from vegetarian sources; and takes up to the daily recommended dose of vitamins, as long as she maintains a balanced diet that includes a variety of fresh fruits and vegetables (see Chapters 13 and 14). If she decides to eliminate all dairy foods from her diet, I would not object (even though I would not recommend it), as long as she consumes adequate amounts of vitamin D and calcium from other sources. I think juicing large amounts of carrots and wheat grass is acceptable as long as her diet is otherwise balanced. I strongly favor vitamins in food over vitamins in capsules or pills.

If a patient is experiencing significant stress and anxiety, I encourage her to seek comfort and support from music, massage, meditation, visualization, distraction, yoga, acupuncture, support group, and, if indicated, individual counseling and antianxiety medications. If she is experiencing noncancer-related back pain, I recommend anti-inflammatory and pain agents, complete bed rest followed by appropriate back-strengthening exercises, massage, acupuncture, and, if indicated, chiropractic management. Cancer-related back pain can also benefit from mind-body techniques and acupuncture, in addition to the conventional therapies, radiation, and pain medication (see Chapter 23).

If a patient asks me what I think about detoxification with coffee enemas, I must admit this makes me uncomfortable. Although it's important to have regular bowel movements, I question the safety of frequent bowel manipulations that can result in trauma and chemical imbalance. I think the best way to have regular bowel movements and minimize your exposure to toxins (and optimize your nutrition) is to eat large amounts of organically grown fruits and vegetables, and drink eight glasses of water a day (a challenge in itself).

When you interview a complementary care practitioner, ask practical, direct questions. "What experience do you have with my type of diagnosis? What is the therapy? How does it work? How will your treatment help my problem? What are the treatment goals? How long will treatment take? How much will the full course of treatment cost? Will my health insurance pay for this therapy? Will you communicate with my primary care physician and my oncologist about your treatment of my condition throughout the period of my therapy with you?" Then listen very carefully to the answers, and take notes.

However uninformed your primary care physician may be about complementary therapy, *it is absolutely vital* to your health that you keep her or him informed about whatever therapy you are engaged in, particularly if it involves any kind of medication. Statistics claim that seven out of ten people who seek help from alternative medicine practitioners do not tell their physicians about their "other" therapy. This lack of communication can be dangerous. Herbs, potions, and pills may sound harmless and natural, but they can be harmful, even fatal, especially if taken in large enough doses. Popular herbs can alter the effects of your standard medication; in excess doses, they may cause liver or kidney damage, or worse. So you and your doctor should know what medication you're on, what it does, and what dosage is safe.

Be wary of quacks. There's no sure-fire way of spotting one, but there are important warning signs to look for. If you encounter any resistance on the part of your alternative therapist to connect with your primary care physician, any vagueness, evasion, anger, mystery or secrecy, exaggerated claims of miracle cures, or surprisingly high fees, beware!

Most unproven therapies are based on anecdotal information. Keep in mind that anecdotes are about one person, who may or may not have biopsy-proven cancer, whose cancer may be very different from yours, whose stage of cancer may not be substantiated by objective evaluation, or who may be taking effective conventional therapies concurrently with complementary medicine, making it hard to attribute results to any one treatment. I've heard of a nutritionist who starts women on wheat grass immediately after they finish chemotherapy and then performs serial measurements of their fighter T cells to gauge results. The blood tests show improving T-cell counts, which he attributes to the wheat grass. But your immune system normally rebounds after chemotherapy with increasing T-cell counts, wheat grass or no wheat grass.

Inform yourself. Ask for credentials, experience, and references. Call the relevant professional society—for example, The Acupuncture Society of Pennsylvania—and ask for a recommendation. Call a local women's health center, The American Cancer Society, or The Wellness Community, for their recommendations. Go to the library and the bookstores, and get on the internet. Read, find out about therapies that interest you. Ask your friends and fellow patients. Ask your doctor. Stick to licensed practitioners of the discipline that intrigues you. Be sure, whatever you decide, to tell your primary physician about your plans and to keep him or her informed as you go along.

Chinese Traditional Medicine

Many of my patients have used a range of Chinese medical therapies during and after breast cancer treatment to help restore their physical and emotional wellness. A Chinese woman I take care of explained: "When I get really sick, I go to my Western doctor for treatment; then I go to my Chinese doctor to get back my health and energy so I can stay well." I have seen and been impressed by the benefits my patients have obtained from Chinese medicine: relief of nausea, stress, and pain; improved energy, mood, and equanimity; personal empowerment from active control of their own care. This form of therapy has a track record of thousands of years, keeping millions of people feeling well, with few side effects, at reasonable cost. In the last few decades, Chinese medicine has entered the mainstream of medical treatment in the Western world, informing us and enriching our ultra-scientific, high-tech methods. I welcome its benefits with an open mind.

The underlying philosophy of Chinese traditional medicine is that illness results when Xi (pronounced tchee), the vital energy or life force, ebbs, alters, or gets stuck in one region of the body. Wellness is restored by returning Xi to its normal healthy force and balance. The state of Xi is determined by pulse (the doctor may monitor different body pulses for ten minutes or more), patterns of breathing, and the appearance of the tongue (practitioners of Chinese medicine must memorize 200 tongue patterns).

Traditional Chinese medicine does not employ surgical intervention; healing is accomplished with acupuncture (discussed later), acupressure, herbal medicines, and physical movement. Chinese medicine may have seemed quaint and old-fashioned to twentieth-century doctors at one time, but more and more conventionally trained physicians (and lay therapists) are receiving training in this ancient method of treatment, which can complement Western-style medicine. In fact, Western-style medicine now dominates medical care in China, which has over a million MDs and about 350,000 traditional Chinese-medicine practitioners. The two systems can and usually do work smoothly together.

Proponents of traditional Chinese medicine say it can be particularly useful for cancer therapy in the areas of stress reduction, concentration, wellness, pain relief, and the easing of side effects from conventional cancer therapy. The efficacy of Chinese medicine by itself as cancer therapy has not been tested with clinical trials. The intuition, strong belief, and centuries of patients' stories that serve to recommend Chinese medicine are persuasive and promising, but they need to be formally assessed. If enough Americans find relief through Chinese medical principles, its popularity will undoubtedly increase, and studies will be performed to establish its value by modern medical standards.

This form of therapy requires dedication and commitment to a lifestyle that includes meditation, relaxation, formal exercise, and extra time to shop for fresh ingredients to prepare herbal brews—perhaps several times a day. (See the section on herbal remedies later in this chapter.)

Acupuncture is an aspect of Chinese medicine that is designed to relieve pain and illness by the insertion of hair-thin needles in any of 400 or more specific points of the body along meridians, to adjust the internal wind or energy of the body and restore balance and health. Only disposable needles should be used. (Laser acupuncture is a recent innovation.) The process can be mildly uncomfortable. "I think you have to have a bit of pain so you know the right spot has been hit. When my acupuncturist inserts the needle, she always asks if I can feel it."

Benefits from acupuncture include relief of nausea, pain, headache, anxiety, fatigue, and depression; side effects are minimal or nonexistent. Results are impressive: I've seen major brain surgery performed with acupuncture as the sole anesthesia. The perceived benefit may also be caused in part by the placebo effect: positive results from receiving treatment the patient *believes* will help, even if the treatment has no clear therapeutic content. "I was very skeptical: I thought it was a bit of baloney, and I didn't want to go—but I trusted this friend and I figured I should give it a try. I plugged into it immediately. I feel very calm when I leave after treatment. It gives me real balance and peace of mind, and I sleep better than ever I can remember. It's not humbug—I'm an intelligent, reasonable person, I've tried and benefited from traditional therapy, but this—I only have good things to say about it."

Thirty percent of acupuncture practitioners in this country are MDs. An acupuncture physician should have a minimum of 200 hours of training; a nonphysician trains for years and should be properly licensed or registered in your state or should have passed the National Commission for the Certification of Acupuncturists exam. Referrals from friends you trust may be the most important credential for you.

The first visit, lasting from thirty to sixty minutes, is for evaluation of your state of health. About ten sessions comprise the usual course of treatment, and costs per session range from $25 to $100. Most insurance plans do not cover these expenses, but that is changing as benefits weigh in and lower costs relative to conventional treatment impress the business managers of insurance plans.

Acupressure is a kind of massage, relying on the same focal points of the body that acupuncture does. The practitioner exerts finger (or hand or arm) pressure on these points, massaging and manipulating the internal energy, Xi, to relieve symptoms. There should be no side effects.

Xi Gong and *Tai Chi Chuan* are traditional Chinese therapeutic, meditative exercise disciplines. They enhance and promote the healthy flow of Xi throughout the body, preventing blockage or unduly high or low energy in one place or another, which would lead to pain and illness. The Xi Gong master manipulates the power of the inner Xi in an intense, directed design, sometimes resulting in a quasi-hypnotic state. Tai Chi is much more widely practiced: the centuries-old stylized patterns of slow circular and stretching motion and balanced positioning of the body are performed by millions of people daily in the parks of China. My patients have reported the following benefits: improved muscle tone, strength, and agility; improved ability to concentrate; increased appetite and energy level; sounder sleep; greater interest in sex; and fewer hot flashes. They have reported no unwanted side effects.

Ayurvedic Therapy

Ayurveda, an ancient Hindu approach to healing and life enhancement, has close parallels to Chinese medicine. Dr. Deepak Chopra has popularized the therapy in this country within the last few years through lectures, books, and TV appearances.

According to Ayurveda, three doshas—vata, pitta, and kapha—are the forces that control your biological functioning; consciousness and the flow of the mind through the body are the focus of therapy. The balance of your doshas, your well-being, is achieved by appropriate diet, living habits, yoga, meditation, massage, herbs, and enemas (detoxification). A reporter from *The New York Times* went to an Ayurvedic-type institute and came away singing its praise: "A miraculous two-hour treatment (mostly massage and steaming) left me stressless—and cost a mere thirty dollars."

The spiritual and dietary recommendations provide benefits similar to those of other complementary therapies with similar approaches.

Herbal Remedies

Some anticancer herbal therapies are already part of mainstream Western medicine, identified and tested by conventional medical research protocols: vinblastine and navelbine. The antinausea ingredient in marijuana has been incorporated into the antinausea prescription drug Marinol. Aspirin was originally derived from the bark of the willow tree; now it's made synthetically.

Herbs are the favored route to healing in Chinese medicine. Doctors of traditional Chinese medicine spend years learning the thousands of individual herbs and combinations used to treat the range of patients' complaints. They believe that herbal therapy should not produce any side effects.

Herbal remedies (readily available at many local drugstores, including the giant CVS chain) have become very popular in this country, and their use is growing each year. Unfortunately, there is no FDA supervision of the production, content, or safety of these products. The respected publication *Consumer Reports* (November 1995) gives a detailed discussion of what to watch for and what might be helpful. "You have no way to be sure whether a plant's active ingredients, whatever they might be, have actually ended up in the herbal pills you buy, whether a supplement's ingredients are in a form your body can use, whether the dosage makes any sense, what else is in the pills, whether the pills are safe, whether the next bottle of those same pills will have the same ingredients." Workers who pick these herbs have sometimes misidentified plants or picked what turns out to be a poisonous part of an otherwise desirable herb. Unless you can perform your own laboratory testing or you have a reliable source, there is no way for you to know what's in the supplements you buy. You are on your own in a sea, or fieldful, of choices.

It's best to pursue herbal therapy under the direction of a reputable herbalist. Don't rely on the clerk behind the counter. Remember, these are medicines. If you must proceed on your own, get some good books on the subject. I recommend *Between Heaven and Earth* by Beinfield and Korngold, *Chinese Herbal Medicine* and *The Complete Book of Chinese Health and Healing*, both by Daniel Reid, and *Healing Wise* by Susun Weed. (See the Selected Readings section of this book.)

Try only one herb at a time, use it for one to two weeks, and stop immediately if you develop side effects (something unpleasant that's new or different). Use extreme caution with any herb with which you have had no experience. Remember to keep your doctor informed, as you do for other forms of complementary therapy, about any herbs you plan to try.

Despite little scientific evidence of its value, ginseng has been promoted as beneficial for "stress, hypertension, ulcers, diabetes, atherosclerosis, depression, edema, memory problems, anemia, and menopause." There are also claims for it as an aphrodisiac and as a tonic for extending life. Because of its purported ability to ease hot flashes, ginseng is thought to contain an estrogen-mimicking substance, referred to as a phytoestrogen. There is a wide variation in the amount of ginsenoside concentration in the various commercial brands of ginseng; some contain as much as twenty times more than others.

Dong quai, evening primrose oil, and black cohash are also thought to have estrogen-mimicking properties, but because they may have questionable, perhaps harmful side effects, check with your doctor before you try them.

Other herbal remedies that may improve your quality of life have been reviewed by *Consumer Reports,* from the research of Varro Tyler of Purdue University and Norman Farnsworth of the University of Illinois. They include chamomile (helpful for indigestion and menstrual cramps), *echinacea* (supposed to enhance the immune system, although some people may prove allergic to it), feverfew (useful for migraine headaches), ginger (fresh or crystallized, for nausea), *Ginkgo biloba* (supposed to enhance blood circulation, in particular to the brain), hawthorn (purported to lower blood pressure), milk thistle (may help protect the liver against various toxins), and valerian (believed to possess tranquilizing properties, good for sleep problems). Don't take any of these herbs, particularly hawthorn or milk thistle, without your doctor's approval.

Tyler and Farnsworth warn against chaparral, comfrey, ephedra, lobelia, and yohimbe; they have all been associated with deaths related to their use.

Nonherbal Remedies

Melatonin is a hormone, now available synthetically, released by the pineal gland (located in the brain) that controls sleep patterns. It has recently been publicized as a way of controlling the effects of jet lag and as a potent antioxidant, or neutralizer of free radicals. It has also been touted to help Alzheimer's disease, AIDS, autism, Parkinson's, cancer, sexuality, and even aging. Some have called it the body's natural wonder drug.

I would approach the use of melatonin with great caution. The only studies we have so far are experiments with mice. These studies indicate that melatonin actually inhibits sexual activity; other studies suggest melatonin may have a booster effect on the immune system (as a free-radical neutralizer), but this was in mice. For human beings, there is no solid proof of melatonin's value as a neutralizer of free radicals, and no proof of its value as anything other than a sleep enhancer.

Dr. Dan Orrin of the National Institute of Mental Health worries about careless use of this hormone. He explains that our body is very delicately balanced, and that it produces this important substance only in the dark and generally in small amounts; there must be a reason why it's not in the body at other times. Playing with melatonin levels may bring on effects you're unprepared for (such as experiencing intense nightmares or getting drowsy at odd times), as the body clock gets shifted away from its normal setting.

Melatonin can't be patented, so drug companies aren't rushing to do expensive studies to evaluate its efficacy. And there is no FDA regulation of melatonin.

Melatonin itself has no known toxicity, but that doesn't mean it's harmless, especially in large doses, taken over a long time. Animal studies are all we have at present; human studies are ongoing. Dosage levels are uncharted. There are groups of individuals who are advised to avoid its use (e.g., pregnant women, people with autoimmune disease, and people on steroids). Use this hormone only after consultation with your physician.

Chiropractic

Chiropractic is a method of treatment that involves manipulation of the spine by a trained practitioner to ease pain and compromised function by relieving pressure on nerves and ligaments. Chiropractic manipulation is recognized therapy for back pain, accepted by mainstream medicine, and generally reimbursed by medical insurance. In a survey of back pain treatment and results in the October 1995 *New England Journal of Medicine,* chiropractic and conventional medical therapists were equally effective, but chiropractors' total charges amounted to more than twice as much as those of primary care physicians, not quite twice as much as those of orthopedic surgeons.

Everyone gets back pain, including women with breast cancer, but a woman who has had breast cancer worries that the pain means something more. If you develop new back pain that is persistent and progressive, without a precipitating event such as moving furniture or performing vigorous exercise, and if it doesn't go away within two weeks with rest and medication, you should check with your oncologist. Most back pain is caused by muscle or ligament injury, less commonly by metastatic disease that has reached the spine—but in the latter case, chiropractic manipulation can be harmful.

In general, you should avoid radiographic evaluation in a chiropractor's office (even some orthopedists' offices); equipment may not be up to hospital standards for high resolution or low radiation exposure, and your chiropractor may not be professionally trained to read x-rays for the presence of cancer.

Hands-on Therapies

The touch of someone who cares, who is ready to help you feel better, is valued in every culture. You know the expression: the magic touch. Whether as Swedish massage (rubbing, kneading, patting), Shiatsu (an ancient approach to healing through massage), Reiki (the Japanese version of laying-on-of-hands [more a *resting* of hands] to cure), or plain old hugs (an expression of the love and support of another human being), the immediate touch of hands and body results in an easing of tension and a sense of well-being. These touch therapies are gentle and should be safe.

Shiatsu and *Reiki* concentrate on the internal energy of the body, the source of wellness and health. Shiatsu practitioners manipulate prescribed surface points, (meridians) of the body to affect the inner Xi, vigorously at times, to reach down to deep internal muscle. Reiki practitioners rest their hands quietly on different areas of the body to serve as a conduit for "the healing force that is everywhere, that stimulates the subject's internal energy, to achieve natural healing." Reiki is a gentle approach to inner energy control, kind to the tender parts of women treated for breast cancer.

Conventional or *Swedish massage* is more and more popular and accessible. "I went to this masseuse—I was very nervous, I didn't know what to expect. It was very, very relaxing—especially when she did my feet, with the oils and music. " But Kelly had yet to tell her husband. Maybe it was too off-beat, too intimate, she wasn't sure, but she did know she wanted to do it again.

An expert masseuse knows how to get you to relax, how to gently ease away stress and tension. Massage was a godsend to Dell throughout her cancer care. "It was fabulous, really healing, a place to get away from all the emotional baggage of my life. I was in the middle of chemotherapy, having nightmares, feeling wretched, and I'd go for massage after the chemo—and sleep like a baby, like nothing was wrong. I couldn't believe the difference it made. I've kept it in my life, I love it so." Massage can restore confidence in the goodness and pleasure of your body.

Hugs are simply an intuitive and natural way of helping you heal. When someone hugs you, that person wants to convey hope for your well-being in as direct a way as one human being can communicate to another. "When Edie was so sick, she and her children were hugging and holding each other all the time. It was so important. I held back— I wish I hadn't."

Homeopathy

Homeopathy is a method of treatment that employs "a hair of the dog that bit you": It advocates the use of minute doses of medicine that in larger doses would bring on symptoms similar to those of the disease you are attempting to cure. (The opposite, *allopathy,* uses treatment that produces effects that contrast to those the disease produces, such as taking cold medication to dry up the nasal fluids.) The best known application of the homeopathy concept is how we treat allergies; minute doses of the allergen—say, pollen—are administered to the person allergic to pollen, to desensitize her to the plant.

Homeopathic desensitization has not been fully accepted by conventional medical practitioners, who claim that medications are administered in such dilute amounts that the effects are meaningless. There are no reliable studies to show any cancer remissions or cures from homeopathic cancer therapy.

Mind over Matter

Meditation, hypnosis, biofeedback, massage, yoga, and other relaxation techniques can diminish stress, exhaustion, fatigue, pain, and possibly illness. The techniques focus on a relaxation response that promotes concentration, energy, hopefulness, self-confidence, release from pain, and well-being. The relaxation response can slow metabolism and heart rate and lower blood pressure and muscle tension, in contrast to the "fight or flight" effects of stress, fear, and anxiety. You practice relaxation techniques in a quiet, familiar setting; as you become more skilled, you may be able to achieve that desired state even when buffeted by noise and activity.

Mind over matter: How do you enlist your mind to promote your well-being? Do you have any doubts about the power your mind can muster? Think about what happened when you were given that original breast cancer diagnosis. You felt pretty normal and healthy and balanced till those words slipped out of your doctor's mouth. A few words—and it was as if a load of bricks had landed on you. Or maybe you felt sick to your stomach, drained of energy, verging on tears, your sense of well-being transformed in an instant. Your mind brought on that overwhelmingly negative scenario. And this state of uncertainty, stress, and fear persists. Now it's up to you to alter this unpleasant mind-set, to get away from the constant burning issues of your treatment, to give yourself a break and rest, to achieve a measure of well-being—albeit in the face of a tough reality—by imagining, visualizing, and fantasizing good health and freedom from illness. It *will* help you. Here are some suggestions.

Meditation, or relaxation via mind manipulation, occurs with the repetition of word or nonword sounds, prayer, and thought. You know how hard it can be to get a melody out of your mind. That's the kind of mind-set you want to achieve with meditation: the insistent repetition of sounds that leads to concentration on the internal center of your being. "I wonder if I would have made the recovery I did without meditation. It was a tremendous help," Clara reflected.

It's very easy to work at relaxing—and find yourself asleep when you had planned to meditate. (If you fall asleep after a period of satisfying relaxation, that's fine.) To keep alert and awake, splash cold water on your face and sit in a position that will keep you alert and attentive. (Don't meditate in bed—my constant mistake.) Move your arms about in a rhythmic pattern. Focus and concentrate on an important thought. To learn complete techniques of relaxation, try Jon Kabat-Zinn's books.

Hypnosis is a kind of ultimate relaxation, usually requiring the direct assistance of another person to achieve that distinct, profound altered state of consciousness, something like a trance, something like sleep. The mechanism, again, is repetition of a controlled, monotonous action or sound. While you are under hypnosis, positive suggestions can be therapeutic: "When you wake up, you will feel less pain, you will feel energized and at peace." Some people find hypnosis the only way to get relief from pain.

Self-hypnosis can be taught to receptive individuals, who learn to put themselves into that altered state, suspending their connection with the distractions of their daily life, promoting relief from stress and illness, and securing some measure of control over trying symptoms.

Biofeedback was one of the first mind-body techniques accepted by conventional medicine, as a means to control high blood pressure. Biofeedback is a technique that uses the mind to control your body's physical response to stress and anxiety, resulting in reduced heart rate, blood pressure, or other responsive, measurable, body functions. While you practice a relaxation technique—say, meditation—heart rate and blood pressure are monitored by a trained practitioner to determine how well your body is responding to the relaxation effort.

Visualization, or *imagery,* is an imagining of precise or general visions to enhance peace of mind and body function. Writers can create worlds with words; film artists do it on celluloid; you can do it in your head. I tell my patients, "Visualize your immune system, your T cells consuming cancer cells, eliminating them from your body." One patient called me back the day after I saw her: "It worked for me: I created this image of Pac-Man eating the cancer cells. Maybe it's silly, but it gives me back some sense of control." "I imagine a huge vacuum bag—and I throw in anything that's bothering me."

Imagine yourself in a calm, peaceful place, like the countryside, or floating serenely in a beautiful lagoon in the midst of a romantic encounter, or drifting through a magnificent clothing shop, trying on ravishing gowns: personal movies to reduce stress and tension. Pick a place you can totally control—like an island—and take along whatever and whomever you want: your own chef, exercise guru, sex partner, entertainment center. Escape for a short break whenever you're having a hard time.

If you're the pragmatic type and aren't given to flights of fancy, think about real events, past and future. Maybe you'd like to rerun the "movie" memories of a family wedding, or picture the wedding you hope to put on for your daughter or son one day.

Visualization, fantasy, and daydreaming provide crucial distraction, escape, and relief from the focus on disease and distress—if only for a few restful minutes.

Humor was comfort therapy for Gena. "The night before my surgery, we watched this hysterical movie. I was still laughing about it on the way to the hospital, still feeling silly. It was very therapeutic for me." Edie had just received a devastating diagnosis; she needed time out from thinking about it. Elaine May and Walter Matthau took over her head for a couple of hours in the old movie *A New Leaf.* "I can't talk to you now," she told a friend, "I'm laughing too hard." Later she told her friend, "The movie was such a relief: I totally forgot about how sick I was." Her husband kept up her spirits with daily jokes from *The Big Book of Jewish Humor* that came from a thrift shop near the hospital.

Amy: "It's been years since my operation, but I still tell a joke each day, for myself and for the people I help out through my church." Ever hear the one about the woman who tells her doctor her husband's developed a passion for dog biscuits? "Tell him to stop. They'll kill him!" Six months later, they meet and the doctor learns she's a widow. "I told you those dog biscuits . . . " "No, no," she says, "he didn't die from the biscuits. He got run over chasing a car!" Or: This seventy-five-year-old woman comes back from Italy where she went to get pregnant with their new techniques. She has the baby, and her friends come over to see him. They wait, and they wait, and she says, "Soon, soon." Finally one says, "We're old, we can't wait anymore. We just want a peek." "Look," says the old new mother, "in a few minutes, he'll wake up, he'll cry—and then I'll remember where I put him!"

The Wellness Community, an organization dedicated to the interests of cancer patients, regularly holds joke fests. They are packed. Sessions in Boston had to be moved to Faneuil Hall, there were so many participants. People rolled in the aisles. "Some jokes were raunchy, even filthy—anything to make people happy, boost the immune system. I never slept better," reported a Wellness member.

Movement: Exercise and Dance

Body movement, control, and discipline have always been integral parts of Asian medicine. Western medicine has increasingly developed and promoted the therapeutic value of exercise and dance. Tangible proof of the benefit of exercise has been found with the discovery of endorphins, a substance produced by the brain, that measurably increases following exercise. Endorphins are similar in effect to opiates (i.e., morphine), reacting with the opiate receptors in the nervous system to raise tolerance of pain and increase the sense of well-being.

A program of exercise or dance allows for gradual strengthening of the body, providing, in addition to the esthetics and endorphins, the feeling of control over your body and your health. After recovering from her mastectomy, Gena worked out on her Nordic Track. "I got out a lot of my anger, striding on that machine. I did it naked and blindfolded, first to music, now in silence. It's powerful and primeval therapy for me—it makes me feel so strong." Tina had been regularly running eight miles a day when she was diagnosed with breast cancer. "I'd be bonkers, crazy, if I didn't run—you wouldn't want to be around me. I had to give it up for a couple of months and I'm still only back to about four miles a day. It's a life thing for me. When I run I feel powerful!"

You may not be up to quite that much vigorous activity. But you don't have to knock yourself out to get the benefits of exercise; any regular, moderate program will do. Tai Chi is gentle movement, as is interpretive dance. Dance can be self-expressive movement or a group routine, or it can be programmed routines in a group with a teacher or therapist. Dance therapy has been gaining ground and approval; it's such a pleasing activity, and for many individuals it allows them to dance out feelings that have been difficult to express verbally. If you can free yourself to move about in dance patterns of your invention, you may find benefits in relaxation, flexibility, muscle tone, and increased self-esteem.

Swimming is kind to the joints, and it can be leisurely or vigorous; classes in water aerobics, water walking, or dance are offered at many high schools or Ys. Or try walking, considered the ideal exercise by enthusiasts and exercise experts. Go with a friend, a group, or alone, listening to talking tapes or music. Your choices are limitless. What you choose should be something you enjoy and look forward to, so you'll keep it up for life.

Music Therapy

Deforia Lane, herself a breast cancer survivor of many years, is a doctor of music therapy who works in a hospital setting, treating people with cancer. She brings them her music and changes the atmosphere of illness, breaking through depression, anxiety, and fear—if only for a brief interlude. "I come in with my omnichord and get my patients to try it. (I even go into the operating room.) I make the sound go fast or slow, play harp or drums or whatever. Their bodies respond whether they want to or not. Music will allay anxiety—or nausea."

Dr. Lane talks to her patients and takes their ideas, their feelings, their thoughts, and puts them into song, right then and there. Not every song is poignant. "I've written songs about diarrhea, constipation, gas, enemas. Whatever my patients want songs about, we do. We laugh a lot, too." Dr. Lane's book, *Music as Medicine,* tells more.

Music reduces pain perception, helping to divert the mind. Some therapists are convinced it bolsters the immune system. (Studies of an enzyme in the saliva are trying to demonstrate this theory.) If nothing else, it can add hours of pleasure and distraction to your life. Rock and roll, blues, pop, rap, chamber music, symphonies, opera—take your choice, and let it take you away. "When I'm listening to an opera I love, I can *feel* the pleasure travel along my nerve pathways. It can overwhelm my senses, obliterate pain, make me forget the bad things in my life."

Postural Therapy

Yoga is a Hindu philosophic discipline of mind and body that seeks to achieve mental liberation from the tangible world. Postures, or positioning of the body, and breathing methods help the mind achieve this suspension of involvement with the "real" world; add calming background music, environmental sounds, or chants, and you can erase distracting thoughts from your consciousness and get to inner peace.

Disciplined breathing is an established form of relaxation. Singers and actors have been doing it for centuries; women have been doing it in delivery rooms for decades.

"It's a way of stepping outside yourself, getting a perspective on your problems," Dell explained. If you are successful, a kind of oblivion to worry and pain results: nirvana. Dell prefers doing her yoga in a class. "There's a connection with everyone there that I appreciate, even if I don't know each person. And you're away from distractions like the phone or family. The teacher adds soothing instructions as well. This is a gentle, easy discipline—we're not competing against anyone, especially not against ourselves. Sometimes I do it with my eyes open, sometimes with my eyes closed. Yoga helped me navigate not only through breast cancer, but through my divorce before that."

Spirituality

The support system to beat all: belief, faith, hope—whatever we all lean on when our souls reach out to a greater spirit, whether it's God, Allah, Shiva, Buddha, the Unknown, or Humankind. Amy, a devout churchgoer, organized a prayer chain to help herself and other cancer survivors; their names are part of a list, and church members pray for each of them in church on Sunday or at home. "God hears us wherever we pray. My name went on a list round the world when I first had breast cancer. I believe in prayer, and in doing something for others: I'm on wheels all day, taking people to the hospital and back. It's part of my faith, and part of what keeps me well."

Novella Lyons, breast cancer survivor and community leader, created a support group in her church: Women in Faith and Hope, which emphasizes spiritual healing as well as emotional support and education.

Spirituality is not necessarily religion. It calls on your inner being, on who you are, on a holistic idea: oneness of body and soul with a universal spirit. "I tell my patients to choose a spiritual guide whom they can call on, act through, imagine as their agent in the spiritual world," says Milly Fink, massage and Reiki specialist. "It can be your grandmother, a saintly person from the past, someone you love very much, whom you invest with your hopes and wishes, who helps you with your healing." Milly's patients in guided spiritual imagery say she's a minor miracle, and they stay with her for years.

Support Systems

We've known for many years that support groups help patients deal with the problems in their lives, but it wasn't till the late 1980s that we were given provocative evidence that support groups can actually help extend the lives of cancer patients. As I mentioned in an earlier chapter, Dr. David Spiegel conducted a ten-year controlled study of eighty-six women with metastatic cancer, half of whom had been enrolled in a weekly support group, the other half of whom had not. Over the ten-year study period, women in the support group lived twice as long as women without support and experienced a higher quality of life. Linked by their special bond, sharing their hopes and fears, laughing and crying together, encouraging each other to keep up healthful practices, and having the interest and attention of the professional group leader and Dr. Spiegel were factors that Dr. Spiegel believed made the difference. In addition, he felt these women handled pain, sadness, and even death with more equanimity than did the women without support.

Support therapy forms an essential backbone of many women's posttreatment experience. "The people in my life had heard enough. I couldn't unload any more on my kids or husband. This is the only place to talk and share, with women who *know*. A shared problem becomes so much easier to handle. It's been five years for me, twice a month. It's a lifeline."

Therapies within Easy Reach

Many of you have discovered your own ideas for adding positive, therapeutic programs to your life. One told me about the alternative therapy she had invented for herself. "I've started an organic vegetable garden. I find some interesting parallels to cancer and healing. Pulling weeds is ridding the body of uncontrolled cancer growth. Removing stones from the soil is getting rid of old attitudes and feelings that get in the way of healing. Adding compost and watering is practicing good nutrition to strengthen the body. And working in a garden provides a quiet time for true healing. It reconnects me with the earth and with my soul."

Pets can have a distinctive positive effect on people under stress; stroking a dog or cat can actually reduce blood pressure. For someone sick and stressed out, that simple, repetitive motion can work like meditation. Hospitals and nursing homes now have visiting pet programs for patients. The vivacity, the unswerving devotion, and the company a pet offers are other compelling reasons for bringing a pet into your life.

Therapies on the Fringe

Other therapies that sound compelling at first may fail to produce adequate results. In fact, some can be harmful. You need to balance hope with reality and take advantage of the therapies that will truly help you. What worries doctors most is that a patient may put off sound methods of treatment for breast cancer, and lose critical time and money, by experimenting with unproven, perhaps questionable, perhaps harmful, therapies.

Laetrile (or apricot pit therapy) contains cyanide in small amounts and is supposed to stop cancer growth. There are no studies to show its efficacy; the scattered, unverifiable case reports are not sufficient to make a case for treatment. And Laetrile can be harmful: High doses are poisonous. Furthermore, believers may put off proven therapies.

Shark cartilage: The book *Sharks Don't Get Cancer* (in fact, they do) has popularized shark cartilage as an anticancer agent. Proponents of the therapy say you have to take very large amounts to achieve the effect. In the laboratory, both shark and cow cartilage demonstrate the ability to limit the growth of new blood vessels that feed tumors, but that's in a lab, not in the body, not even in the body of a mouse. The theory is under investigation by the Office of Alternative Medicine at the National Institutes of Health. In the meantime, if you want to try cartilage therapy, it's not known to be harmful, but it is expensive and some people say it causes them to smell quite peculiar: strongly fishy if you settle on shark; no data on how you fare with cow.

Diet doctrines: Specific therapy diets can have healthy aspects, but the more defined and rigid they are, the smaller the population willing to adhere to their restrictions. The macrobiotic philosophy, for instance, which seeks to balance yin and yang, harmony and relativity, mandates a modification of lifestyle as well as diet. The macrobiotic diet has many healthy aspects to it (it's lower in fat than traditional American diets, for one), but the restriction against *all* animal protein and dairy products, sugar, flour, iced foods, tropical fruits, spices, and raw foods makes it trying for many people who otherwise find it has merit. (It can also create vitamin or mineral deficiencies.) "I tried all kinds of diets, and the Zen macrobiotic diet was one of the hardest to stick to—plus it was so bland and boring, compared to all the flavorful foods I grew up on in the American diet; I felt like I was being punished. I gave up the strict macrobiotic approach, but I did remain a vegetarian." The macrobiotic diet is supposed to be followed exactly for any purported anticancer benefits to occur. (Strict adherence to the diet requires a great deal of time shopping and preparing fresh and unusual foods.)

Gerson diet: This diet relies on purges with castor and linseed oil laxatives and coffee enemas to "detoxify" the body of carcinogens that are produced within our bodies or that come from the environment. The purge theory hinges on the idea that toxic elements should be cleared from our system as quickly as possible. Other aspects of the diet are elimination of almost all dietary fat, restriction of salt, and concentration on a vegetarian menu, except for liver—a rather mysterious inclusion, because the liver tends to concentrate by-products that are considered toxic by Gerson standards.

If taken to an extreme, the purge theory is particularly worrisome, because it can result in dehydration, malabsorption of essential nutrients, and chemical imbalances, which can be harmful and even cause death. A more prudent approach to the elimination of waste and toxins from the body is to consume generous amounts of fibrous foods that keep the bowel moving and healthy. I think a strict Gerson diet is radical and unsafe, and it should be avoided.

Other detoxification regimes: Detoxification of the bowel with a more moderate dietary and enema approach has become popular. Some women pursue these treatments, regularly or intermittently, at home or at a specialized health center.

Juicing large amounts of fresh vegetables and herbs, such as carrots and wheat grass, is the basis of vitamin and detoxification therapies, purported to boost your immune system and protect your body from toxins. These fluids are supposed to be consumed throughout the day; large quantities of fresh carrots or wheat grass are processed in a vegetable juicer to get the freshest juice possible. One therapy uses wheat grass juice as an enema tonic, to detoxify the bowel. "I felt just wonderful—and everyone, even the skeptics in my family told me how great I looked (especially my skin) when I came back from the California Health Institute." These detoxification methods are not proven to be harmless, helpful, or harmful. I don't recommend them.

Stanislaw Burzynski, M.D., Ph.D., discovered what are called antineoplastons: proteins your body excretes in urine. Burzynski claims antineoplastons correct the aberrant behavior of cancer cells, particularly those of prostate, lymphoma, pancreas, and brain tumors in children, as well as breast cancer, and that antineoplastons also help in the treatment of AIDS, lupus, multiple sclerosis, arthritis, skin disorders, and baldness. Antineoplaston action is not considered part of the immune system (which protects the body against foreign cells or substances); rather, it purportedly protects against damaging effects of substances formed within the body itself.

At one time part of mainstream research and medicine, Burzynski now operates independently in Houston, Texas, using fees from his patients to sustain his research. The cost of treatment can be extremely high, and it is not generally covered by insurance. Actual case results are hard to identify and properly interpret. Clinical studies have been meager, and it is difficult to establish actual therapeutic value. The antineoplaston theory remains largely unsubstantiated and controversial.

Joseph Gold claims hydrazine sulfate extends life by preventing the weight loss associated with widely metastatic breast cancer, called cachexia. He believes that widely metastatic cancer cells steal food and energy from the patient, making it difficult to function, and eventually to live, and that hydrazine sulfate halts that drain from the patient if given at the outset of treatment. Scientific studies, however, do not confirm Gold's claims.

Conclusion: Caveat Emptor

When you are diagnosed with breast cancer, you want the best therapeutic approach possible, one that combines your inner resources and the best of conventional and complementary medicine. Pursue your care in an open-minded, thoughtful, and critical manner. Reevaluate your choice of therapies periodically, and be prepared to modify your choice as needed.

Favor treatments with solid track records that have weathered critical studies. Your doctors worry about unsubstantiated cures, leading you to put off proven treatment for one that is unproven, losing precious time, funds, and the opportunity to effect a real cure or long-term disease remission. The American Cancer Society provides a list of unproved cancer therapies for anyone interested in unconventional cancer treatments, in an attempt to evaluate safe and sound options.

There are many choices in the compendium of complementary therapies: relaxation response, meditation, massage, herbs, chiropractic, traditional Chinese medicine, Ayurvedic, yoga, music, dance, and support systems. Once you've completed the conventional medical pathways, one of these therapies may improve your quality of life, offering comfort, relief, support, a sense of well-being—and, just maybe, prevention of recurrence and an extended life span.

If you have metastatic cancer and are seeking unconventional therapies after exhausting conventional medicine, or as a complement to conventional medicine, it's important to periodically reassess your response to this therapy with your sense of well-being and also with objective tests such as x-ray studies. I have a patient diagnosed with metastatic cancer who refused conventional medicine. She decided, having gone through conventional therapy some years before, to seek alternative therapies only: detoxification (coffee enemas) and vitamin therapy. Despite x-rays that showed continued progression of disease, she was determined to follow her choice of alternative therapy. Although I respect her taking charge of her life, establishing control when she was so vulnerable to forces beyond her control, I worry about her decision, and I find it very hard to take care of her.

Whatever your choice of treatment, once it stops working, it's time to stop doing it and try something different.

FIVE

The Threat of Recurrence

20

Can You Live Cancer Free?

It's not enough to say you're alive—it's the quality of your life that counts. Like the weather, I have sunny days and cloudy ones. I try to live as well as I can, and worry about as little as I possibly can—but not a day goes by that I don't think about cancer.

"How do I shake the ever-present fear of recurrence so I can live my life like a normal human being?" You respond in your own way to the challenge of this breast cancer experience. One woman insists on having a mammogram every six months; another has her eyes shut tight—has never had another mammogram and refuses to discuss anything that refers to cancer. One woman prints out a transcript from an audio tape she makes of every visit and telephone call to me, another woman seems to tune me out and doesn't appear to hear a word I say. Mary Catherine has not looked at her chest in the twelve years since her mastectomy. Betty's hand is always straying to her armpit, probing and checking for anything out of the ordinary. And Jane always calls me the morning after a "new" treatment is announced on TV or in the press.

As every woman who is living beyond breast cancer knows, even though doctors assure you of an excellent prognosis and you feel healthy and "cured," you are never rid of the knowledge that you had breast cancer and that it can happen again. Remember the whale in the living room that doesn't go away and can't be ignored? Sometimes shrinking to the size of a magazine rack, and, sometimes swelling up to fill your whole room? That's breast cancer fear.

Your Attitude

Are you stuck with a dark inner conviction that "I caused my cancer"? "Was it choosing hormone replacement therapy, the painful divorce, the loss of my job, eating junk food, smoking, not doing breast self-exam?" I can tell you with certainty, you did not bring on your cancer. It doesn't work that way.

But your attitude about yourself, your disease, and what you do after treatment make a big difference to how the rest of your life takes shape. Having a bad attitude or being depressed doesn't bring on the disease, but being depressed, with a paralyzing fear of breast cancer, might keep you from leading a healthy life, effectively managing lingering side effects, continuing with your medications and remedies, recognizing and acting on signs of early-stage breast cancer (new or recurrent), or taking charge of your relationship with your doctor to get the best care possible. In *that* sense, yes, your attitude matters very much. Work on ways to feel more positive about life. Search out productive, life-enhancing experiences. Accept yourself as the person you are, and put a positive "spin" on your attitude.

Your family, friends, doctor, and nurse can help by focusing on the challenges, joys, and simple routine aspects of your life, reinforcing the fact that you are more than your cancer. And it's empowering to learn about the latest discoveries in cancer research and to plan a course of action that incorporates nutrition, exercise, and mind-body therapies. This holistic approach puts your mind where it should be: in command of your own well-being.

If you are still convinced that cancer lurks in every corner of your body, your true risk of recurrence is probably a lot lower than what you perceive it to be. Your doctor can tell you the statistics: five-year survival for stage-one disease is 80 to 95 percent; for stage two, 60 to 80 percent; for stage three, 40 to 60 percent; and for stage four (metastatic), 0 to 20 percent. The chance of developing a new breast cancer (unrelated to the first) is about 1 percent per year, or about 10 percent over ten years.

The value of statistics is limited, of course. They're reassuring when the odds are in your favor. But even when your diagnosis is grim, you may be able to beat out the odds.

21

Recurrence: When Cancer Comes Back

I had my first mastectomy when I was thirty-four years old. Twenty years later, I had my second—and in a way it was an enormous relief—I had always expected that second breast cancer. I never thought I'd reach forty, and here I am pushing sixty-five.

My lung mets [metastases] have been stable for three years now—but I keep waiting for them to go away completely—I wish. When I get my checkup every six months, I'm always a little relieved, and a little disappointed—but I'm not complaining.

Is this the chapter you flipped to first in this book—or the one you avoided till last? The Big Unknown? "It's always on my mind—sometimes it's a banging drum; other times it's background music. The slightest pain and I think it's come back." "Recurrence—the word is like cold fingers on my heart."

It's Back

"I think there's a problem. . . ." If your doctor has just made this announcement, after your original breast cancer had come and, you thought, gone, all those early chaotic feelings surge back over you, and you're devastated. It's worse than the first time, most of my patients say.

When "I think there's a problem" is followed a few days later by "The tests show it's cancer," questions you're too frightened to ask stick in your throat. That terrifying disease is back. It's beyond unfair: double jeopardy, fury of the gods.

How could this have happened—after working so hard to do everything right, following every doctor's recommendation, eating all the right foods, drinking all that strange juice, exercising to exhaustion. "I just can't believe it. The first time was more frightening, the second I was angry! That first surgery was to have prevented the second!" There's a lot of anger that hovers over this crisis: anger at your doctors for their failure to cure you, anger at yourself for not beating the disease, anger at your body for betraying you yet again.

Then comes angst over the things you did or didn't do: "Maybe I should have had the mastectomy." "Why did I stop the tamoxifen when I did?" "I knew I should have gone for the adriamycin instead of the methotrexate." "That second opinion was right, God help me." "How could I have waited so long when I felt that lump—I was sure it was just scar tissue." All this second-guessing gets you nowhere, but it's not easy to let it go. You're trying to make sense of something that makes no sense, pin blame where there isn't any. Maybe it helps to unload your distress *somewhere,* but torturing yourself does you no good. After the shock waves settle down, it's time to go on.

Recurrence is not a death sentence. No matter how grim your circumstances, there is *always* something that can be done to help you. Local recurrence may be curable, and metastatic disease may be put in long-term remission. Your prognosis depends on the type and pattern of recurrence: local, regional, or distant recurrence; number of areas involved, specific organ involvement, size of recurrence; interval since original treatment; and the particular cancer treatments you've already had. All of these facts and the circumstances of your situation as it is now need to be reviewed carefully, and only then can you work out a plan of action. "I knew I beat the odds the first time. I just figured I'd do it again."

Your relationship with your doctor is more important now than ever. You need kindness, compassion, accessibility, and attention in giant-size doses. " 'We're going for total cure.' My surgeon looked so bright and positive, I burst out: 'If you're going for total cure, then so am I!' " If your doctor is repeatedly not as there for you as you'd like, or if you have serious misgivings about your relationship or his or her expertise, maybe it's time to address these issues, and see if you can work it out to your satisfaction, and, if not, consider a change.

You need good friends at this time, but you may find that some friends, even some women who have also had breast cancer, may be unable to listen or talk with you about this news. They may pull away—their cancer worry, their fear that it can happen to them, gets wrenched to the surface. Now is a time that a support group can be very helpful, a safe place to share your concerns with other women in a similar situation. (See Chapter 2.)

How Breast Cancer Recurs

When cancer comes back, it is a regrowth of the cancer you were previously diagnosed with, the cancer your doctors and you believed was eradicated or put into remission. Cancers from other parts of the body, such as the colon or endometrium, rarely spread to the breast or to the chest wall area where the breast used to be. Metastases to the lung, liver, bones, and brain are more likely to have come from your prior breast cancer than from a new and different cancer.

How could this have happened? It's hard to make sense of this diagnosis, particularly if your original cancer was completely confined to the breast (with or without lymph node involvement), your chest x-ray, blood work, and bone scan were all normal, and your surgeon assured you: "I got it all."

Tests can detect a growth of one half to one centimeter, but they are not currently sensitive enough to detect a small collection of cancer cells visible only under a microscope. Since your original diagnosis and completion of treatment, those breast cancer cells that somehow escaped destruction remained undetected and then grew to a size that is now detectable by x-ray, or big enough to be felt or to cause symptoms, at the site of the original breast cancer or elsewhere in your body.

Type and Site of Recurrence

Breast cancer can return in three ways: local, regional, metastatic. Local recurrence occurs in the breast where it started, or in the skin and underlying tissues where the breast used to be. Regional recurrence shows up in the lymph nodes next to the affected breast. Metastatic cancer is cancer that has spread beyond the breast area and the immediately adjacent lymph nodes.

Local cancer recurrence in the previously treated breast develops from cells that weren't removed by surgery or weren't successfully eliminated by radiation or chemotherapy. When breast cancer develops in a completely separate part of the same breast or in the other breast, it is usually a new cancer, unrelated to the first. That is, it is not considered a *re*-occurrence, but another *first* occurrence.

After mastectomy, cancer that recurs on the soft tissues of the chest, where the breast used to be, grew from breast cancer cells close to the skin or behind the breast area against the muscle of the chest wall; this is referred to as a chest wall recurrence.

In rare cases, a "brand new" breast cancer can develop following mastectomy from one of the few remaining normal breast cells that adhered to the skin lying over the breast or along the muscle behind the breast. These cells that remained after surgery were presumably normal at the time of the mastectomy, but later they developed into a cancer. A careful review of the tissue biopsy by an experienced pathologist can usually differentiate this kind of new breast cancer from a recurrence of a previous one. The prognosis of this type of chest wall breast cancer may be more favorable than a true chest wall recurrence.

Regional recurrence is the term used for cancer that grows in lymph nodes adjacent to the breast from cells that were presumably present but undetectable at the time of original surgery, or from cells that recurred in the breast and then later spread to lymph nodes. The immediately adjacent lymph node groups include the axillary region (underarm) (some, if not most, of these lymph nodes were probably removed during diagnosis and treatment of the original breast cancer); the internal mammary region (under the chest wall, along the length of the breastbone); and the infrapectoral region (under the pectoralis muscle that goes from your shoulder to your chest; these lymph nodes are also called Rotter's nodes).

Metastatic recurrence is disease that develops in another part of the body, such as the lymph nodes at the base of the neck, or in the lung, liver, bone, or brain. Twenty to 30 percent of all women who are first diagnosed with cancer limited to the breast eventually go on to develop metastases from cancer cells that presumably were present but undetectable at first diagnosis. Thirty to 60 percent of women with lymph node involvement at initial diagnosis eventually develop metastases; their risk depends largely on the number of positive lymph nodes and other characteristics of the tumor.

When Does Recurrence Happen?

Cancer recurrence most often develops within the first five years after treatment. The median time for developing local and regional recurrence after initial treatment for breast cancer is three years; the median time for developing distant recurrence is two years. (*Median* is the middle point in a range of intervals, roughly similar to the concept of an *average*.)

But breast cancer also can come back twenty-five years after the original treatment, in the same place where it started or in some other part of the body. When this happens, the cancer cells have been in your body all along—they just grew very, very, very slowly.

Local Recurrence

When a recurrence is suspected, initial tests—generally including a biopsy—are performed to establish the diagnosis. If recurrence is confirmed, additional tests are performed to define the nature and extent of the cancer before appropriate treatment can be defined and implemented (just as was done at the time of the initial diagnosis). (See Chapter 5.)

About 80 percent of the women who develop a recurrence in the breast have no documented metastases before or at the time of the breast recurrence; about 40 percent have lymph node involvement. About 80 percent of breast cancer recurrence limited to the breast can be completely removed by surgery.

The type of cancer that comes back after radiation therapy can be invasive or noninvasive. Two thirds of the breast cancers that come back in the same breast come back in the same place or right next to the original cancer.

One third of breast recurrences are found by mammography alone; one third by physical exam alone; one third by both (see Chapter 5).

If you had a lumpectomy, with or without breast radiation, for your original breast cancer, local recurrence is suspected when you and your doctor find a new, persistent, and enlarging lump or a discrete area of new thickening in the breast; or when the mammogram detects a distorted area of the breast that is worrisome, a new mass, or a new cluster of small calcifications.

Don't panic if you find a lump in your breast at the site of the original tumor. Within the first year of completing your cancer treatment, it is common to have a smooth, flat firmness within the area around the scar where the tumor used to be, the same area where the surgeon operated and where the radiation boost was delivered. As radiation-related swelling of the whole breast resolves, you and your doctor may find that this firmness feels relatively more prominent. This probably is normal scar tissue, but should be evaluated further if you or your doctor is more concerned.

A discrete lump in the area of the scar soon after surgery is most likely one of two things. It may be fatty tissue that disintegrated because of the effects of treatment (called fat necrosis), which can produce irregular hard lumps of various sizes that stay the same or gradually get smaller over time. The second possibility is that it is a suture granuloma along the scar, a very small (about three millimeters or one-quarter inch), hard, smooth, beadlike nodule consisting of scar tissue wrapped around a little stitch your surgeon tied when sewing the area back together. This, too, does not get bigger with time.

An uncommon example of local recurrence after lumpectomy, with or without radiation, is when the whole breast swells up. The skin becomes thick and looks something like the skin of an orange, with part of the area having a reddish-pink color, with or without an underlying mass; this may be an inflammatory breast cancer recurrence. This condition can sometimes be confused with breast infection, called mastitis, which is much more common, benign, and responsive to antibiotics.

If you had mastectomy for your original breast cancer, with or without reconstruction, local recurrence can also be felt or seen on the skin where the breast used to be, in the soft tissues that remain on the chest wall, or in the reconstructed breast. After mastectomy with reconstruction, suture granulomas can form along the incision; when tissue reconstruction is also done, lumps and fat necrosis are fairly common (much more common than after lumpectomy). Again, these are benign, not cancerous. How do you tell the difference? A new, irregular, firm to hard, pearly pink to red, fleshy, usually nontender nodule within or under the skin, with or without ulceration, is strong evidence of recurrence. The nodule is most likely to occur along the scar, but it can also occur in the general area where the breast used to be. "I have a lump on my chest now, over my mastectomy scar. I've had it for two weeks. I keep denying it, but I'm going to have it checked today." Evaluation is done by biopsy. Mammography is not usually performed on a tissue-reconstructed breast (although I've seen it detect recurrence in a number of women), and it can't be done on implant reconstruction (see Chapter 5).

A red velvety rash with swelling of the skin can be an infection or an inflammatory type of recurrence. But if the rash has areas of ulceration, it is almost certainly cancer.

Regional Recurrence

After mastectomy or lumpectomy (with or without radiation), you may develop regional lymph node recurrence: a hard, persistent, and enlarging lymph node in the armpit or at the base of the neck, which may cause new swelling of the arm on that side.

Regional recurrence in lymph nodes under the arm alone is rare. Fewer than 5 percent of women treated for breast cancer have recurrence that happens this way. Most regional recurrences are associated with breast or chest wall recurrence, rather than by themselves. Recurrence in the lymph nodes under the arm (axillary) is more common than recurrence in the lymph nodes above the clavicle or collarbone (supraclavicular lymph nodes), which in turn is more common than lymph node involvement below the clavicle (infraclavicular), or in the internal mammary chain. The relative rarity of reports of internal mammary recurrence is partly because these nodes are nonpalpable and rarely seen on a chest x-ray. Even when they are enlarged, they don't usually cause symptoms of new and progressive chest pain until they erode the overlying sternum (the breastbone). The supraclavicular and infraclavicular lymph nodes are considered metastatic sites of disease.

Metastatic Recurrence

I suspect metastatic disease if my patient develops a new, persistent, and progressive symptom in a particular part of her body. For example, if a woman comes to me with persistent (more than two to three weeks) and progressive back pain, I order a whole-body bone scan, with or without plain bone x-rays of specific areas (see Chapter 5). If there is evidence of cancer in the spine, I order a magnetic resonance imaging (MRI) test to better understand the extent of the disease in the back and its relationship to the spinal cord, which lies in the spinal canal within the spine. If the tumor is growing near the spinal cord, emergency treatment must be given to avoid irreversible spinal cord injury.

If a woman comes in with new headaches, changes in vision, unexplained persistent and progressive nausea, a specific area of numbness or weakness, personality change, confusion, or new seizures or falling episodes, I order a computed axial tomography (CAT) scan or an MRI to evaluate the brain for possible metastases.

Abdominal discomfort that is persistent and progressive, and isn't explained by history or physical examination, is evaluated first with blood work, then with plain x-ray, ultrasound, and/or CAT scan of the abdomen.

The development of persistent and progressive cough, shortness of breath, or chest pain beyond what can be explained by history or physical examination, is first evaluated by obtaining a chest x-ray; if called for, further evaluation with a CAT scan of the chest may follow. When breast cancer involves the lung tissue, it usually affects both sides, showing up as round ball-like masses. Less commonly, it can appear as a hazy area (an infiltrate) along the lymphatic and blood vessels, called lymphangitic spread. For a cough producing blood or other signs of airway obstruction, bronchoscopy will be recommended to further evaluate your condition and to obtain a biopsy. Cancer cells can grow in the space between the lung and the inside surface of the chest wall, which causes an accumulation of fluid in that space, called a pleural effusion.

Sometimes metastatic disease is detected on routine medical evaluation without any symptomatic clues. Routine blood work might show an elevated cancer marker CEA (carcino embryonic antigen), elevated liver function enzymes, or high levels of calcium or alkaline phosphatase. A routine bone scan (ordered by some oncologists) might light up in new places, indicating cancer.

Biopsy to Confirm Recurrence

The purpose of a biopsy is to establish a definitive diagnosis of recurrent breast cancer, and to rule out other, noncancer causes of the problem. Knowing what you are dealing with is the first step in knowing what to do.

Biopsy is always done if there is anything that makes your doctor suspicious about local or regional recurrence, or about possible metastases in an accessible area such as a lymph node at the base of the neck. If there is strong evidence that cancer has spread throughout the body, a biopsy of the most easily accessible abnormal cancerous region is performed. If tests show a problem limited to the liver or to lymph nodes in the abdomen, or if the problem is limited to the lung and there is not a more accessible lesion to biopsy, a biopsy of the abnormality can be done under ultrasound or CAT scan guidance (to direct the biopsy needle to the correct spot). A needle biopsy is the preferred biopsy procedure because it is the least invasive. (Chapter 5 describes the various biopsy techniques.)

Lung lesions near the center of the chest may also be biopsied through bronchoscopy, and fluid around the lung can be removed by thoracentesis and analyzed for the presence of cancer cells. (In thoracentesis, a hollow needle is inserted between the ribs; fluid is drawn off and sent to a laboratory for analysis.)

Biopsy is not usually recommended in the following cases: (1) The radiographic (x-ray) findings are clearly consistent with metastasis, as are test results of other parts of the body; (2) the affected part of the body is difficult to reach safely for biopsy (such as the brain, spine, or eye); (3) biopsy would cause undue side effects, and results would not alter treatment; (4) breast cancer metastases have been established, and a new site of involvement may be presumed to be caused by the same cancer.

You and your doctor will decide whether to biopsy or not, which area to biopsy, and which biopsy technique to choose.

Once the biopsy is obtained, the tissue is examined under a microscope and compared with the cells of the original breast cancer. (Your prior pathology slides are stored in the pathology department's archives.) The appearance of the two cancers is usually very similar, if not identical. But occasionally the metastatic cancer does not resemble the original, raising the possibility that a new kind of cancer such as colon or uterine cancer may have developed. Additional studies are then done to identify the type of cancer that is present, so the appropriate treatment can be implemented.

Stop and Take a Breath

You must be exhausted by all the tests you've been put through, and by gathering all the bits of information coming in from different directions—the tests, your doctors, this book—but you are also exhausted by all of the uncertainty, fear and anxiety, and isolation. I believe the sooner you and your doctors figure out what your problem is and decide on a course of action (even if your prognosis is grim and requires aggressive treatment), the sooner you can begin to restore your energy, do what needs doing, and get on with your life.

(If you have not had a recurrence but are just reading this section to keep informed, it's likely you'll shortly develop highly suspicious symptoms. This is a very natural reaction.)

Once the diagnosis of recurrence has been confirmed, meet with your doctor to fully define the extent of the problem, figure out what it means, and consult with other doctors on your team. Together you will establish a battle plan. All this takes time; these are not discussions that can be rushed.

You know your doctors from before and you are probably more comfortable asking for what you need and want than you were the first time. Take your time; get the information and attention you need, even if it means extra office visits and phone calls to go over some things again, not because you forgot, but because fear and shock blurred what you heard at that first go-round. New information has to be added to the picture, and family members are seeking clarification. Gather your strength and confront the challenge. Let's move on to the battle.

Managing Local and Regional Recurrence

"I had two primary cancers, one in each breast; then I had the first recurrence, and then the second. I had to find someone I could talk to, who had at least as many nodes involved as I had—not five or six, but *seven*—or more. When I found her, I would call whenever I needed a support 'fix.' 'Get rid of the garbage in your life,' she'd always say. We still talk every now and then. She's been more than sixteen years 'out,' and I'm eight from that last recurrence."

Defining the Problem

If you find you have local or regional recurrence, how do you assess your prognosis and determine your treatment? Doctors rely on a list of predictive factors, or prognosticators, that help describe the cancer's character, or personality. Prognosticators for recurrence, which mirror those in the original diagnosis, are most meaningful when considered together.

The prognostic factors that most strongly and reliably predict the cancer's nature and your outcome include the following:

1. Invasive or noninvasive breast cancer: Is your cancer confined to the breast structure where it started or has it started to break through barriers, invading normal surrounding breast tissue (a sign of invasive breast cancer)? Noninvasive tumors are more favorable.
2. Interval between original treatment and recurrence: How soon after your original treatment for breast cancer was the recurrence discovered? Did your cancer come back within two years of finishing treatment for your first cancer or after two years?
3. Lymph node involvement: Has the cancer in your breast spread to lymph nodes? Which lymph nodes? How many lymph nodes? (Removal of lymph nodes as part of your original treatment for breast cancer may make it harder to reliably assess your lymph nodes now. There will be fewer lymph nodes left to evaluate, and lymphatic drainage of the breast area has probably been altered.) Having no lymph node involvement is more favorable. If lymph nodes are involved, the fewer involved, the more favorable the outlook.

Prognostic indicators of moderate significance include the following:

4. Size of recurrence: Is the size of the in-breast recurrence more than one centimeter, more than two centimeters, or over five centimeters? Does it involve the skin? Is the recurrence after mastectomy on the tissues where the breast used to be small or diffuse (rashlike)? The smaller the cancer, the less likely it has traveled elsewhere and the more likely that it can be removed completely.
5. Hormone receptors: The presence of hormone receptors in the breast cancer cells, where the cells interact with estrogen and progesterone, has prognostic and therapeutic significance. If hormone receptors are present, the prognosis is more favorable than if

they are absent. The higher the level of receptor activity, the better the response to hormone therapies such as tamoxifen.

6. Rate of growth: What proportion of the cancer cells are growing and reproducing? If more than 6 to 10 percent (the number depends on which laboratory and test are used) of the cancer cells are proliferating, the rate of growth is considered high and less favorable. Two tests measure proliferation rate: S-phase fraction and Ki-67.

7. Grade: When the pathologist looks at the cancer under the microscope, does it look high grade (angry, disorganized, irregular, with many cells in the process of making new cells)? Or does it appear low grade (calm, well organized, with few cells reproducing)? Moderate grade is the middle of the spectrum. The lower the grade, the more favorable the expected outcome.

8. Lymphatic and vascular invasion: When the pathologist looks at the cancer under the microscope, has it invaded the normal lymphatic channels and blood vessels within the breast tissue? The presence of invasion is considered a sign of an aggressive cancer.

9. Number of chromosomes: Do the cancer cells have a normal number of chromosomes (diploid) or do they have an abnormal number (aneuploid)? Diploid cancers are more favorable than aneuploid cancers, but this difference in outcome is small.

10. Prior chemotherapy: Recurrence soon after conventional chemotherapy indicates a "clever" tumor that was able to hold out against the original treatment and is more likely to resist new treatment.

11. Age and menopausal status: If you are premenopausal and younger than forty, your cancer may behave in a more aggressive manner than that of a woman who is beyond menopause.

12. New cancer, not recurrence: If your cancer occurs in an area of the breast or in tissues of the chest wall entirely separate from where your initial cancer was located, particularly if more than five years have elapsed since your initial diagnosis, then your current cancer is more likely to represent a new cancer rather than a recurrence of the prior cancer. The prognosis for a new cancer is generally, but not always, more favorable than a recurrent kind.

Treatment of Local and Regional Recurrence

Treatment for local and/or regional recurrent breast cancer has two possible approaches: *local regional treatment,* which treats your entire breast or breast area, and/or adjacent lymph nodes; and *systemic treat-ment*—chemotherapy and hormonal therapy—which treats your whole body, or system. Every woman diagnosed with recurrent breast cancer needs local treatment. Although not every woman needs treatment to her whole system, if you have a recurrence, you should discuss the pros and cons of systemic therapy for your particular condition with a medical oncologist.

Recurrence in the Breast

Local treatment is directed at the whole breast. Your original treatment choices were mastectomy (removal of the whole breast) and lumpectomy (removal of the portion of the breast that contained the cancer, with radiation to treat the remainder of the breast). Your current options are more limited.

If your original treatment was lumpectomy with radiation, then mastectomy is now the only proven option for treatment of the whole breast. Radiation is no longer an option because the breast has already received its maximum allowable radiation dose. It's questionable whether less surgery—complete removal of the recurrent lump only—is a medically equivalent alternative, as the remainder of the breast would not be treated. Doctors in France and Switzerland have published several studies describing results of lumpectomy alone in women who developed a single site of cancer recurrence in the breast. There were more repeat recurrences of cancer in the breast (roughly one third more) when women were treated this way than when they were treated with mastectomy, but it appears that women treated either way live equally long.

I recommend mastectomy for recurrence for three reasons: (1) its effectiveness is most clearly established, (2) I have more experience with this approach (this is how I was trained and how other doctors I work with have been trained), and (3) most of my patients feel uncomfortable watching and waiting for another local recurrence, for which they'd be at even higher risk if they elected lumpectomy alone. Mastectomy makes it unlikely that they'd have to face the same news again: "Your mammogram shows a problem." Rarely has a woman I've taken care of for recurrence refused a mastectomy and insisted instead on a lumpectomy alone to keep her breast.

If you had lumpectomy alone for your first breast cancer (without radiation), and now you have a breast cancer recurrence that is present only at the original site of the first breast cancer, if it is four centimeters or less, if it is completely removable, and if mammography is otherwise clear, you do have a choice of local therapies: mastectomy, or lumpectomy and radiation.

Regardless of your previous local treatment, if you develop an in-flammatory breast cancer in the same breast, associated with a persistent and progressive red rash on the skin and enlargement of the breast, with or without an underlying lump, your doctor will recommend a mastectomy. Systemic treatment—chemotherapy and hormonal therapy—should be given first, followed by mastectomy. If no radiation was given for the original breast cancer, then radiation should also be given, after chemotherapy, coordinated with the mastectomy.

Local treatment also involves an assessment of possible lymph node involvement at the time of mastectomy. There are certain circumstances, however, when lymph node removal may not be done: (1) if there are few lymph nodes left under the arm after your original breast cancer (unless your original breast cancer was not invasive and your lymph nodes were not removed), (2) if your doctors judge the risk of lymph node involvement to be very low, (3) if your recurrence is noninvasive, (4) if the results of the removal will have no impact on treatment decisions, or (5) if you have significant arm edema or are at high risk for it as a result of prior treatment.

The role of systemic treatment for the management of recurrent disease is based on your relative risk for developing metastatic disease. That risk is based on the prognostic factors discussed at the beginning of this chapter. These factors, and the chemotherapy options that are available to you, are discussed in the last section of this chapter.

Limited Chest Wall Recurrence

When cancer recurs after a mastectomy in the area where the breast used to be (commonly as one or a small cluster of nodules just beneath the skin surface, which may be pink or red), the best initial management is surgery. The area of visible and palpable tumor is removed, then radiation to the chest wall is begun, provided the area involved is discrete and removable, and you have not had radiation after your original mastectomy. Radiation therapy starts when the incision has healed (about two weeks after surgery).

If you have already had radiation, a moderate dose of additional radiation (about 3000 centigrays [cGy]) may be effective and relatively safe when combined with direct heat therapy (hyperthermia) or chemotherapy. You and the radiation therapist must make the decision whether to give additional radiation, even a limited dose, and very carefully. The additional radiation therapy increases the risk of side effects from your prior radiation, including breakdown and non-healing of the skin, rib fractures, excess scarring of the muscles, and possibly even heart problems if the left side of the chest is the side that receives the additional radiation.

If you had reconstruction of the breast with either a tissue flap or an implant, your doctor may recommend removal of the reconstructed breast, depending on the extent of the recurrent cancer, the length of time between your original cancer and its recurrence, and how aggressive the tumor seems to be.

Systemic therapy is likely to be recommended in addition to local therapy to the chest wall area, to improve control of the local site of cancer and to eradicate any cells that might have escaped beyond the local area. Your risk of wandering cells is significant; at least half the women who develop chest wall recurrence after a mastectomy develop distant metastases along with, or relatively soon after, the chest wall recurrence. An exception to this is the postmenopausal woman who is many years beyond her initial mastectomy and who has a small removable recurrence on the chest wall.

Diffuse Chest Wall Recurrence

Definitive treatment for diffuse chest wall recurrence involves radiation (assuming you did not have it before) and chemotherapy. If the nodules are widely scattered in or under the skin where the breast used to be, or if you have an enlarging red rash, the recurrence is unlikely to be removable.

I believe it is a mistake to try to remove the area of the diffuse rash even with the skills of the best breast cancer surgeon and plastic surgeon. The operation is extremely long, the convalescence can take many months, and some areas may simply not heal because of tension of the skin that has been sewn back together or because of tumor regrowth along the new incisions. Furthermore, the initiation of more effective treatments (radiation and chemotherapy) is delayed because of the length of recovery and inadequate healing. The patients I have taken care of in this situation are invariably exasperated; they are unable to get on with other therapies they know they should have, and cancer regrowth along an open, nonhealing incision causes symptoms, and is an ever-present reminder of the cancer.

Unfortunately, even with effective radiation and chemotherapy, a diffuse chest wall recurrence is likely to come back again, in the same area, or extending away from the breast area to the other breast, down along the upper abdomen, or to the back area. The skin recurrence can produce a stiff feeling to the involved skin (called *en cuirass* recurrence, French for leather-like). Some areas may grow into nodules or mounds; the tumor can break through the skin, weep fluid, and bleed (so it sticks to your clothes and may become infected and smelly); and you may have pain. Additional radiation may be given to the specific problem areas, with or without hyperthermia or radiation-sensitizing chemotherapy.

Hyperthermia has gone in and out of favor for many years. However popular or unpopular it is at the moment, it does make a moderate dose of radiation act more like a high dose ("a bigger bang for the buck") at least for the first few months, which may mean important short-term relief. It is available in relatively few centers, however. I have had several patients who were helped by combined radiation therapy and hyperthermia. Chemotherapies, such as fluorouracil, Taxotere, and Taxol, can also act synergistically with radiation.

Simultaneous Breast or Chest Wall Recurrence and Metastases

A significant group of women experience both chest wall recurrence and distant metastases; a smaller number of women experience both recurrence in the breast and metastases. The two groups need different approaches.

If you have both a chest wall recurrence and distant metastases, local treatment and systemic treatment for metastases are both important. The next chapter helps identify the appropriate roles of local and systemic therapies.

Although it is true that hormone therapy and chemotherapy can help control the cancer on the chest, I also recommend surgical removal of a limited chest wall recurrence and radiation therapy as soon as possible (assuming the place to be treated falls within a manageable treatment area). These local therapies are the most effective means of preventing or postponing an out-of-control chest wall recurrence.

Local therapy can be given at the same time as any hormonal regimen, but it cannot be given at the same time as all types of chemotherapy. If your chemotherapist is pushing to get started with an adriamycin-based regimen immediately because of rapidly progressive metastases, extensive liver involvement, or diffuse lung involvement causing shortness of breath, proceed with the chemotherapy first and hold off the radiation till later. Radiation is not usually given together with adriamycin because of excessive side effects. If your doctor is recommending Taxotere or Taxol instead of adriamycin for the above problems, it may be possible to give concurrent radiation, depending on the dosage of the drugs and the seriousness of your other problems.

Inflammatory breast cancer recurrence diagnosed along with metastatic disease is treated with chemotherapy first. Whether you have surgery and radiation depends on how you respond to the chemotherapy in the breast and in the rest of your body, and on your general medical and psychological condition.

If you have metastatic breast cancer as well as an asymptomatic localized recurrence in the breast without skin involvement, you need systemic therapy first, with local treatment delayed as long as the cancer is in remission or is not causing local symptoms. These are my treatment recommendations; your unique circumstances and your own doctor's judgment may lead to a different plan of action.

Radiation Therapy for Chest Wall Recurrence

Radiation is an essential part of the definitive care of chest wall recurrence, controlling local disease on the chest wall area. A dose of 5000 cGy over five to five and a half weeks is given to the soft tissues of the chest wall area, but a higher dose may be necessary if there are still nodules on the chest wall tissues, or if the nodules were removed with positive margins (cancer cells along the edge of the surgical boundaries). The dose doesn't usually exceed 6600 cGy. Radiation to the lymph nodes may also be recommended.

The procedure that maps out the radiation fields to be treated is called simulation. If you have had a reconstruction, the reconstructed breast will also be within the treatment field. Your plastic surgeon may tell you to have your radiation therapist treat only the area of recurrence and leave any other reconstructed area alone, but that is simply not possible.

The area at risk for chest wall recurrence includes the actual site of recurrence as well as the whole area where the breast used to be. The goal of the radiation planning process is to maximize the dose to the areas that need to be treated—the skin and immediate underlying tissues, because this is where the cancer cells are lurking—and minimize the dose to the normal surrounding tissues. Radiation to the chest wall eventually results in a brisk, tender, red skin reaction, with possible areas of wet peeling (like a blister) or dry peeling (like an old sunburn). A brisk skin reaction is associated with a better response to treatment because it is direct evidence that a therapeutic dose of radiation has in fact been delivered to the tissues at risk.

It takes a few weeks to develop the pinkness, then redness, and the area usually becomes sore and itchy. The discomfort and itching respond nicely to aloe vera (in a fragrance-free, alcohol-free preparation, or directly from the plant), Aquaphor, A & D ointment, or 1 percent hydrocortisone cream. Aloe and Aquaphor may carry you a few weeks, but eventually you'll have to use cortisone, applied lightly three times a day. The 1 percent cream is usually enough (available over the counter), though some women do need the 2.5 percent strength, which requires a prescription. Tylenol (by pill) can help with the soreness of the area. By the fifth week, the skin is mostly red. Any open skin areas that develop need to be kept clean with a half-and-half solution of hydrogen peroxide and water, two to three times daily, followed by Aquaphor or A & D ointment (A & D is a lot cheaper and more readily available). Some women like Bag Balm, meant for cow's udders (moo cares; it works).

These skin reactions can really frighten you, but believe it or not, they all heal. New skin grows to cover the open spaces, migrating from the edges of the area, forming pale, pearly white circles of new skin that eventually coalesce to cover the entire chest space. Within a few weeks of ending radiation, the area should be completely healed. It may take a little longer for the skin to return to something more like its normal color, and its not uncommon for the skin to remain somewhat pinker or tanner than the skin on the other side of your chest. You might be scared by shooting twinges of discomfort and stiffness of the chest wall that may occur randomly, but it's just inflammation of the tissues of the chest wall, and it responds nicely to anti-inflammatory agents, such as Tylenol.

Radiation therapy to the chest wall can affect an existing reconstructed breast or the options for future reconstruction. If you have a breast implant beneath the skin and muscle of the chest area at the time of radiation for local recurrence on the chest wall, radiation can cause some stiffening of the skin overlaying the implant, and it can increase the scar-tissue capsule that forms around the implant. The chance of developing a hard capsule that becomes painful and distorts the shape of the reconstructed breast is about 20 percent. Radiation to a tissue-reconstructed breast, such as a TRAM flap, may make the tissue stiffer, but it rarely if ever jeopardizes the viability of an established flap.

If initially you had a mastectomy without reconstruction, and then you had a local recurrence that was treated with radiation, you can still have reconstruction, if that's what you want. But your options may be somewhat limited. The success of a tissue expander/permanent implant may be limited because the radiation-induced scar tissue makes the skin thicker and stiffer and thus harder to expand. A tissue flap can usually be performed without much difficulty.

Treatment of Regional Lymph Node Recurrence

The treatment of lymph node recurrence depends on the region involved, the presence or absence of local breast and chest wall recurrence and distant metastases, and how your original cancer was treated. Both local and systemic treatments are usually required.

A recurrence confined to the *axillary* lymph nodes is treated locally with lymph node removal. If there is a simultaneous in-breast recurrence, a mastectomy is also performed. Radiation also may have an important role.

The appropriate treatment for lymph node recurrence in the *supraclavicular* area (above the collarbone) depends on whether or not the recurrence is limited to that area. An isolated supraclavicular recurrence is treated by surgical removal of the lymph node(s) when possible, followed by radiation (assuming the area had not been irradiated before). Chemotherapy also has a role. If a supraclavicular recurrence is accompanied by other sites of metastatic disease, it is usually treated with chemotherapy alone, with radiation added just to relieve symptoms. If supraclavicular recurrence is accompanied by an in-breast recurrence, chemotherapy is given first. If both respond to chemotherapy, and if no distant metastases have developed, your doctor may recommend mastectomy and lymph node removal, followed by radiation (again, assuming the area was not previously irradiated).

An isolated recurrence in the *internal mammary lymph node chain* is usually quite large when discovered because it produces symptoms only when it is large enough to burrow into the sternum (the breastbone). Treatment depends on the extent of lymph node involvement, the size of the lymph nodes, the interval since original treatment, the presence or absence of distant metastases, and the severity of symptoms. Very little data are available to guide your doctor to the best approach for this particular form of recurrence.

The goal of treatment for isolated internal mammary nodal recurrence is to control local disease and prevent metastases. Radiation alone for significant lymph node disease over one centimeter is unlikely to provide long-term control. A combination of surgery and radiation would provide the best local control, but if surgery is not possible, a combination of radiation and chemotherapy may result in local control that is nearly as effective. Systemic treatment is usually also needed.

If metastatic disease is also present, chemotherapy is the main form of treatment. Radiation therapy may be added to relieve the pain that is associated with tumor involvement of the immediately adjacent bone and nerves.

Systemic Therapy for Local-Regional Recurrence
If you have a local-regional recurrence without metastatic disease, you still have a very real possibility of achieving a cure. Systemic treat-

ment, consisting of hormone or chemotherapy, may have a key role. The goal is to eradicate any cells that might have traveled to other parts of your body and also to improve control of local disease in the area of the breast or the chest wall. (See the next chapter for a discussion of specific chemotherapies and hormonal therapies.)

"Will local therapy be enough, or do I need systemic therapy?" To answer this vital question, you need a full assessment of the prognosticators that estimate your risk for developing metastases. Your risk is based on the same factors that were used to assess the role of chemotherapy at the time or your original breast cancer diagnosis. Your doctor will weigh the significance of all your prognosticators, your general medical condition, and, of course, your preferences for treatment. His or her treatment recommendations will also be based on a gestalt of his or her practice experience in oncology and treatment guidelines from the literature. There are no randomized prospective clinical trials evaluating the correct local or systemic treatment for women with local-regional recurrent breast cancer—but you and your doctor can still come up with an effective treatment strategy that is best for you.

Although there is no clear consensus on who needs systemic treatment, all oncologists would surely recommend systemic therapy for any woman whose risk of developing metastases is close to 50 percent or higher. This is considered a high-risk group.

Your type of recurrence would fall into this *high risk group* if the cancer you have fits in one of the following categories:

1. Invasive and recurring within the first two years after original treatment.
2. Involving multiple lymph nodes, especially more than four (as well as can be interpreted in view of prior lymph node removal).
3. A tumor measuring over two centimeters, with one other aggressive feature, such as absence of hormone receptors, presence of rapid proliferation, or high grade.
4. A tumor over five centimeters.
5. An inflammatory breast cancer.
6. A combination of negative hormone receptors, high proliferation rate, and high grade.
7. Recurring on the chest wall within five years of mastectomy.
8. Recurring soon after adriamycin chemotherapy.

Some oncologists would also consider a recurrence at a young age, forty or under, without any of the above criteria, a high risk.

If these descriptions apply to your cancer recurrence, your doctor will probably recommend systemic therapy. The choices are hormone therapy alone, hormone therapy with chemotherapy, chemotherapy alone, or participation in a clinical study of high dose chemotherapy with bone marrow/stem cell transplantation. Which treatment you need will depend on your individual circumstances. You may find yourself in one of the following general treatment categories:

1. If you are premenopausal and at high risk for recurrence, chemotherapy would definitely be recommended. Adding hormone therapy may be advised, but only if your cancer is estrogen-receptor positive.
2. If you are postmenopausal and your cancer is estrogen-receptor positive, and if your risk is at the high end of this high risk category, your doctor would probably recommend a combination of chemotherapy and hormone therapy.
3. If you are postmenopausal and your cancer is estrogen-receptor negative, chemotherapy would be recommended.
4. If you are postmenopausal, your cancer is strongly estrogen-receptor positive, and your risk is at the lower end of the high risk group, and if the recurrence did not occur while you were taking hormone therapy, your doctor may recommend hormone therapy alone. If, however, the recurrence occurred while you were on hormone therapy, chemotherapy may be recommended as well as another type of hormone therapy. Whether chemotherapy is also necessary for a postmenopausal woman at moderate risk is controversial.
5. If you have more than ten positive nodes or you have a recurrence of inflammatory breast cancer, you need chemotherapy and you may be eligible for bone marrow transplantation.

Your cancer might fit into a *middle risk group* of roughly 20 to 40 percent risk of developing metastases if your cancer meets one of these criteria:

1. Size between one and two centimeters.
2. Involvement of one site of removable chest wall recurrence five or more years after original diagnosis.
3. Being estrogen-receptor negative alone, or high grade alone, or high proliferation rate alone.
4. Only microscopic involvement of less than three lymph nodes.

Again, most medical oncologists would recommend systemic therapy for this level of risk. The same choices apply, except for bone marrow/stem cell transplantation. If you are premenopausal, chemotherapy would probably be recommended. If you are post-menopausal, tamoxifen would probably be recommended for a hormone-receptor-positive cancer and chemotherapy for a hormone-receptor-negative cancer. There may be some crossover, with some premenopausal women whose cancers are hormone-receptor positive also taking hormone therapy, and some postmenopausal women also taking chemotherapy. Again, it's a very individual decision, one that you and your doctors must work out together.

You would be included in the relatively *low risk group* if your cancer is without the high risk factors listed above, and the following are true:

1. It is less than one centimeter.
2. It has no lymph node involvement.
3. It appeared in the breast after five years without any other recurrence.
4. It involves only one site of a removable chest wall recurrence, ten years or longer after initial treatment.

If your cancer fits this description, local treatment may be sufficient. But the role of systemic management still should be assessed by a medical oncologist.

If you developed an entirely noninvasive cancer in the previously treated breast, your risk of developing metastases is extremely low—less than 5 percent. No systemic therapy is indicated for this level of risk.

What's Going to Happen?

Most women who develop a local-regional recurrence after treatment for breast cancer get a good second chance at life. If you have a recurrence limited to the breast, with or without axillary lymph node involvement, and have been treated with mastectomy (with or without chemotherapy), your chance of living five years ranges from 60 to 85 percent. If your recurrence is limited to the chest wall, five-year survival has a large range, between 10 and 85 percent, depending on whether lymph nodes are also involved and whether or not the chest wall disease is controlled. If the chest wall disease is controlled and there is no lymph node involvement, survival can be at the top of the range; if chest wall disease is not controlled, survival is closer to one-third, and if there is significant lymph node disease, survival is at the bottom of the range. Survival after treatment for a supraclavicular re-currence remains poor.

When I talk to a patient with recurrent cancer, I try to present the information that you have read in this chapter and to provide a general idea of what her chances might be, using terms such as "a very aggressive problem," or "moderately aggressive," or "looks pretty favorable," or "seems very curable." I stay away from quoting specific numbers to predict her outcome because I don't think it's helpful. No one can see into the future. She is an individual. If she is one of the women who will do well, it's 100 percent for her; if she doesn't do well, it's also 100 percent for her.

Don't get caught up in a numbers game. No matter where your prognosticators point, there's always something that may help you in a significant way.

22

Living with and Managing Metastatic Cancer

I have a true appreciation now for what time is, having been lucky enough to get a second chance. All your priorities shift. But I don't fantasize about growing very old; I figure I'll die much earlier than I thought—whether it's twenty years from now or two. It's much more difficult having death in your face. It does highlight the preciousness of the moment. Looking at my husband and son with their heads together at the bird-feeder—I never would have looked at that scene with such joy (and sadness), soaking it all in. A great moment. I know now when and if the time comes—they'll be so fine together.

Metastatic disease can respond well to treatment, and it can go into remission for a long period of time. Treatment goals are to extend life as long as possible with the best quality of life possible. This means relieving your symptoms, putting the cancer into remission by arresting its growth, and eradicating the cancer cells if possible, with therapies that produce the fewest side effects. Many women can live for years, with metastatic cancer in remission. I believe there is genuine hope for a significant response to treatment that can provide a meaningful period of life, as well as an effective reduction of unwanted symptoms.

What Is Metastatic Disease?

Breast cancer that grows *beyond* the breast and its immediately adjacent lymph node regions is considered metastatic. Once breast cancer cells get into the bloodstream, they can travel to other parts of the body. Most cancerous cells are destroyed by your immune system or they simply can't survive on their own. But some may manage to lodge in a particular spot and begin to grow. Most often, they grow in the lymph nodes at the base of the neck, or in bone, liver, lungs, brain. Even if you know of only one site of metastasis, it's unlikely that it is the only place the mobile breast cancer cells have settled. Most likely, there are other places that haven't as yet manifested themselves in symptoms, physical signs, or x-ray tests.

Metastatic cancer is usually diagnosed within the first two years after initial treatment for what was thought to be localized disease, but metastases can also be diagnosed after two years. Only 10 to 15 percent of women already have known metastatic disease when they are first diagnosed with breast cancer.

All types of metastatic disease can respond well to treatment. How you respond to treatment depends on the unique features of your original cancer and the nature, number, and distribution of the metastases, as well as the kind of treatment you've already had, how you responded to it, and how long ago it took place. Metastatic breast cancer is most likely to respond to treatment in the following situations:

1. No organs are involved. Metastases to the liver and brain predict a less favorable outcome than metastases to the bone.
2. Hormone receptors are present in the recurrent cancer cells, predicting a better response to an anticancer hormone therapy (effective medication with relatively few side effects).
3. No prior adriamycin, Taxol, or Taxotere was given.
4. Three or fewer areas are involved. (One is the most favorable.)
5. There is no spinal cord compression from cancer in the back growing and compressing normal nerve tissue.

Conversely, if your recurrence (1) involves organs, (2) has no hormone receptors, (3) has already been treated with effective chemotherapies, and (4) has many sites of cancer involvement, the nature of your cancer is more aggressive, necessitating more aggressive treatments. There are still many treatment options available to you; it's just a matter of deciding which one you should choose.

Once a full evaluation has been performed to determine the extent of cancer that is present and the nature of the problem, you, your family, and your doctors need to sit down together and talk about treatment.

You and Your Doctor: Sharing the Treatment Decisions

The doctors on your team may include a number of specialists: a *medical oncologist,* who specializes in the delivery of chemotherapy and hormonal therapies; a *radiation oncologist,* who specializes in the use of radiation therapy to treat specific sites of pain or bleeding, painless bone metastases in weight-bearing bones (which could result in fracture), neurologic compromise, and chest wall recurrence; a *surgeon,* who performs a biopsy, removes a single metastasis, and performs other procedures; and a *radiologist,* who obtains and interprets diagnostic studies, including mammograms, computed tomography (CT) scans, magnetic resonance imaging tests (MRIs), bone scans, and ultrasounds, to evaluate the extent of cancer at diagnosis and to help assess your response to treatment; and a *pathologist,* who reads the biopsy material. Make sure these doctors are on your team in a truly active capacity (see Chapter 3). You may also have to affirm your access to each of these specialists with your health insurance plan (see Chapter 26).

You and your doctor should agree about the approach to your care. This is a very important issue. Let your doctor know how aggressive or unaggressive you want to be. Even if your perspective is very different from that of your doctor, he or she should respect your wishes and help take care of you in a manner acceptable to you. For example, if your doctor recommends aggressive treatment, but you want supportive care only, you both need to listen carefully to each other—but in the end, he or she should honor your decision. However, if you choose alternative treatments that your doctor is uncomfortable with, he or she should tell you that. You may be able to agree on how to work together, but if you decide *not* to work together, find another physician who can be open to your philosophy.

How you make decisions about treatment when you are well may be very different from how you make decisions when you have metastatic breast cancer. A study from England reported that patients with cancer indicated they were willing to accept highly toxic treatment for just a 1 percent chance of cure, whereas participants in the study who were without disease said they would need to have a 50 percent chance of cure to accept the same high toxicity level.

Furthermore how you make choices may change over time, as your medical situation, symptoms, family issues, and financial concerns evolve. Patients with advanced metastatic breast cancer rarely choose hospice care first if they know there are untried treatment options still available with some prospect of diminishing the tumor, easing symptoms, and extending their lives. There's always something more to celebrate, a life event that must be witnessed: a graduation, a wedding, a birth. Many mothers of young children choose continued aggressive therapy almost to the very end for the chance to live as long as possible for their children.

For other patients, relief of pain is the first priority. Chemotherapy and radiation—and sometimes surgery—are therapies that can provide very important palliative benefits (directed solely at relieving and preventing suffering). The most effective treatment of liver pain caused by metastasis, with the fewest side effects, is not morphine but chemotherapy. The most effective way to treat brain metastases is to give radiation and steroids, rather than pain medications alone.

Not every patient wants to push all the limits. I have patients who tell me, "I want to preserve as much quality of life as possible, and since I'm going to die soon anyway, I don't want my last days ruined by suffering from the side effects of treatment."

I urge you to keep an open mind on therapy choices, and to communicate to your doctor clearly and firmly exactly what you have in mind. Then bounce the decision back and forth, so you know that your doctor knows exactly what you want and you fully understand his or her recommendations. Don't leave any room for misunderstanding.

Treatment for Metastatic Disease

Metastatic breast cancer is a cancer involving various parts of the body connected within a "system." Chemotherapy and hormone therapy are "whole system" approaches to treatment. (I refer to most drugs by their commonly used names—whether brand names or chemical names.) Your treatment plan may also require treatment for specific pain or blockage problems, using radiation, surgery, and interventional x-ray procedures.

During your treatment for metastatic breast cancer, your doctor needs to periodically assess your response to treatment. Your doctor's ability to assess your *cancer's* response to treatment depends on the results of appropriate tests: for example, a bone scan to assess bone metastases. When you have surgery or take radiation or a drug, however, you and your doctor also want to know what *your* response is going to be.

Your response to a local treatment is measured primarily by reduction of symptoms—pain relief, increased activity levels, easier breathing—and less by repeat radiographic studies. Each chemotherapy or anti-estrogen therapy, alone and in combination, has been studied to determine just how effective it is in groups of women with breast cancer. Response to a particular chemo- or hormone therapy by a group of women treated in a similar manner may help you and your doctor understand the value of a therapy for you. Your doctor may say, "This chemotherapy has a response rate of 30 percent," meaning that 30 percent of the women who take this particular chemotherapy regimen have a 50 percent or greater regression rate of their disease, lasting three months or longer (the measured duration of the response).

Response to treatment can be described as follows: (1) complete response (complete disappearance of cancer, complete remission), (2) partial response (greater than or equal to 50 percent tumor regression), (3) minimal response (less than 50 percent regression), (4) stabilization (cancer remains the same), or (5) progression (cancer is growing). A complete or partial response needs to last at least three months to qualify. The better your response to chemotherapy, the better your outcome.

Local Treatment

You may have signs or symptoms at a particular site of metastasis that are causing, or threatening to cause, an immediate problem. Your doctor will consider using a local form of treatment to relieve the symptoms and to control the disease at that site. For example, radiation therapy might be used for specific sites of pain and bleeding, or surgical placement of a needle to remove fluid from around the lung that is causing severe shortness of breath.

Metastatic disease that compresses the spinal cord is another emergency. Symptoms usually include progressive back pain, and may also include numbness or weakness in a particular part of the body; and a change in bowel or bladder activity, but only when there is significant spinal cord compromise. Most commonly, these symptoms indicate a metastasis in the backbone that is squeezing the spinal cord housed within the spine; less commonly, the problem is caused by a metastasis directly involving the spinal cord (without bone involvement). Treatment includes immediate use of steroids, usually Decadron, and radiation therapy directed at the area of involvement. Rarely, surgical decompression of the spinal cord pressure is necessary.

Brain metastases also require rapid initiation of treatment. Symptoms of brain metastases can include headache, first-thing-in-the-morning nausea that eventually progresses to all-day nausea, loss of strength (or weakness) in a particular part of the body, change of behavior, confusion, seizures, and loss of consciousness. Steroids are started first; whole brain irradiation is next. Surgery may be considered for a solitary lesion that shows up after a long disease-free interval between initial diagnosis and time of recurrence; surgery may also be necessary if a solitary metastasis is causing severe pressure in the brain that is not responding to noninvasive treatment.

When cancer cells get into the fluid that bathes the brain and spinal cord (a condition called cerebrospinal carcinomatosis), cancer cells may grow on individual nerves causing a very specific alteration of sensation or function. Carcinomatosis is treated with steroids, and chemotherapy drugs are sometimes instilled directly into the fluid. Uncommonly, radiation is given to the entire brain and spinal cord if this is the only area of metastasis present, because it results in excessive suppression of your immune system, making it difficult to give chemotherapy within the most desirable time frame. Radiation to the whole brain or a specific area of nerve involvement can be given with less toxicity.

If you're in pain, you need immediate attention. (Pain management is addressed fully in Chapter 23.) Radiation provides significant or complete pain relief from bone metastases in over 85 percent of people for a significant period of time, without the side effects of pain medications. Radiation can also effectively relieve pain from cancer growth in enlarged lymph nodes pushing on adjacent normal tissue and structures, and from headache caused by brain metastases and increased pressure.

Bleeding from a skin recurrence in the breast area or from tumor involvement in an airway will respond quickly to radiation.

Metastases to weight-bearing bone (legs and hips) can weaken and destroy the structural strength of the bone, making it more vulnerable to "pathologic" fracture (a broken bone resulting from an underlying problem, not just trauma). After radiation eradicates the cancer, and the cancer cell debris is removed by blood and lymph cells, the bone can rebuild and strengthen itself. If a bone in the leg or arm (occasionally in the back) is extensively weakened and at risk for imminent fracture, an orthopedic surgeon may recommend first placing a metal rod into the bone to give it strength and to reduce the chance of pathologic fracture. Then radiation is given to destroy the cancer so the bone can heal. (Bone cannot heal if cancer cells are in the way.)

Radiation is usually performed with a linear accelerator machine that directs radiation into the body (called external beam radiation). Radiation treatment can also be provided by placing a radioactive source directly into the area where the tumor is located (e.g., into the airway to shrink a tumor growing in the esophagus). This is a local form of treatment; radiation to one specific area of metastasis does not affect an existing cancer at any other site. Nor does radiation reduce the chance of developing a new site of metastatic disease.

Side effects of radiation depend on the site being treated. Brain radiation causes transient loss of hair on your head, scalp irritation, fatigue, and a stuffy sensation in your ears; it can also cause a loss of short-term memory. Radiation to an area of the arm or leg causes minimal if any side effects, but if the area near your stomach is treated (e.g., the upper lumbar spine), you may experience nausea. This side effect can usually be prevented by taking antinausea medication forty-five to sixty minutes prior to treatment. (I usually recommend Torecan or Compazine, for starters.) Radiation of the upper spine can irritate your esophagus (you'll feel a transient lump in your throat, followed by pain with swallowing); radiation of skin recurrence causes temporary redness, tenderness, and itching.

If you develop shortness of breath and your chest x-ray shows fluid around the lung, preventing the lung from expanding normally, the fluid can be removed with a needle, but if it keeps accumulating, a surgeon can insert a tube into the chest cavity and drain the fluid. To prevent fluid from reaccumulating, a substance is placed within the cavity; the lining of the cavity is irritated by the material (antibiotic or talc can be used) and scar tissue forms between the surfaces of the cavity, eliminating the space the fluid was able to collect in. (The process can be quite painful for a day or two or three.)

Liver pain, caused by tumor expansion of the liver and stretching of its capsule covering, is best treated with chemotherapy. But if no chemotherapy or pain medication appears to be working, radiation to the liver can be effective at reducing pain.

Diffuse, painful bone metastases that persist despite chemotherapy and pain medication, and that can't be readily treated with localized radiation (the area that needs to be treated is too big), can be treated with a medication called Aredia or with the injection of strontium-89 (a radioactive material) into the bloodstream. The strontium is taken up by bone cells, the radiation gets delivered into cancer cells around the bone cells, and pain relief follows. If one or two or three of many sites of bone metastasis are producing severe pain, but your pain is otherwise being controlled, localized radiation can be given to those one to three sites, and strontium can cover the rest.

Hypercalcemia (an excess of calcium in the blood), which may result from the tumor itself, from its effect on bone, or as a side effect of cancer therapy, requires immediate attention to prevent medical complications. Treatment includes extra fluids, with or without medications (depending on the cause and degree of the elevated calcium).

Aredia, which inhibits the loss of calcium from bone, is used to reduce the high calcium that can result from bone metastases.

Systemic Whole Body Treatment

Ground Rules and Guiding Principles for New Regimens

Some treatments work faster than others. Treatments that are slower to act are not necessarily less effective in the long term. Anti-estrogen therapies may take a few months until you get a full response; at least two cycles of chemotherapy are given before your doctor repeats tests to evaluate the cancer's reaction.

But you may require a treatment that works quickly. If you have symptoms of a life-threatening condition that requires immediate attention while the hormone or chemotherapy is in the process of kicking in, your doctor will need to find a treatment that will work immediately, such as steroids, radiation, or surgical decompression.

You and your doctor must reevaluate the cancer's response to treatment on a regular basis. After a treatment has been given a fair chance to see if it works, act on your findings. In most cases, if your cancer is not responding to treatment, your doctor will want to put you on a different drug regimen. If your cancer was able to grow despite recommended doses of a hormone or chemotherapy, it is assumed that that particular hormone or chemotherapy was unable to eradicate or stop the growth of your cancer cells, and the surviving cancer cells have probably developed a resistance to the treatment. More of the same medication would be unlikely to elicit a favorable (to you) response from those cells.

The next drug your doctor recommends should have a different mechanism of action, with a better chance of being effective against your cancer. For example, if you developed metastatic disease while you were taking tamoxifen, it would mean that tamoxifen failed to prevent the growth of your particular cancer. It is no longer effective for you and it should be discontinued. Perhaps a different attack, using another type of anti-estrogen therapy or a chemotherapeutic regimen, will work instead.

You must be informed of the potential benefits and side effects of all treatments. Prior to having any procedure or starting any kind of treatment, you are asked to sign a consent form. You have the right to refuse a procedure or treatment, and you have the right to stop a treatment at any time, even when it is in progress.

TABLE 22.1. Therapies for metastatic breast cancer

Type of therapy	Name of drug or procedure (brand name)	Response rate (duration of response)	Most common side effects (rare effects)
Anti-estrogen	tamoxifen (Nolvadex)	30–80% (6–18 mo)	Hot flashes, vaginal dryness or discharge, irregular periods, nausea (blood clots, endometrial cancer)
Aromatase inhibitors	anastrozole (Arimidex)	25–70% (6–16 mo)	Hot flashes, vaginal dryness, nausea, diarrhea, weakness
	aminoglutethimide	30–50% (6–16 mo)	Lethargy, imbalance walking, rash, nausea, loss of appetite, depression of blood counts, low blood pressure
Gonadotrophin inhibitors	goserelin acetate (Zoladex)	not used as a single agent	Hot flashes, cessation of menses, vaginal dryness, depression
Progestin	megestrol acetate (Megace) medroxyprogesterone acetate	25–70% (6–16 mo)	Hot flashes, weight gain, fluid retention, vaginal dryness (high calcium, rash, high blood pressure, low blood counts, depression, low platelet count)
Androgen	fluoxymesterone (Halotestin)	5–50%	Increases facial and body hair, libido, deepens voice, stimulates aggression
Estrogen	diethylstilbestrol DES	5–50% (6–10 mo)	Nausea, vomiting, fluid retention, change in skin pigmentation, urinary frequency, vaginal bleeding (blood clots)
Surgery	ovary removal (oophorectomy)	30–80% (6–10 mo)	Rapid onset of early menopause, surgical risks
Radiation	ovary ablation	30–80% (6–16 mo)	Rapid onset of early menopause

This table includes basic information on these drugs. It should not be considered all inclusive, particularly with respect to side effects.

Stick with treatment that has been working and has acceptable side effects. Abandon what is not working, and try something that, according to your doctor, has the potential to do the job you need.

First Choice: Anti-estrogen Therapy

Anti-estrogen therapy can be the most effective weapon against metastatic breast cancer, with the fewest side effects. Anti-estrogen therapy, therefore, should be the first treatment of choice for the following groups of women: (1) those whose cancers are hormone-receptor positive, (2) those who have never had hormone therapy before or who have had a prior good response to first-line hormone therapy (tamoxifen), (3) those who have unknown hormone receptor status (and maybe even for postmenopausal women who have negative hormone receptors, who still have a 10 percent chance of responding), and (4) those who have metastases limited to bone, skin and underlying soft tissues, and lymph nodes; early lung involvement; or involvement of the lining around the lung (the pleura).

The presence of estrogen and progesterone receptors in your breast cancer tumor cells predicts a good response to tamoxifen and other hormone therapies; the more receptors, the better your response. If both estrogen and progesterone receptors are positive, your chance of responding to hormone therapy is about 70 percent; if only the estrogen or the progesterone receptor is positive, there is a 33 percent chance of response; if neither receptor is positive, there is a 10 percent chance. The chance of a favorable response also increases if you are older, and if there was a long disease-free interval after your original cancer diagnosis.

Hormone-receptor-negative tumors, tumors involving the liver, and diffuse involvement of the lung are unlikely to respond significantly to anti-estrogen therapy. Chemotherapy is a more appropriate approach.

Hormone therapies work in a number of ways: (1) by blocking the attachment of estrogen to the estrogen receptor (tamoxifen or Halotestin, which may work as an anti-estrogen), (2) by blocking the conversion of the male hormone androgen (made by the adrenal glands) into estrogen (Arimidex, aminoglutethimide), (3) by eliminating ovarian estrogens (removing ovaries surgically or stopping estrogen production with radiation), (4) by reducing available estrogens, the number of estrogen receptors, or estrogen's effects on cancer growth (progestins such as Megace, medroxyprogesterone acetate; Halotestin), and (5) by reducing the brain's stimulation of ovarian production of estrogen in pre- or perimenopausal women (Zoladex, and maybe Halotestin).

Tamoxifen (which benefits both pre- and postmenopausal women) is the first anti-estrogen medication that should be tried (if you have not already been on tamoxifen therapy), because it has the highest response rates and it produces *relatively* mild side effects (see Chapter 7). If you have metastatic disease and respond to tamoxifen, you should continue with it as long as it is working for you, even ten years or more.

If, however, your cancer recurred or progressed while you were taking tamoxifen, it should be stopped. Sometimes, discontinuing the tamoxifen alone can be therapeutic; the cancer cells may have learned to thrive on the presence of tamoxifen, so stopping it may be equivalent to starving the tumor.

If you did respond to tamoxifen, at least for a while, and you have just been advised to discontinue it because it is no longer working, your doctor will probably suggest a different anti-estrogen therapy, as long as there is no involvement of the liver or brain, or lymphangitic involvement of the lung (a spread of cancer cells alongside blood and lymphatic vessels of the lung). Other anti-estrogen therapies include Arimidex, Megace, Fareston (a "new kid on the block"), Zoladex, Halotestin, aminoglutethimide, DES, ovary removal, and ovarian ablation.

Response rates and duration of response to therapies are relatively similar, so your doctor will recommend a hormone therapy for you based on the treatment you have already tried, and on side effects, cost, and convenience of administration.

Specific Options

Table 22.1 contains information about hormone therapies, but be aware of its limitations. The reported response rates depend on the particular group of women whose responses were measured, and there are many things we just don't know. What was the status of their hormone receptors? Was the treatment being used for women who had already progressed on other hormone therapies? Did the same proportion of women have organ involvement? Also, side effects vary considerably. Your response to a particular drug will depend on the type of cancer you have and your previous treatment.

Megace has been second in line to tamoxifen for many years (i.e., it is used after tamoxifen has stopped working), and it is effective in both pre- and postmenopausal women. But the women I've taken care of who are on this drug have been less than thrilled with its side effects of weight gain and fluid retention; they also feel inconvenienced by having to take pills four times a day. Now, however, there is Arimidex for women beyond menopause and for women who have had their ovaries removed. Arimidex and Megace have similar response rates, but Arimidex has fewer unpleasant side effects and is taken only once a day. Arimidex and aminoglutethimide both reduce the relatively large amount of estrogen that is derived from adrenal gland androgens in postmenopausal women (in contrast to premenopausal women, in whom most estrogen comes from the ovary). Arimidex is preferable to aminoglutethimide because its action is more precise and it has fewer serious side effects. Aminoglutethimide needs to be taken with steroids, because it lowers your adrenal gland's production of steroids to below normal levels. You don't want to be without adequate steroids during times of stress and danger, when your body normally produces an instantaneous surge to help you through the normal "fight or flight" reaction to stress. If you have experienced progression of breast cancer while on Arimidex, Megace may still be effective.

Ovary removal (under general anesthesia, through two small incisions, with or without a laparoscope) or cessation of ovarian hormone production with a short course of radiation are as effective as tamoxifen in arresting the production of estrogen. Either of these procedures was the treatment of choice before tamoxifen came on the scene, and both remain quite effective for premenopausal women. They are both one-time procedures, they work quickly, and they avoid the need to take pills on a daily basis. However, ovary removal is a surgical procedure requiring anesthesia, and it causes sudden and complete premature menopause—with all of the attendant effects (see Chapter 18).

Halotestin is a male hormone that has proven anti-breast-cancer activity. Its average response rate, however, is only about 20 percent. Because it tends to be less effective than other options, and because the masculinizing side effects are unacceptable to many, Halotestin is not commonly used. "My voice deepened, the hair on my face was awful, and the sexual tension was not to be believed—I can now understand what drives men to rape. And then migraines. I was screaming at everybody in sight. I had to get off it—the side effects were worse than the disease."

Zoladex suppresses the brain's stimulation of the ovaries' production of estrogen; it is usually prescribed in combination with another form of hormone treatment: tamoxifen or Arimidex. It is particularly effective in premenopausal women.

Rarely prescribed these days is DES, which is actually a type of estrogen that, when given in high doses, can suppress breast cancer growth, although how it works is not understood. (DES is probably best known to you for the birth defects it produced when women took it years ago to prevent miscarriage.) The side effects of DES are greater than those of other options.

The role of combined hormone therapies to give more complete reduction of estrogen in the body theoretically offers benefits over the use of one agent—like the addition of Zoladex to tamoxifen in premenopausal women, or Arimidex to tamoxifen in postmenopausal women. Whether there is in fact any added benefit to this combination is unclear, and the question is under study.

All hormone therapy can cause a "flare" reaction, a transient initial exacerbation of pain and/or high calcium levels, as the tumor reacts to being starved of what it needs to grow. Good for you, bad for the cancer. This may happen in about one third of the women on this therapy.

And remember, the pharmaceutical industry is actively investigating new and effective drugs for tomorrow, including a more effective tamoxifen with fewer side effects.

I've known many women with metastatic breast cancer who have done well for long periods of time on tamoxifen followed by other hormone therapies. One of my patients originally had CMF chemotherapy (see below), and then she developed a single painful metastasis in her back. The tumor was hormone-receptor positive. Her treatment includes systemic therapy with tamoxifen and local radiation to the area of pain in her back. As long as her disease is controlled with tamoxifen and she is pain free, she won't need additional chemotherapy and pain medications; she will enjoy the best possible quality of life with closely supervised minimal therapy.

There usually comes a time with metastatic disease—months from now or many years from now—when the cancer progresses and chemotherapy is required. Some women continue with their hormone therapy and add chemotherapy to the regimen, or hormone therapy is stopped when chemotherapy is started.

Chemotherapy: How Much? Alone or in Combination?

There is a huge selection of chemotherapies to choose from: all kinds of drugs, given singly or in combinations, in various doses. Whether your situation is favorable or grim, there is hope of remission. You have many options.

Don't automatically jump to the most aggressive approach. More is not necessarily better, and using more agents means having more side effects. A higher dose of chemotherapy is better only if the cancer responds to the same chemotherapy at standard doses.

TABLE 22.2. Chemotherapeutic regimens

When to try	Regimen	Response rate
Anytime, usually first or second	CMF CAF FAC AC adriamycin paclitaxel (Taxol) docetaxel (Taxotere)	30–75%
Later	VATH MitoC/Vinca 5-FU vinorelbine (Navelbine) gemcitabine (Gemzar) Mito X/5-FU/Leuk M/Leuk	10–40%

C, cytoxan; M, methotrexate; F, 5-fluorouracil; A, adriamycin; V, vinblastine; T, thiotepa; MitoC, mitomycin; MitoX, mitoxantrone; Vinca, vinca alkaloid class of drugs, which includes vinblastine, vindesine, vincristine, vinorelbine; Leuk, leukovorin.

Single agents generally offer a response rate of 20 to 47 percent, lasting three to eight months; combinations of drugs can produce a response rate between 50 and 70 percent, lasting one year. You can start with one regimen, and if that doesn't work, you can always step up the aggressiveness of your attack and pull in the heavier guns. But you just might be the individual who does very well on that single agent.

The ideal combination chemotherapy regimen (1) attacks all the different kinds of cells in your breast cancer (cancer is heterogeneous, made up of different kinds of cells that may respond differently to any one drug), (2) uses drugs that work in complementary fashion, without overlapping benefits or side effects, (3) works by a mechanism something that is too tricky for the cancer cells to figure out and overcome, and (4) has an acceptable level of side effects.

If you have already had chemotherapy at initial diagnosis, or you have been treated previously for metastatic disease and are looking for your second, third, fourth, or nth chance, your doctor will try to find something new that works by a different mechanism, something that

TABLE 22.3. Walk-through chemotherapy

PRIOR TO TREATMENT

Initial Consultation and Follow-up Appointments with Medical Oncologist:
History and physical: review of all lab and x-ray results.
Treatment recommendations are laid out.
Benefits and side effects of recommended chemotherapy are explained.
The consent form is carefully reviewed and signed.
Your appointment is scheduled for start of treatment, timing dependent on
 your individual situation.

DAY OF TREATMENT

Initial Steps:
Register at chemotherapy center.
Meet nurse or chemotherapy technologist who will administer your
 chemotherapy.
Vital signs are taken: blood pressure, pulse, respiration rate, temperature.
Your height and weight are measured to calculate the appropriate doses of
 chemotherapy.
Intravenous catheter is inserted. If you have an intravenous port, it is
 prepared for use.
Complete blood count is obtained at the time that intravenous access is
 established.

Meet with Medical Oncologist:
Medical evaluation.
The amount of chemotherapy you need is calculated, prescribed, and
 ordered.
The pharmacy prepares the chemotherapy. Processing can take up to an
 hour. (Chemo orders may be written prior to your first day if the plan is
 set and your blood counts are adequate.)
Pre-chemotherapy medications to prevent side effects like nausea, anxiety,
 and inflammation are given, usually through the intravenous line. Fluids
 are also given as indicated by the type of chemotherapy, some of which
 (such as cytoxan) require ample hydration before medication is
 administered.
Chemotherapy drugs arrive; your name, the drug name, and the dosage are
 verified before treatment begins.

Duration of Chemotherapy:
Chemotherapy is administered—via an intravenous pump "push"
 mechanism within a short period of time, or via a slow intravenous
 infusion drip taking up to several hours.

Continued on next page

A nurse or doctor supervises the push process, to be sure the medication (such as adriamycin) goes into the intravenous line properly and does not leak outside the vein (extravasation), where it can cause a burn.

Some chemotherapy involves a combination of intravenous infusion and pill form. (CMF can be delivered this way; methotrexate and 5-fluorouracil are given intravenously. Cytoxan is taken as a pill with a large glass of water).

On Your Way:

At the end of chemotherapy, when the intravenous catheter is removed and your vital signs are stable, you are given instructions on what side effects to expect, and medications and instructions are provided on how to manage the side effects. If you develop any significant symptoms, such as mouth sores, uncontrolled nausea, diarrhea, or fever, you are instructed to call your doctor. (Obtain the telephone number of your doctor's answering service.) You are then free to leave.

is non-cross-resistant: Your cancer learned to resist the anticancer effects of previous treatments, so the next drug you choose should work in a different manner so that the cancer's familiar bag of tricks can't elude the new drug's method of action.

Chemotherapy is generally given intermittently, such as once a month. (Some drugs are given by continuous infusion over several days, once a month.) Intermittent therapy usually produces fewer cumulative side effects, and it gives your normal tissues time off to repair themselves. Occasionally, a drug such as 5-fluorouracil alone may be given continuously by pump for an extended period of time—a few days—but the level of drug in the bloodstream at any given time is a lot lower than when it is given intermittently, causing a lower level of continuous side effects.

Chemotherapy Side Effects

Perhaps the most important thing for you to keep in mind is that, regardless of how you feel during and after chemotherapy, your cancer cells will feel much, much worse. Everyone responds differently to each chemotherapy drug, and the exact nature of the side effects you will experience cannot be predicted. You may be unable to use a drug that most other women tolerate easily, because of how the side effects hit you, or you may cruise through every regimen without even a single bout of nausea.

Many of the chemotherapies given in combination have an acceptable level of side effects (that's not to say that they are anything less than unpleasant). Almost all drugs cause nausea, fatigue, suppression of the immune system with an associated risk of infection, and partial or complete hair loss. Some drugs also cause diarrhea or constipation, inflammation and ulceration of mucous membranes, fluid retention, rashes, infertility, menopausal symptoms, and liver inflammation. Most of these symptoms can be prevented or managed so that they are fairly well tolerated, and most of them are temporary.

Individual drugs have unique serious, but rare, side effects. Adriamycin can weaken the muscle of the heart; Taxol/Taxotere can cause irreversible loss of nerve function; cytoxan can irritate the bladder; mitomycin can cause inflammation and irreversible scarring of the lung. A tiny but real risk of developing a treatment-induced leukemia is associated with the use of methotrexate (less than a 1 percent risk). It's just about impossible to give you a good notion of the specific side effects of every medication in any reasonable way, because how you experience one drug is strongly influenced by what you've already been through and what other drugs you are taking at the same time. Your doctor can give you the most realistic sense of what to expect.

What Chemotherapy to Try Next, and Next, and Next . . .

Chemotherapy should be initiated if your cancer is growing despite various hormonal therapies, or if your cancer is hormone-receptor negative, or if your cancer involves the liver, or if it involves your lung tissue in a diffuse manner (lymphangitic spread). This may be your first treatment for metastatic disease, or you may be coming back for a fourth try or more. It's true that there are quite a number of different regimens that have significant response rates, so even if this is your fourth try at chemo, you still have a chance to respond to a new treatment (see Table 22.2). You may not have had a significant response to one chemo regimen, but that doesn't mean you won't have a significant response to subsequent ones.

Remember, quality of life is important. Think carefully about choosing what you think is "the strongest" therapy if it has the highest side effects and if you could just as well try something less toxic first. Save the strongest in case you need it later on. Who knows, you might have a good response to a regimen that *doesn't* make you feel sick.

If you have never had chemotherapy before (see Table 22.3 for a typical day of treatment), your medical oncologist might choose a tried-and-true combination of drugs, with response rates ranging from 35 to 60 percent: CMF (cytoxan, methotrexate, fluorouracil), CAF or FAC (C and F as above, A for adriamycin; the two regimens differ by dose and frequency of administration), AC, or AT (T for one of the two taxane drugs, docetaxel [Taxotere] and paclitaxel [Taxol]), or he or she will choose a single agent such as adriamycin or either Taxotere or Taxol (response rates 30 to 60 percent).

If you have already had CMF, your doctor will probably recommend a regimen that uses adriamycin or one of the taxanes, or a combination: CAF, FAC, AC, AT, or VATH (V is vinblastine, A is adriamycin, T here is Thiotepa, H is Halotestin). With recent studies showing a better response rate to a taxane than to adriamycin as a single agent, with less nausea, vomiting, and mouth sores, many oncologists are choosing to use a taxane first. (As a single agent in women with metastatic breast cancer, Taxotere had a response rate of 47 percent compared with a 26.5 percent response rate to adriamycin.) Taxol and Taxotere are highly effective drugs for the treatment of metastatic breast cancer. Taxotere requires that steroids be administered (by pill at home) the day before treatment begins, then Taxotere is given by intravenous infusion for just over an hour. Intravenous premedication for Taxol takes one hour and is followed immediately by a three-hour infusion of the Taxol.

If you prefer a somewhat less aggressive approach, and you are willing to accept the tradeoff—a little less effectiveness for a lot fewer side effects—you can choose between two drugs: vinorelbine (Navelbine) and gemcitabine (Gemzar). Each can be used as a single agent to help keep the tumor and its associated symptoms under control without causing too many side effects (including less hair loss). The range of response is 20 to 40 percent, lasting about eight months. Navelbine is recommended for the older patient, gemcitabine for the younger woman; both can work well even if you have other illnesses, such as diabetes.

If you have already had an adriamycin-containing regimen, most doctors would recommend one of the taxanes, with impressive response rates averaging around 30 percent, and ranging between 15 and 60 percent. CMF might also be considered, but probably as a second choice. You might also consider Navelbine and gemcitabine.

If none of these regimens works, additional regimens can include mitomycin and vincristine (or another drug from the same class of vinca alkaloid drugs); 5-fluorouracil (5-FU) by continuous infusion or in combination with leucovorin (response rates range from 10 to 40 percent); mitoxantrone (Novantrone), 5-FU, and leucovorin; high dose methotrexate and leucovorin; or a new unknown-at-this-moment experimental regimen.

Most of the regimens considered here can be used to stave off the cancer and preserve the most reasonable quality of life. Careful use of steroids can reduce side effects and improve your appetite and how you feel; Megace can be added to any regimen to improve your interest in food.

As you try one regimen after another, you may continue to respond, or you may find that you are reaching your limit and you're tired of trying so hard, while the cancer, with a second wind, has "learned" how to resist the power of the therapy. The result: Your response to subsequent regimens may start to decline.

Bone Marrow Transplant
Dose: How High Do You Go?

The dose of chemotherapy that is prescribed for you is based on a balance of benefits and side effects. If you could give enough chemotherapy to kill all the breast cancer cells in any woman who has the disease, the associated side effects would simply be too great. The most actively growing parts of your body are the most sensitive to chemotherapy, so cells and body tissues in your gastrointestinal tract, your immune cells, and your hair follicles are hardest hit. Of these, your immune system is the most sensitive to chemotherapy, and this is what limits how much chemotherapy you can safely take (one exception is adriamycin, which is limited because of rare, but potential, heart effects). Your immune system is depressed by standard doses of chemotherapy, but it recovers. Excessive doses of chemotherapy, however, could eradicate your immune cells completely.

The only way your doctor can possibly give you a higher-than-standard dose of chemotherapy is by removing your immune cells from your body before therapy (referred to as harvesting) and replacing them when it's finished. This clever procedure, combining high dose chemotherapy and immune cell replacement, is called bone marrow transplantation or peripheral stem cell transplantation if the immune cells are harvested from the bloodstream. For simplicity, I will use the term "BMT" when referring to this procedure.

Bone marrow transplant is a technique that removes the marrow, the soft spongy material that is one of the major sources of blood and immune cells, from the center of your pelvic bone and sets it aside for transplant back into your body (autologous) later on, to allow for short-term high dose therapy. Autologous transplant avoids the risk of rejection, a major concern for nonautologous transplants.

Not every woman is eligible for BMT: Women under sixty-five years of age, who have a relatively healthy heart, lungs, kidney, and liver, are generally eligible. Women with metastatic breast cancer or women with more than ten positive lymph nodes or with inflammatory breast cancer without metastases may also be eligible. If you go this route, consider taking your treatment as part of a research study, so that you can help provide better answers to important questions about the effectiveness of high dose chemotherapy plus transplantation relative to standard dose chemotherapy.

There are two ways to approach high dose chemotherapy with bone marrow or peripheral stem cell transplant. Most protocols start with the initial standard dose chemotherapy; if you're responding well, you proceed to high doses of chemo, either with the same agents or with new drugs (but not usually high dose adriamycin, because of heart toxicity effects). Gaining favor, but still less common, is another approach. Go to high dose chemo right away, after harvesting the bone marrow or peripheral stem cells. The "best" approach has not yet been fully defined, nor is bone marrow transplant proven to be more effective than standard dose chemo at this time and the benefits are uncertain for many. Furthermore, a BMT can be a life-threatening procedure.

You must have a full discussion of the side effects of the procedure, as well as a comprehensive review of alternative methods of treatment, *before* you sign informed consent forms and take the next step. (This is assuming you have received the okay from your health care plan for the bone marrow transplant; some insurers have rejected coverage for this procedure. See Chapter 26.)

If you and your doctor decide to go ahead with high dose chemotherapy that exceeds the normal tolerance of your immune system, arrangements must be made to harvest your bone marrow or peripheral stem cells. (The steps are outlined in Table 22.4.) Stem cells are immature immune cells that have the potential to develop into a wide range of different mature immune cells, depending on which type your body needs most. Once a stem cell receives an "assignment," it commits to becoming the assigned cell and matures accordingly. These stem cells are most concentrated in the bone marrow, but they also circulate throughout the bloodstream, looking for an assignment, a job to do against agents that can do you harm. Both "free agent" stem cells and "committed" immune cells are harvested. Transplantation requires a high proportion of stem cells in the harvested immune cell mix. Harvesting is usually scheduled for about two weeks after the end of standard chemotherapy, after your counts come back up but before giving the high dose chemotherapy. Your blood counts are usually high enough when they're above 1500—and if they meet the treatment protocol specifications. The steps for high dose chemotherapy and transplantation are carefully timed.

Harvesting immune cells from your bone marrow, which has more

TABLE 22.4. Steps of bone marrow transplantation

Steps	*Purpose*	*Place and order of procedure*
Standard dose chemotherapy	To eradicate the cancer and to test the cancer's response to chemotherapy	Out-patient or in-patient setting
Harvesting bone marrow	To remove immature immune stem cells and mature immune cells before they are damaged by high doses of chemotherapy.	Bone marrow collection takes place in the operating room; later, you go to recovery area for observation. You may be released that day or the following morning.
Harvesting peripheral stem cells	Same as above	Peripheral immature stem cells and mature immune cells are collected by apheresis, as an outpatient procedure. Each apheresis takes 2–6 hours; about 2–4 procedures are required.
Processing and storage of immune cell sample	To filter the immune cell mix. Purging of cancer cells is performed if necessary. Samples are frozen.	Liquid nitrogen freezers in hospital or other appropriate facility.
High dose chemotherapy	To more effectively eradicate cancer cells, not possible at lower, standard doses	Special isolation rooms in the hospital or in an adjacent hotel when blood counts are critically low, to reduce your risk of infection; when counts are above a critical level, you may go home with special precautions.

Continued on next page

Steps	*Purpose*	*Place and order of procedure*
Restore the immune system, with reinfusion of immune cell mix	To reinfuse immune cell mix to restore your immune cells after high dose chemotherapy.	Reinfusion done in hospital.

immature immune cells than your bloodstream, takes place while you are under general anesthesia. The medical oncologist (who specializes in bone marrow transplant) inserts a large hollow-centered needle into the bone marrow space in the middle of each of your hipbones where you have the largest supply of stem cells, and the marrow is sucked out, or aspirated; two doctors usually perform the procedure, one at each hip. Several cups of thick bloody material containing the immune cells are removed through the needle; this represents less than 10 percent of your total marrow. The material is then filtered and frozen. The procedure leaves you with sore hips and a few black-and-blue marks.

The alternative to this arduous process is to collect stem cells from your bloodstream, which contains more mature immune cells than are present in the marrow. This process is called apheresis. Apheresis is an out-patient procedure, anesthesia is not needed, and, except for the needle stick, it's not painful.

An intravenous catheter is placed into each of two separate veins; blood is removed from one vein, circulated through a closed system of plastic tubes, then passed through a cell-sorting centrifuge that separates the stem cells from the rest of the cells. Your blood, minus the stem cells and the more mature immune cells, is then returned to your bloodstream through the second intravenous catheter. The collected cells are stored in a freezer at a very low temperature. Your blood circulates continuously in this fashion until enough cells have been harvested. The process can take three to six hours, and it may need to be repeated if your blood count is so low that an insufficient number of stem cells is harvested. (Samples of the harvested cells are checked for stem cell number, so your doctors know just when they have collected enough.) The full process can take up to three days of outpatient visits.

Apheresis is usually the preferred method of harvesting stem cells from your body, because the committed immune cells in your blood that are collected along with the stem cells are more mature and prepared for action than the mix of immune cells and stem cells taken from your bone marrow, and your immune system therefore recovers faster.

If you have ever had evidence of breast cancer in the bone marrow, most medical centers "purge," or remove, any cancer cells from the immune and stem cell collection. This may seem like an essential step in the process, but it's not yet standard procedure at every center because the purging process is not fully reliable and various studies have come up with conflicting evidence of its usefulness.

Your frozen stem cells are stored until you are finished with your high dose chemotherapy, at which point your immune system is weak and needs refortification. That's the time for the transplantation, the step that gives you back your defrosted stem cells, through an intravenous transfusion.

It takes an average of one month for your transplanted stem cells to perk up, start making new cells, and reach a critical defensive squad of 500 cells per cubic millimeter, at which point they are just about able to protect you from infection. For some women, the full recovery of their immune system can take many more months. Side effects of the whole BMT procedure can be severe, and depend on which chemotherapy agents and blood products are used. The biggest risk is a severe infection that can result in death.

The high risk of life-threatening infection continues as long as the immune cell counts remain below 500; until the transferred stem cells have recovered to 1500 or above, your body's defenses are still tenuous. Special growth factors such as Neupogen and Epogen/Procrit may be given to stimulate faster recovery and proliferation of the stem cells. Transfusion of someone else's immune cells may be necessary. Antibiotics are commonly given at the very slightest hint of infection. Relative isolation from sources of infection is standard policy.

Despite these intense efforts, up to 10 percent of transplanted immune cells don't "take," and death can occur from bleeding or infection. (The chance of dying during the actual bone marrow transplantation is generally less than 5 percent with current techniques.)

But Does It Work?

The relative effectiveness of bone marrow or peripheral stem cell transplantation compared with standard conventional chemotherapy is being studied in different ways throughout the world. Each study focuses on a slightly different group of women, employing different combinations of drugs and dosages, and using varying definitions of survival and quality of life.

At the present time, bone marrow or peripheral stem cell transplantation doesn't seem to have a survival benefit over standard treatment for women with metastatic disease. However, women who have had a partial or complete response to the initial cycles of standard chemotherapy prior to the high dose phase of the process *may* obtain a survival benefit from bone marrow transplantation. Women who go right to high dose chemo and have an excellent response may also have a measurable survival benefit. Neither regimen cures metastatic breast cancer, even in women with the most positive results.

A woman who has had a partial or complete response to initial chemotherapy has a choice: proceed to high doses of chemotherapy with transplantation or continue the same drugs at standard doses that do not require bone marrow rescue. It is difficult to offer you definitive answers in this book, because results depend entirely on your individual history and response.

New and Experimental Therapies

There are several new therapies that may help boost your immune system. They offer exact instructions for fighting each individual breast cancer and provide extra immune system weaponry: antibodies, fighting proteins made to target a particular abnormal gene that's contributing to the growth and development of the cancer. Two such genes are HER-2/*neu* and EGFR (epithelial growth factor receptor).

New drug therapies currently under study for their effectiveness in battling breast cancer include Amonafide; anthracylines (related to adriamycin, but cause less heart damage); antifolates (related to methotrexate); anthrapyrazoles (related to mitoxantrone, similar to losoxantrone); and camptothecins (a class of drugs with proven efficacy against ovarian cancers; Topotecan is an example).

Nutrition and other complementary therapies that augment your immune response are currently under study, with major financing from the National Institutes of Health (see Chapters 13 and 19).

One day soon you may be offered tomorrow's newest discovery—and tomorrow can be as soon as one day away. The Natural Products Division of the National Cancer Institute studies 40,000 to 70,000 new natural substances each year for their potential efficacy against breast cancer. A breast cancer vaccine has been worked on for years, and one of these days it will be real and available. Participating in a study gives you faster access to these therapies and helps determine what tomorrow's treatments will be. It's an important way to make a difference and to hasten discoveries that may save lives.

Research on the function of the breast cancer genes and the proteins they encode may lead to a new group of important therapies, such as the injection of normal breast cancer gene protein into your bloodstream to replace the damaged breast gene's protein, restore control, and eliminate any cancerous cells—prevention and cure in one fell swoop.

Treatment On and Off

"It's a crap shoot, really. What works for one doesn't mean it'll work for all. I'm still pushing along. I'm fighting the battle. I know I'm not going to win the war, but I would rather go down fighting. I'm going to do it my way. As it is, I'm not supposed to be alive so many years after this all started."

If you have slowly progressive metastatic disease and your quality of life is good, you may decide to stop treatment, enjoy your life without treatment, and reevaluate your decision periodically. "My quality of life was much more important to me. 'Take a holiday from your medications,' my doctor said, so I dumped 'em all out. My body was so happy to be done with that crap!" Evelyn was able to live comfortably for almost two years with slowly growing metastatic breast cancer involving bone, without treatment. When her cancer progressed further and she developed significant pain, she returned to her physician and decided to try chemotherapy again. Her disease and her pain are under control again now that she is on chemo, nine years after she was first diagnosed with metastatic disease.

If you've been off treatment for a while, and you find yourself needing more and more pain medication to relieve a specific site of pain, but the side effects of the pain medications are compromising your quality of life, you may benefit (as suggested earlier) from radiation to the area of persistent and progressive pain. Radiation may allow you to eliminate or significantly decrease all pain medications, reducing troublesome side effects. Discuss this option with your physician.

When Do You Stop Treatment?

There are many women who want to be remembered for having sought absolutely every treatment possible, as proof of their love and commitment to their family and to life. If you are a mother with young children, you probably feel this need most desperately. Even if you develop widespread disease and are simply lying in bed, looking and feeling sick as can be, just being there for your children is reason and meaning enough. A month more of life can be worth the torture, your mind at relative peace even if your body is not.

I was talking to one of my patients who was feeling terribly ill and wondering about preparing her children for what might happen. "If my cancer is what is making me feel this bad, I must be close to death, but if the chemo, the radiation, or the steroids are making me feel this awful, maybe I can look forward to feeling better after treatment is over. Maybe I have a little more time ahead of me. My kids know I am sick, but I haven't told them that I am going to die. Until that happens, why upset them any more than is necessary?" (See Chapter 25.)

Pursuing every last possible form of treatment can come at the price of cumulative side effects and a great deal of misery for you and your family—including an unmanageable financial burden. This can be a bitter time for you, with perhaps your funds nearly gone, and perhaps your health care plan unwilling to pay for one more therapy. Maybe your doctor can help defend your right to additional treatment by negotiating with your insurance company.

But when the cancer is progressing despite all efforts, the physical, emotional, and financial cost of treatment can exhaust you and all those close to you. "Enough," your body and your family may be saying, though not in so many words, and you may sense their feelings. Realizing that you've reached the limit can compound your anger, depression, despair, and confusion. You feel helpless to make your last desperate wishes come true.

For others of you, it is your families who expect too much of you, urging you to pursue every available treatment, signaling their determination to prolong your life. But if you are close to death and you'd just as soon call a halt to your treatment for a little peace and relief at the end of your days, their push may make you feel cowardly and guilty for betraying their love.

Maybe what you need is simple respect for your needs. It's up to you to decide when enough is enough, when it's time to stop treatment— as much as you want to please those close to you. Can you say it, or do you need your doctor or religious counselor to intercede? When the possibility of remission may no longer be real, controlling your care and how you want to live until you die should rest in your hands. You have to do it your way.

End of Treatment

The point will come when your treatment ends. It may come at the moment of death, or you may decide to end active intervention before then. This could be the hardest decision you have ever had to face, or it may be straightforward: the right thing to do. It's not up to your family, but having your family's support for whatever decision you make is crucial.

You may worry about being abandoned by your physicians after you stop aggressive intervention, but they can still be actively involved in your care. However, you will be giving up regular visits to your physicians and the regular tests that assessed the status of your disease; you will no longer be seeing the caring nurses, technologists, and secretaries and you will miss the camaraderie of the patients in the cancer center.

Your care still continues and may even improve when you decide to stop aggressive intervention. At that point, you can get access to a whole new realm of care at a hospice (see Chapter 24). But hospice may not even be an issue for a significant period of time.

"My oncologist told me something that I will always remember. 'You can wake up each morning and worry about dying, or you can wake up each morning and celebrate living. Before you know it, several years may have passed. Do you want to waste that time with mourning or use every minute to celebrate?' "

23

Understanding and Controlling Pain

I was in such pain—and I'm good with pain—but I really needed that morphine. The nurse came in to say, 'We don't have the kind of morphine you need. You'll have to wait till morning. There's nothing more I can do,' and she left. But I couldn't stand it, and I started to cry, and another nurse heard me, and went and found something that helped. That experience was the worst. Later on, I found out that someone always has a key to the pharmacy, but I was in no condition to demand anything. I was just lucky the nurse who heard me understood how much pain I was in.

The Power of Pain

"Anytime something hurts, I think the cancer has come back." Maybe it has and maybe it hasn't, but if you have had breast cancer, there are only two kinds of pain you care about: cancer pain and noncancer pain—and knowing that most pain has nothing to do with cancer may not reassure you. The physical and psychological overtones of pain can be overwhelming. I'm always getting calls from my patients who are worried about a new pain and what it means. I can understand their fear; past experience has taught them that they're vulnerable.

Noncancer pain can result from injury, aging, other medical conditions, and treatment. Treatment-related pain may come from surgery, radiation, or chemotherapy. You might feel breast pain right after breast surgery, skin soreness during radiation, or mouth sores after chemo. Treatment pain may not stir up fear of recurrence as other pain does, because you've probably been prepared to expect it, but it still carries its own psychological weight. It's a persistent reminder of the breast cancer treatment you've been trying to put behind you. And it is *pain,* whatever the cause.

Pain you can't attribute to anything, pain that *might* be caused by cancer, is the pain that really worries you. The fear of cancer recurrence or progression begins to accelerate—and you think about dying. And one of the greatest fears of dying is being in pain, so there you are in a vicious circle.

Both noncancer and cancer pain can be acute or chronic. Acute pain is brief and intense; chronic pain is persistent and ongoing, and varies in degree. Acute pain scares you—then you deal with it and it's over. Chronic pain, on the other hand, can steal away the quality of your life, leaving you weak, helpless, dependent on others for the simplest needs, uninterested in much of anything, and feeling isolated from friends, from places you love, from the pleasant rough and tumble of your normal life. No matter how warm, helpful, even fascinating the people who look after you may be, it's miserable feeling so helpless, especially if you've always been independent and in charge.

If you are deeply religious, pain may shake your faith in God: "Why are You making me suffer this way? What have I done to deserve this? How can this be part of Your plan?" Follow this up with guilt for doubting, and you probably end up feeling depressed on top of everything else. Even if you're not at all religious, you may ask yourself very similar questions, wondering why you are suffering.

You Don't Have to Suffer

But you don't have to suffer. Pain can be treated and alleviated. Pain medications have become increasingly sophisticated and effective, with better delivery systems, new knowledge and awareness of how to use them, and fewer side effects. The options appear limitless, and with proper treatment most people can be relieved of most, if not all, of their pain.

The "old days" of undertreating pain are history—or should be. Fear of addiction and dependency, an "I can take it" stoicism, and contempt for pill-taking self-indulgence are outdated notions. There's nothing virtuous about suffering pain, and addiction is not an issue (especially if someone is nearing the end of life). Get it straight: addiction is "living your life for drugs"; medication—a medical issue—is "using drugs to live your life." People often confuse tolerance, the need to increase medication to maintain pain relief, with addiction. There can be a physical dependence on pain medication, after weeks or months of treatment, that can involve withdrawal symptoms if it is stopped, but these problems can be solved medically, once the pain has been successfully managed.

That doesn't mean you'll necessarily have smooth sailing, that you're not going to run into some resistance. There are still some caregivers out there—doctors and nurses—who can be downright stingy about pain control, who don't fully empathize with the patient's pain, who might not want to give "too much" pain medication, or who aren't familiar with current effective treatment of moderate to severe chronic pain. So nine o'clock at night rolls by and you're in the hospital, in real pain, and the nurse says, "That's all the doctor has ordered for you." "Well, then, find the doctor and have him order more. I'm not leaving my wife's side till she gets more medication. I'm not going to let her suffer all night, and I'll raise hell if necessary." Relating the incident sometime later, Richard confessed he had to bully the staff to get help, but his wife got the medication she needed, and it wasn't really all that much trouble for the staff.

If you are alone in the hospital and need help, and the nurse says she can't give you more medication, politely request that the nurse page the doctor on call—there always is one. If the doctor is tied up, or doesn't answer within fifteen minutes, and the nurse has not proven helpful, demand to speak to the patient ombudsman or patient relations person. You'll be letting the nurses on the floor know how much you're hurting, and that you're not going to let them put you "on hold," that your complaint is not going to disappear. Someone should be able to find a doctor. Sometimes you must be prepared to stand up to intimidation and authority, and insist on the help you need. Make it happen. I can't emphasize this enough. Speak up for yourself. Forget docile. Don't lie there quietly in pain.

If you are alone at home and you have new or uncontrolled pain, call your doctor through his or her answering service or through the hospital, and ask to have a prescription called in to a pharmacy that delivers. (Narcotic prescriptions can't be called in; someone has to pick them up.) If you can't get anybody, and you have new excruciating pain, go to the emergency room. If you're in hospice, call your hospice nurse.

There are other ways of controlling pain besides medication. Radiation therapy offers very effective and durable relief from a wide range of local types of cancer pain. Temporary nerve-blocking procedures (using analgesia) are introduced prior to surgery to reduce postsurgical pain. Other nerve-blocking techniques can alleviate particular points of pain for longer periods of time. Chemotherapy can reduce pain from advanced cancer. Complementary therapies such as hypnosis, distraction, visualization, biofeedback, acupuncture, and massage may do wonders. So does music, in whatever mode you prefer. "I felt best listening to Mozart—it was like healing sunshine—much better than Shostakovich." Try Verdi (sung by The Three Tenors), Van Morrison, k.d. lang, Frank Sinatra, Lawrence Welk—anything that sends you into a state of pleasure and takes your mind off the pain.

Dr. David Spiegel has great faith in self-hypnosis, using a simple form of focused concentration. You might enter an imagined world—floating, perhaps, on a tropical ocean—for a self-altering experience. Or you allocate attention to one or two things, and put everything else in your mind outside your field of concentration. You might focus on the pain itself, either willing it outside the boundary of your concentration field or imagining the part of your body in pain as being warmer—or cooler or lighter. Or you might focus on competing perceptions, such as listening to music you love. You "filter the hurt out of the pain," competing with the pain messages traveling along your nerve cells and bombarding your brain. You alter and reduce pain perception; you don't—you can't—eliminate it altogether. Relaxation is also part of the self-hypnosis process: as muscles relax and tension eases, pain lessens.

This chapter has a lot of information about pain and pain relief: descriptions of common pain problems, names of drugs, radiation and chemotherapy, side effects—but it's not a how-to, do-it-yourself chapter. The information is provided to help you understand the source of your pain and to help you work with your doctor and nurse to best relieve your pain. The more you know, the more confidence you'll have in speaking up for better care. If there is a symptom in this chapter that seems to apply to you, or there is a medication that you think may help you, ask your doctor or nurse about it. *Don't take any of these medications without your doctor's close supervision.*

Taking an active role in your care by reporting all symptoms, asking about new treatments, and making suggestions helps your doctor and nurse help you. If you feel your doctor is not taking your pain seriously enough, find a doctor or a pain management team who will. Many hospitals have established or are in the process of establishing special pain treatment teams and centers.

Communication Is Crucial

Communication is the first step toward pain relief. If you don't tell your doctor that you are in pain, your doctor can't help relieve it. Don't let personal scorn, intimidation, or embarrassment about "complaining" keep you from telling your doctor or nurse where and how it hurts. Reporting or describing pain is *not* complaining! You also need to be sure you and your doctor fully understand each other; either of you may use words that mean different things to the other. A patient might say, "I don't have any pain," but if I ask whether she has any aches or discomfort, she'll say, "Yes."

Communication also means listening, with an open mind, to what your body has to tell you. Don't let cancer fear warp your thinking, convincing you that your pain comes from recurrent or progressive disease. Many types of pain have nothing to do with cancer. Pain is a by-product of life's wear and tear and is often a side effect of cancer therapy. If you think about what you've been doing in the past few weeks, you'll realize the ache in your lower back probably comes from all the standing you did preparing for Thanksgiving or the vacuuming you did when you were cleaning up for Christmas.

If you experience side effects from pain treatments, let your doctor know, and indicate which side effects you are willing to tolerate and which ones you find unacceptable. For instance, all morphine and codeinelike products cause constipation and lethargy. One patient may say, "I'll accept a little sleepiness if I can get complete pain relief." Someone else may insist on a clear mind above all, pain relief being secondary.

Don't be embarrassed to tell your doctor or nurse if you're having trouble paying for your medications—you can usually get effective medications to fit your budget. And tell your doctor exactly what you are physically capable of doing. If you are able to take care of yourself and to swallow without difficulty, you can handle pills. But if you are bedridden and have limited assistance, pain medication in a patch that gets changed once every three days, or that is delivered automatically by a subcutaneous pump managed by your caregiver, makes a lot more sense.

Continuous communication is essential to sustained pain relief. Tell your doctor and nurse if: (1) the pain medication isn't working, (2) you have symptoms such as nausea, constipation, or excessive sweating, or (3) you develop trouble breathing or a rash or itching (these may be signs of allergy and you may need to stop the medication immediately).

If your care is transferred from one group of doctors to another, or from one hospital to another, the new team must to talk to the old team. Jane lived in a rural area and had always sought treatment from a university hospital two hours from her home. As her condition worsened, the trip into the city became formidable, so she transferred her care to her community hospital and a new team. "The change was upsetting and scary until I found just the right doctor for me, who cared enough to read through all my records and call my two doctors from the university hospital to get the full scoop on my condition."

Communication defines your care, makes your relationship with your doctor and nurse more meaningful, and helps keep you in control of your well-being.

Understand Your Pain

Your pain is always unique. Before an effective treatment plan can be designed for you, you must be able to describe and characterize your pain for your doctor and nurse as accurately as you can. And you and your doctor and nurse must reevaluate your pain periodically to continually maintain and improve your pain management.

Your caregivers can better understand your pain if you can provide answers to the following questions:

1. Where does it hurt? Does it start in one place and stay there, or does it move around to other spots?
2. What does it feel like? Sharp, dull, hot, cold, aching, throbbing?
3. Were there any precipitating events? A fall, discontinuation of long-term steroids, resumption of activity after prolonged bed rest, or strain from compensating for a problem elsewhere (such as sore shoulders from using a walker)?
4. How bad is the pain, on a scale of 0 to 10? Zero for no pain, ten for the worst pain you can imagine.
5. How long does the pain last? When does it start? Is it constant, intermittent, fleeting, the same throughout the day, or worse at a particular time?
6. What makes it get worse? A certain position or movement, particular foods, lying on a hard surface, cold or rainy weather, feeling upset?
7. What makes it get better? A particular position, time of day, medication? When your mother or mother-in-law arrives—or leaves?
8. Do you have any other symptoms associated with the pain? Sweating, anxiety, palpitations, depression, insomnia?

Once you are satisfied that your caregivers understand your answers to these questions and appreciate your symptoms, circumstances, and living situation, your doctor will examine you and order appropriate tests to further understand the cause of your pain. (See Chapter 5.)

All of the information that your doctor gathers leads to a hypothesis and a working theory of what causes your pain, which is undoubtedly complex and multifaceted. For example, you may have had recent breast surgery, and your job involves moving small boxes from place to place. This activity is increasing your discomfort in the area of your surgery and worsening minor but persistent muscle pain. Or, you may have a swollen arm (lymphedema) as a result of your treatment, producing a heavy, uncomfortable, persistent ache in your arm and shoulder, which in turn stresses your neck and back. Or, you have metastatic disease to the spine that is causing you bone pain, nerve pain, and muscle soreness, leading to anxiety and depression (psychological pain). Each of these important issues must be addressed and analyzed by your caregivers.

A Strategy for Pain Management

The next step is to define the solution to your pain problem. There is a large and evolving armamentarium of pain therapies that can effectively relieve pain, alone or in combination. Specific sites of pain suggest specific treatments; diffuse pain requires general treatment.

The best way to treat limited pain and get the fewest side effects is to treat the underlying cause of pain in the part of the body where the pain is located, and leave the rest of the body alone. This is possible only if the pain is localized in a small area of the body, and pain medications can be added or removed as needed. The best way to treat diffuse pain and get the fewest side effects is to combine local and general therapies.

Effective use of pain medications should operate on the following principles:

1. Combine medications to take advantage of the synergy between medications and to address the multifaceted nature of the pain.
2. Start medications in the low end of their therapeutic range; then increase the dose based on symptomatic response.
3. Plan for continuous round-the-clock pain relief, rather than intermittent, "as needed" pain relief.
4. Change medication if it fails to relieve your pain after you have used it to its therapeutic potential. Try any subsequent medication for at least a few days before you give up on it and try another. If you are taking a combination of pain medications, try to change only one at a time.
5. Treat or prevent side effects. Address other medical and psychological conditions that can affect how you experience pain.

6. Keep the solution to your pain problem simple, within your budget, and compatible with your lifestyle.

Make sure your doctor knows about any allergies you may have, so you can avoid any medication to which you are allergic. In fact, it's a good idea to mention your allergies whenever your doctor is about to prescribe any medication for you. Allergies to codeine and morphine are not uncommon. Bear in mind, however, that there is a significant difference between an allergy and a difficulty in tolerating the side effects of a particular medication. For example, nausea is a side effect, not an allergic reaction.

The simplest and cheapest way to take medication is by mouth. If you are unable to swallow or you have nausea, you will probably have to use another method of delivery. Avoid medications that must be given intramuscularly: it hurts, it's inconvenient, and absorption into your system is unreliable.

Getting Started

Most pain regimens start with a nonsteroidal anti-inflammatory drug (NSAID) and add (not substitute) a narcotic or an opioid. NSAID dosages have an upper limit, because too much can cause kidney and liver damage, or worse. Narcotics can be given in increasing doses, side effects permitting, without a comparable "ceiling." There are many choices of medications in each group (see Table 23.1). Your doctor and nurse must monitor you closely to balance benefits and side effects.

Mild Pain to Moderate Pain

NSAIDs include over-the-counter and prescription drugs. These are the NSAIDs that I usually use, listed by their chemical and trade names: acetaminophen (Tylenol), ibuprofen (Advil, Motrin), aspirin compounds (Trilisate), and ketorolac (Toradol). Among NSAIDs, I usually start with acetaminophen. Don't exceed the maximum dose recommended by the manufacturer. Mild but persistent discomfort, such as breast and underarm surgery pain, can usually be managed by NSAIDs alone.

If NSAIDs are unable to control all your pain, the next level of medications combine an NSAID with a narcotic, offering more pain relief through synergy between the drugs, with fewer side effects than if you took a narcotic alone to control your pain. Combined medications within this group are all fairly similar, and which one you start

TABLE 23.1. Pain Medications

MILD TO MODERATE PAIN
NSAIDs (nonsteroidal anti-inflammatory drugs)
    acetominophen (Tylenol and generic brands)
    ibuprofen (Advil, Motrin)
    aspirin (aspirin, trilisate, Ecotrin, Excedrin)
    ketorolac (Toradol)
    entodolac (Lodine)

Narcotic and NSAID combinations
    acetaminophen and oxycodone (Percoset, Tylox, Roxicet)
    aspirin and oxycodone (Percodan)
    acetominophen and propoxyphene napsylate (Darvocet)
    acetominophen and hydrocodone (Vicodin and Lortab)

MODERATE TO SEVERE PAIN
NSAIDs
    as described above, taken in combination with one of the following

Narcotics Alone
    morphine (sustained release preparations: MS Contin, Oramorph,
       Kadian; immediate release: MSIR, Roxanol)
    hydromorphine (Dilaudid)
    oxycodone (sustained release: oxycodone; immediate release: Roxicodone,
       OxyIR)
    fentanyl (Duragesic patch)
    meperidine (Demerol)
    methadone (Dolophine)

with depends on what your doctor and nurse recommend and what you accept. Percoset and Tylox both contain acetaminophen and oxycodone (Tylox has 500 mg of acetaminophen, Percoset has 325 mg), Percodan contains aspirin and oxycodone, Darvocet contains propoxyphene napsylate and acetaminophen, and Vicodin and Lortab have acetaminophen and hydrocodone. You can also take codeine and acetominophen in separate pills to get the combined relief.

Of these various combinations, I like to prescribe Percoset because I've been using it for years, it works, and I'm comfortable with it. I usually avoid aspirin, because it prolongs bleeding. Codeine is a reasonable choice if you have mild pain and you also need a cough suppressor. Otherwise, it causes too much constipation, nausea, and sedation for the amount of relief it provides. How you, your doctor, and your nurse choose one medication over another depends on various factors, discussed in the next few sections.

I increase the dose of Percoset (or other combined tablet) until the pain is controlled or until the maximum dosage of acetaminophen is reached. The dosage of combined pills that you can safely take is limited by the amount of acetaminophen or aspirin they contain. Once you get to that point, if pain persists or progresses, I give my patients a choice: (1) use the maximum dose of acetaminophen and separately increase the oxycodone (Percoset, plus extra oxycodone [Oxycontin], or acetaminophen and oxycodone taken separately), or (2) use acetaminophen and a stronger narcotic, such as morphine or Dilaudid.

Moderate to Severe Pain

There are many choices for relief of moderate to severe pain, all of which have significant side effects proportional to the amount of medication you take, including constipation, lethargy, nausea, and dry mouth. But these side effects are usually more tolerable than the pain.

Morphine is very effective and versatile. It comes in many forms: immediate-release; twelve- and twenty-four-hour extended-release; pill, liquid, suppository, and intravenous. Hydromorphine (Dilaudid) is a good alternative to morphine and is also available in various forms, but usually requires more frequent dosing: every four hours. Fentanyl (Duragesic) is an effective pain medication that comes in a patch, which is worn on the skin and changed every three days. Methadone is good for persistent pain, but the dose has to be adjusted slowly because it is long acting, so it's easy to overdo an increase and get excessive side effects when blood levels of the drug and its active metabolites (breakdown products) accumulate.

The essential difference in treatment of moderate and severe pain is the dose of narcotics you take for relief. I usually increase the amount of narcotic to improve pain control, and I keep the dose of the NSAID the same.

Let your doctor know your preference: medication every four hours, twice a day, once a day, or every three days. Your goal should be round-the-clock pain relief without having to get up in the middle of the night to take any medicine. There are some people, however, who prefer taking pain medication on an as-needed basis, preferring to *treat* pain rather than *prevent* it. Others don't want to take unnecessary medication, so they wait to be sure they have pain before they treat it.

If your pain is likely to improve on its own in relatively short order (e.g., immediate postoperative breast surgery pain; bone marrow or liver biopsy pain), your doctor will probably select a short-acting medication like Demerol or Dilaudid, or a short-acting morphine.

If the pattern of your pain is variable and no set dose works, your doctor may suggest one of these options to cover the background mild to moderate pain: (1) a variable dose of one narcotic like Dilaudid; (2) a longer-acting morphine (every 12 hours, like MS Contin or Oramorph; every 24 hours, like Kadian); or (3) a Duragesic patch; and for all three options, adding in a short-acting morphine for the episodic, more intense breakthrough pain.

Persistent, steady, predictable pain is easier to control; the choice is among the extended-release morphine preparations, a fentanyl patch, or methadone.

If your pain worsens and your condition declines, you will need an augmented but simplified regimen. Under these circumstances, I prescribe the longest-acting oral morphines, the fentanyl patch, or continuous morphine by intravenous drip or subcutaneous pump.

No matter how significant your pain becomes, you and your doctor should always attend to the other aspects of your physical and emotional health that can affect how you experience pain. Are you nauseated? Constipated? Depressed? Paying attention to and managing these other symptoms can make treatment of your pain much more effective, at lower doses, with fewer side effects.

To ease depression, apart from pain relief, stay in charge of the manageable responsibilities and activities in your life that you care about; find comfort in family and friends; call support lines sponsored by breast cancer organizations; participate in a support group; seek individual counseling; stay connected with your place of worship; talk to your rabbi, priest, or minister; and talk with your doctor about a full range of effective antidepressant medications (Prozac, Zoloft, Pamelar, etc.).

Treatment of nausea and constipation is discussed later in this chapter.

Management of Common Pain Syndromes

Your pain management may fit into one of the following common pain syndromes, each of which requires a different approach.

Painful Mucous Membranes, or Mucositis

A lump in the throat and painful swallowing are common symptoms of treatment-induced mucositis, which is characterized by inflamed and ulcerated linings of the mouth, throat, rectum, and vagina. Vaginal mucositis causes pain, discharge, and sometimes itching. Mucositis can be caused by yeast infections, certain chemotherapies (such as 5-fluorouracil), and unavoidable radiation to the esophagus. Yeast infections are caused by suppression of the immune system or by the use of steroids or antibiotics, and they can be recognized by a cottage-cheese-like coating of the mouth or discharge from the vagina.

A combination of diet changes, medications, and common sense is the most effective approach to relief. Diet recommendations include avoidance of hot (temperature), spicy, and acidic (tomato sauce, orange and grapefruit juices) foods, and caffeine. Cold milk products are most comfortable. Try cold sour cream just before meals to coat the passageway and ease discomfort (if you don't like the taste, you might like adding sugar and vanilla extract or fruit syrup). Avoid big pills, or try swallowing them mashed in applesauce.

Medications include nonsteroidal anti-inflammatory agents in liquid form; carafate suspension; 2 percent viscous lidocaine mixed half and half with Maalox or Mylanta, and swallowed slowly before meals or as needed to numb the mouth and throat. Liquid Tylenol with codeine is also helpful. Your doctor may have his or her favorite throat-numbing "cocktail."

Oral yeast infection is treated with antiyeast medicine (Diflucan, Nystatin, or ketoconazole). Vaginal yeast infection may respond to medications (Terazol 3 vaginal cream, Diflucan) or to plain yogurt with active acidophilus culture introduced into the vagina. (Some women use a turkey baster [you can snip the tip to make the hole bigger]; others just maneuver the yogurt in with their hand or a spoon.)

Underarm, Breast, and Chest Wall Pain

After surgery under the arm and around the breast, many women experience a strange mixture of numbness and pain in the area of the surgery because of nerve injury. Small nerves were unavoidably bruised, stretched, or cut during surgery. Radiation can add to the tenderness of the nerves, skin, muscles, and soft tissues of the breast.

The region of the shoulder, arm, armpit, and adjacent chest is a very busy area that you normally pay little attention to. But if asymmetry and pain develop, you may be constantly aware of this area of your body, and the symptoms may become an insistent reminder of your condition.

As nerves regrow, you may experience a weird crawly sensation, itching, and a supersensitivity to touch. Your discomfort may resolve on its own, or it may persist but you find you can adapt to it.

Radiation-induced skin soreness responds nicely to hydrocortisone cream (I start with 1 percent and move up to 2.5 percent as needed), pure nonalcohol-based aloe vera ointments, and avoidance of very hot showers and hot tubs. Don't use antiperspirants or fragrances within the sensitive area until it has healed. (If you must use an antiperspirant, and cornstarch doesn't work, ask your doctor for a prescription for Drysol. An application once a week is usually sufficient.)

Narcotics are usually unnecessary; NSAIDs are generally adequate to resolve this type of pain.

Management of a tender, swollen arm caused by lymphedema is described in Chapter 10.

Recurrent cancer on the chest where the breast used to be can cause significant pain, which can respond to radiation and chemotherapy combined with pain medication.

Bone Metastases

When breast cancer spreads to the bone, it destroys the scaffolding of the bone, irritates nerve endings, and causes pain.

If there is one or just a few areas of significant bone pain, the most effective way to relieve the pain is to eradicate the cancer that is causing it. Local external beam radiation therapy is the most effective treatment of painful bone metastases, providing substantial or complete pain relief in over 85 percent of people for a significant period of time, without the sedation and constipation associated with narcotics.

Radiation can cause fatigue and is inconvenient. (You have to go to a hospital for treatment five days a week for a period of about thirty minutes a day.) Depending on what site is treated, radiation can cause other side effects: nausea, if the area near your stomach is treated (upper lumbar spine), or irritation of your esophagus with transient lump-in-throat discomfort and pain with swallowing, if radiation is given to the upper spine. Radiation can be combined with a narcotic and an anti-inflammatory agent.

Pain from diffuse bone metastases is best treated with a narcotic and an anti-inflammatory agent. Chemotherapy or tamoxifen can be very effective at eradicating cancer cells in all areas of bone involvement. External beam radiation therapy can be given to one or just a few areas that are causing the most pain. Diffuse pain can also be treated with a medication called Aredia or an intravenous injection of strontium-89, a radioactive substance that is taken up by bone-making cells throughout your body; its dose is then delivered to the adjacent cancer cells, easing pain. If no other therapy works, external beam radiation therapy can be given by machine, to half of the body at one time. If, for example, you have diffuse painful metastases of the pelvic bones and legs, the lower half of your body can be treated with one large dose.

Immobilization of a painful area is sometimes helpful. For example, a sling can be worn until radiation to a painful shoulder metastasis has been completed. (See Chapter 22.)

Nerve Pain

Surgery can cause nerve pain in several ways: when scar tissue entraps nerves or when nerves are cut, stretched, or bruised. Breast cancer can cause nerve pain by growing around, along, and into nerves in both the central nervous system (in the brain, at the base of the skull as nerves leave the brain, in the spinal cord, next to the spinal cord) and the peripheral nervous system of the body (in nerves that branch off the spinal cord, such as the shoulder area's brachial plexus).

Nerve pain may respond best to a combination of therapies. First, steroids may be initiated to relieve some of the swelling and pressure on the nerve tissue (Decadron). Then, radiation therapy is given to shrink and eradicate the cancer that is pressing on the nerves—treating a bone metastasis in the back that is pushing on a nerve, or whole brain radiation for brain metastases, or radiation of lymph nodes that are sitting on the brachial plexus. If you have a specific site of pain that is mild and persistent, your doctor may recommend trying a TENS (transcutaneous electrical nerve stimulator) unit, a small electrical device that you wear, which emits low voltage vibrations that can interfere with or drown out the pain message your nerves are sending from your body to your brain.

An NSAID is helpful for mild pain; a narcotic may be needed for more significant pain. Many patients also benefit from a special group of drugs that work directly on nerve function: nortryptyline (Pamelor) or amitryptyline (Elavil). It takes one to two weeks for these drugs to start working; your doctor and nurse will need to adjust the dose according to your response.

Noncancer scar tissue nerve entrapment may respond to surgical release of the nerve if the surgeon believes the area of compression is discrete and can be precisely localized. Otherwise, it is treated with the therapies mentioned previously, excluding radiation.

If these specific therapies and pain medications don't give you adequate relief for a specific nerve pain, there are several procedures that can numb the involved nerve. Pain medication can be delivered through an epidural catheter (a small plastic tube) into the fluid that surrounds the spinal cord. This treatment affects the area that's producing the pain and leaves the rest of you alone, avoiding unnecessary side effects. Another approach is to "block" the particular compressed nerve that is causing the pain by injecting a substance such as alcohol around the nerve. These two procedures are done by an anesthesiologist. A surgeon may actually cut the nerve causing the pain, but only if the nerve can be safely sacrificed.

Muscle Pain

Any person who suffers pain from bone metastases as well as nerve pain may overwork and strain muscles to compensate for the pain. If you are holding your back rigid and straight to minimize movement-induced back pain, your back muscles inevitably are going to get sore. If you swivel your right hip each time you walk to take pressure off a painful left hip, the muscles surrounding your right hip will get sore. If you must use a walker to get around because your legs are weak or you have pelvic pain, your arms and shoulders will get sore from all the extra work they have to do. And if you're suddenly released from pain that's kept you from doing things you enjoy, such as tennis or swimming or dancing, you may start up again with such enthusiasm that you overstrain your out-of-shape muscles, and you'll be sore once more.

Back muscle strain responds to a few days of complete bed rest and doctor-supervised use of NSAIDs, muscle relaxants (such as Valium), massage, heat or cold applied to the surface (depending on the type of problem and status of your circulation), and strengthening of the muscle groups with guided exercise.

Shingles

Shingles is a reactivation of the herpes zoster virus (the same virus that causes chicken pox) in a particular nerve pathway, most commonly in the face and chest areas, with moderate to severe pain. This is noncancer nerve pain, but it is not uncommon in women with breast cancer.

The infection shows up as a red rash with small blisters in a band-like area, which becomes extremely painful. The rash may be barely visible (or, on occasion, totally absent), but the pain is still there. Treatment starts with acyclovir (Zovirax) plus pain medications described under nerve pain: steroids, NSAIDs, narcotics, Pamelor or Elavil, as your doctor prescribes.

Abdominal Pain

There are many kinds of abdominal pain. Probably the most common forms of noncancer abdominal pain and discomfort are treatment side effects on bowel function: constipation, gas, and diarrhea. The treatment of constipation will be outlined more fully later. Diarrhea and gas caused by chemotherapy or abdominal-area radiation are managed by the change to a low-residue diet (no fresh fruits or vegetables, limited fiber) and the use of medication such as Pepto-Bismol, Immodium AD, or Lomotil and/or Bentyl. Diarrhea caused by antibiotics needs to be evaluated first with a stool sample, because it may be the result of a *Clostridium difficile* infection that is treated with another kind of antibiotic (Flagyl).

Women who have had the TRAM flap reconstructive operation (see Chapter 6) have abdominal pain, which usually lasts a couple of months, from the tummy tuck that goes with the procedure. Other common causes of abdominal pain are the ones already described: back pain that radiates forward, and shingles.

Obstruction of the bowel caused by blockage by scar tissue or cancer produces crampy belly pain and bloating, followed by nausea and vomiting. This condition requires immediate evaluation and management by your oncologist and surgeon.

Other types of abdominal pain in women with advanced breast cancer include pain in the center of the abdomen from enlarged lymph nodes invading or compressing adjacent organs and nerves. And liver pain, in the upper right and side of the abdomen, which occurs when the liver is distended with cancer, stretching the fibrous capsule that surrounds it. These two kinds of pain are usually addressed with chemotherapy and pain medications.

If abdominal lymph node or liver disease has not budged, or has grown, despite chemotherapy, and if the pain remains uncontrolled and progressive and these one or two areas are the only areas of metastatic disease, radiation can be given to one site or the other, usually one at a time. (If the area is too big, the side effects can be too great.) If you have diffuse metastatic disease, and if pain in these abdominal areas (and other areas) is significant, narcotic pain medication by intravenous drip or subcutaneous pump may be indicated.

Other Pain Syndromes

The preceding descriptions of common pain syndromes and their management with conventional therapies is by no means all-inclusive. If your pain doesn't fit any of these descriptions, it doesn't mean that your pain is bizarre and that there is no way to relieve it. Talk to your doctor and nurse about it, obtain the necessary evaluation to figure out what is causing your pain, and then figure out a treatment plan together that is reassessed at regular intervals.

The treatments I've described are not all-inclusive, either. Conventional treatment combined with complementary medical therapies such as acupuncture, visualization, distraction, hypnosis, Reiki, Shiatsu, and biofeedback can be very helpful in dealing with mild to significant pain. (See Chapter 19.)

Use the information in this section to help you understand your symptoms and to give you the confidence to ask your doctor and nurse for the therapy that you think might help. Exactly which medications will help you depends on your unique experience with pain. Work closely with your doctor and nurse. Remember: Don't use anyone else's medication, and don't use out-of-date medication. Take none of the medications we have talked about without your doctor's specific recommendation. Have one physician in charge of your medications. More than one doctor prescribing pain medications can be confusing and even dangerous.

Commonsense Pain Relief

There's always room for common sense to improve your pain symptoms. Be practical, and consider your lifestyle. Keep your approach to pain control as simple as possible. Avoid complicated regimens with multiple medications that must be taken frequently but at different times of the day; you wind up watching the clock and trying to keep track of dozens of different pills.

If your pain is worsened by a particular movement, try to avoid such motion if you can. Prevent falls before they happen, an important way to prevent additional pain and suffering. The last thing you need is a broken bone, a twisted back, or a disabling muscle spasm. Fix that loose board on the stair landing; always use the stair handrail; never carry packages that block your view going up or down stairs. Tack down loose rugs. Make sure hallways and stairs are well lit. Buy a nonslip bathtub mat. Avoid wide slacks that can cause you to trip. Wear rubber-soled shoes. Always use the brake when getting in and out of a wheelchair. Always look where you are going. Don't ever step onto icy patches—better yet, when the weather report mentions icy conditions, stay home.

There are more ways to save your energy and prevent injury when your mobility is compromised by pain. Keep your telephone, clock, radio, TV changer, tissues, water, medications, and reading materials next to your bed or chair so you don't have to get up unnecessarily or scramble to the phone. If you require help getting to the bathroom, someone should instruct your caregiver to ask you at regular intervals throughout the day whether you need to use the bathroom. This saves you from embarrassment or a last-minute rush, and it helps preserve your dignity. Drink lots of fluid when you take any pills, sitting upright or standing to avoid choking or irritating your esophagus.

Managing Side Effects of Pain Medication

If you encounter side effects with the pain medication you are taking, you can change the medication with the hope of finding a more tolerable drug, or you may decide to continue the drug you're on because it gets rid of your pain and you're prepared to cope with the side effects.

Lethargy

Lethargy that shadows you through the day is a significant side effect of the use of narcotics. Nighttime drowsiness is not the problem; uninterrupted sleep through the night is a blessing. It's the logy feeling in the daytime, robbing you of energy, that can be so discouraging. Lethargy from pain medications tends to improve within a week or two of starting the medication.

In addition to making you drowsy, narcotics may also make you confused. But have your calcium level checked to be sure it's within normal range, since a high calcium blood level is not uncommon in women who have bone metastases, and it can also cause lethargy, confusion, and constipation.

How much lethargy you experience depends on your sensitivity to each individual narcotic; morphine may snow you, whereas fentanyl may just give you a buzz. Your doctor can switch the type of pain medication you are taking to find the one you tolerate best. The way you take the medication can also make a difference. Smaller, more frequent doses of medication usually produce less sedation than higher doses taken less often.

Try to avoid other causes of lethargy: dehydration, heavy foods, depression, not getting out of bed, and not moving around. You will become dehydrated if you are not eating or drinking (particularly if the weather is hot or you have a fever), or if you are not taking in sufficient nutrients and essential chemicals. Signs and symptoms of dehydration include dry loose skin, palpitations, high pulse, dizziness, low blood pressure, dry mouth, and lethargy. (The last four symptoms are also frequent side effects of narcotic use.)

Depression is a common cause of lethargy in people who are approaching the end of their life. Antidepressant medications can be very effective and can help relieve pain at the same time. Prozac, Zoloft, and Pamelor are some examples.

Lethargy can also result from a constant nighttime-like environment. You're tucked in bed all day, curtains closed, quiet voices, low lights, no activity or exercise, no natural light, minimal hustle and bustle, lying half asleep, daydreaming. Bring daytime back into your life. Pull back the curtains and get out of bed if you can. Keep your mind active with conversation, talk-radio, TV, an engaging novel.

If lethargy persists and you are fighting to stay awake, you can drink caffeinated coffee or take caffeine supplements, if your doctor okays them. Other stimulants you can ask your doctor about include dextroamphetamine (Adderall, Dexedrine) and methylphenidate (Ritalin).

Constipation

Constipation is a common side effect of pain itself, and of inactivity, depression, and stress, as well as pain medication. A bloated, stopped-up, heavy feeling can aggravate any other symptom you have. If you become severely constipated, you may even develop nausea because the food you eat has nowhere to go but up.

Contrary to intuition, even if you are not eating much food, your body still makes stool, which needs to be eliminated. (Much of stool comes from sloughed off cells that line the inside of the bowel, which are renewed every three days.) As troubling as constipation can be for you, it is both preventable and treatable.

To avoid constipation when you're on pain medication, drink lots of liquids, keep to a high-roughage diet that includes fresh fruits and vegetables and bran, and use daily stool softeners such as Senokot or Colace. Bulk-formers, such as Metamucil and Citrocel, act a little like sawdust. Once they fill up with water, they help move your bowels, but if you're not taking in much fluid, they can stay put and stop you up. Colace is a lubricant that softens the stool. If you simply can't eat enough roughage and drink enough fluid to move along the contents of your intestinal tract, and constipation develops, you'll need to take the next step.

If you are already constipated, a simple stool softener alone doesn't usually do the trick. But before buying a bagful of expensive products off the drugstore shelf, try to figure out what kind of constipation you have. Is it slow bowel activity or bowel blockage and associated backup? If your bowels have simply slowed to a halt, you need to take something that will get that conveyor belt going again. Start out with a combined stool softener and gentle laxative, such as Peri-Colace or Doxidan. If you still have no bowel movement within one to two days, you can add one of the following medications that stimulate the bowel muscle to move faster: Dulcolax, milk of magnesia, Haley's M-O, or your favorite over-the-counter brand. If there is still no action after one to two more days, ask your doctor if it's okay to proceed with *one* of the following bowel stimulants: Dulcolax suppository, magnesium citrate (looks like a small bottle of soda), senna extract X-Prep Liquid, or lactulose (this one is my favorite for real results). Or use mineral oil, which works as a stool lubricant. A Fleet enema will both stimulate bowel action and lubricate the stool.

If there is still no action, you should have your caregiver perform a rectal exam to see if the cause of your constipation is impacted stool (hard stool plugging up your rectum). If stool is impacted in the rectum, treatment has to be aimed at unblocking the stool. The process of disimpaction starts by softening the stool with a glycerin lubricant suppository and taking a pain medication to ease discomfort. Then a doctor, nurse, or nurse's aide inserts a gloved and lubricated forefinger into the rectum to break up the hard stool so that it can be passed more easily. This procedure is followed by an enema and repeated until the coast is clear. (Take your pick: Fleet, warm tap water, or soap suds; if you still have no luck, a Fleet Mineral Oil Enema will do the trick.)

As soon as you have managed to relieve the constipation, stick to a high-fiber diet, a daily dose of Senokot or Colace to keep your bowels rolling, and maybe even a mild nightly cathartic (Peri-Colace). If you don't stick to this regime, you'll find yourself right back where you were before: stopped up. Work closely with your physician and nurse to guide your choices and to closely watch your blood's chemistry, which can be disturbed by excessive use of bowel stimulants such as lactulose and magnesium citrate.

Nausea

Nausea can be a side effect of pain medication, chemotherapy, and radiation. Loss of appetite or queasiness may be your only symptoms if you have very mild nausea. Mild to severe nausea is usually associated with some degree of vomiting. Nausea may resolve on its own as your body gets used to the pain medication, or it may be reason enough to stop that particular pain medication and try something new. If, however, your pain medication is working really well in all other respects, it's worth staying with it and adding an antinausea medication. Discuss the problem with your doctor and nurse.

Slight nausea may respond to Dramamine, scopolamine, or Benadryl; mild to moderate nausea usually responds to Torecan, Compazine, or Vistaril; for severe nausea, try Zofran first. If you have no luck with these, you may need to spring for the top-of-the-line Kytril.

If vomiting interferes with your ability to hold down medications by mouth, most antinausea medications are available in suppository form (e.g. Compazine). Scopolamine comes in a patch. Others can be given intravenously.

Radiation-induced nausea can usually be prevented by taking an antinausea medication forty-five to sixty minutes prior to treatment (e.g., Torecan or Compazine).

Alternative therapies, such as acupuncture, visualization, and herbal combinations, may also be considered and may be quite effective. And try ginger—in ginger ale, ginger tea you can brew from fresh ginger, or my favorite: crystallized ginger.

Dry Mouth

Dry mouth can be a side effect of any narcotic or antidepressant. It usually eases up somewhat with time, but some degree of dry mouth often persists. Carry water with you wherever you go, avoid dry foods, and drink fluids with your meal to help wash down your food. Sucking on hard candies and chewing gum can turn your saliva on; your mouth moistens and tastes a lot better.

Respiratory Depression

Respiratory depression can be a side effect of high doses of narcotics. If your breathing is slowed and you and your doctor are concerned, this narcotic side effect can be reversed by using a drug called naloxone (Narcan). This medication should be given in small doses, enough to get your breathing within acceptable range but not enough to allow pain to return.

Urinary Retention

A full, distended bladder that you can't empty on your own is a potential side effect of significant narcotic use. This is managed by lowering the dose of the narcotic and using intermittent catheterization to drain the bladder, until you are able to urinate spontaneously.

Reducing Your Costs

Cost is an important factor in choosing pain medications. Pills are generally the cheapest form of medication. Most of the medications available today—MS Contin, Oramorph, Dilaudid, Duragesic, Kadian—cost approximately the same for equivalent pain relief over a defined period of time. For example, one Kadian tablet is approximately twice the cost of MS Contin, but it lasts twice as long. The cheapest narcotic is methadone, which is also very effective.

I give my patients samples to try out any new prescription medication before they fill a big expensive prescription that doesn't work for them. Or, if samples are not available (narcotic samples are very hard, if not impossible, to get), I suggest they ask their druggist to fill only part of the prescription they are going to try; for example, asking for just ten pills of the sixty prescribed. If the pills work, they go back and get the balance.

To save money, you can send away to a bulk-order pharmacy or shop through AARP (the American Association of Retired Persons). But remember, you save money on a bulk order only if you are sure you will use the medications.

The high cost of over-the-counter medications may surprise you. Ironically, over-the-counter medications may cost you more money than prescription drugs because they are not usually covered by health insurance plans. To save at least some money, go for the generic or store brands, such as Thrift Drug's Treasury Brand, or acetaminophen instead of name-brand Tylenol.

Some American Cancer Society chapters will help pay for pain or antinausea medications.

The cost of specific palliative therapies—radiation, chemotherapy, and anesthesia procedures—is generally covered by most health care plans. If you have already elected the Hospice Benefit under Medicare, you should still be able to have palliative treatment *only if* adequate relief is not obtained from pain medication. (The decision to start Hospice Benefit requires that you agree to give up definitive treatments—your health insurance resources are then applied to a full range of supportive care services.) It's best to check with your plan to make sure of its requirements—say, precertification for one of these procedures. All HMOs (health maintenance organizations) are likely to require a strong, clearly defined letter from your doctor to justify the reason for one of these expensive palliative treatments. And be advised: Your hospice business advisers may try vigorously to discourage you from this therapy because the cost of the particular treatment may be subtracted from their fee.

Filling Your Prescriptions

Call your doctor during the workday if possible for pain relief prescriptions, suggestions, complaints, and renewals. Federal law forbids filling most narcotic prescriptions without a form *in hand*. You may sometimes be able to get a twenty-four- to forty-eight-hour supply from a pharmacist who knows you, to hold you over until your doctor mails in the prescription form or until you or your delegate can pick up the prescription from your doctor and take it to the pharmacy.

The law also stipulates no refills on narcotics. So every time you run out of medications, you need a new prescription form in hand. At the least, you can ask your doctor or nurse to call in the prescription so it's ready when you show up with the actual prescription slip, saving you some time and frustration.

If you want to save money by sending away to a bulk-order pharmacy or buying these medications through AARP, you may need two prescription forms from your doctor: one to take to your local pharmacist to hold you over until the larger order arrives, the other to send away for the larger order. You may be able to expedite your mail-away order by asking your doctor to fax the prescription to your supplier.

Conclusion

It's normal for anyone plagued by pain to feel angry, exhausted, and depressed, and to sometimes wonder if life is even worth living. Try not to be discouraged. Pain can be successfully treated. Let this chapter guide you and your caregivers toward achieving relative comfort and independence for you, empowering you to ask for—maybe even demand—the help you need.

Communicate with the people who can help you. Use common sense. Stay open-minded to some of the complementary therapies out there, such as acupuncture, hypnosis, meditation, and distraction, all of which have been relieving pain for centuries. And don't forget: Pain medications work only if you take them, if you take the right ones, and if you take enough of them. Above all, you must have your doctor's prescription before you try any of the suggestions in this chapter.

So get your pain under control, and then shoot for *pain-free*—and get back to feeling more like your old self.

24

Hospice

> I had very little knowledge of hospice when my mother
> was told she had less than six months to live, and we didn't
> know to get started right then. I thought hospice was just
> last-minute help. I lived out of town, and when we finally
> did connect with hospice, I felt awful that my mom had
> missed out on months of care.

How you live is very important, and how you die is very important.
Everyone talks about quality of life, but I feel more people need to
talk about quality of death. Hospice does, and more. It seeks to enhance the quality of dying, to provide physical and emotional support,
in a humane and professional manner. Wherever possible, that service
and support is provided within your own home, so that you may die in
the place you know and love, with peace and dignity, surrounded by
people you know and love. If home is not an option, you can go to a
hospice facility that serves the same purpose. For most hospice workers I work with, this is a calling, not simply a job.

Medical, psychological, and spiritual support are all part of hospice
care. Hospice also provides supportive services for your family. Care
comes from hospice nurses, social workers, physical therapists, nutritionists, chaplains, and volunteers who often have personal experience
with the value of hospice. You can get help with ordinary chores like
bathing, dressing, cooking, and cleaning, as well as with logistical
arrangements for transportation, equipment, nursing care, blood
draws, drugs for pain, and counseling (even help with financial and
estate plans). Hospice workers and volunteers intermesh to bring relief on many levels. Some volunteers provide their most valuable support just by sitting with you or your family, a presence that keeps you
from feeling helpless and alone.

If you are at the end of your life, you may find that hospice care is
the most responsive and effective resource available for providing

pain relief and overall support and for respecting your final wishes. If, however, the idea of hospice is not quite acceptable to you, if you still want to keep open the possibility of chemo or radiation therapy, it is possible to get something similar to hospice care, a step before hospice— "oncology care" at home—but the level of care is not usually as comprehensive as what you get from hospice.

I know families who just don't want strangers intruding on their privacy at this difficult time in their lives, who would rather do the caregiving themselves, and who would rather have their physicians to continue to be in charge until the end. One of my patients strongly objected to the religious fervor of the hospice worker she met. "I don't believe in God and I don't want these admittedly well-meaning zealots coming into my home as I'm dying and talking about life in the hereafter." Some hospice programs are tied to religious organizations; most are not, but even those that are usually do not impose their personal religious beliefs on you.

Many doctors offer end-of-life care rather than referring you to hospice, and they go on seeing you regularly, arranging for home care as needed or hospitalization if required.

When Hospice Starts

When it appears that illness has taken over, that you have six months or less to live and you have decided to give up definitive medical treatment for supportive comfort care only, you qualify for hospice care and can draw on hospice resources twenty-four hours a day, seven days a week. It sounds clear and straightforward in print; it's not. All signs may say you have six months or less to live, but most people are not prepared to give up all hope; most people—as we know from studies and anecdotal material—want to hold on to every shred of hope, want to try one more therapy, get one more chance, which may explain why more people don't use hospice. The point when your doctor tells you that your time is very limited may be the first time you learn about hospice and what it can do.

Starting hospice requires a doctor's referral. "I passed out and they brought me to the hospital. I am feeling fine now—but my doctor has stunned me with the news that I have only a few months to live. I can't believe it, but I'm trying to take in what's happening." Esther's children and family and friends were in shock, but they absorbed the news and acted on it, coming quickly to her side and engaging hospice.

Talk with your physician about hospice care as soon as you feel you can handle it, difficult though this may be. It's very hard to hear one more message confirming the reality of your circumstances. You may feel hopeless, rejected, and abandoned by your doctor, but I find that my patients very quickly get to appreciate the support and care that hospice offers, and they begin to recover some sense of well-being. Hospice has even prolonged the lives of some of the people they have cared for.

If your doctor doesn't talk to you about hospice, you should bring it up for discussion; hospice care has become a widely available service, but less than a third of those people eligible for it use it—in part because they live where it may not be available, or where doctors are not familiar with its value. Ask about hospice as early as possible, to find out whether it's for you, and to receive the maximum benefits possible from this service if you elect to use it. You may want to interview several different hospice groups—if there are more than one available to choose from—to find the one that comes closest to your spiritual beliefs, plans for end-of-life care, and other issues that matter to you; your family should participate in these interviews as well. Most important may be how all of you relate to the particular hospice nurse who will supervise your care.

Who's in Charge

The doctor who refers you to hospice usually agrees to oversee medical decisions presented by the hospice nurse, such as pain medication or intravenous hydration, but your physician's relationship with you does change when you begin hospice care. He or she is still involved in your care, but at a greater distance. You communicate primarily by phone, you seldom go to the hospital or the doctor's office, and it's uncommon for your doctor to visit your home with any regularity, if at all. This distance can often trigger separation anxiety that adds to your stress and sense of desperation. Don't let these feelings scare you. Talk to someone—maybe the hospice nurse, who is most likely to understand and can best help you manage the problem. Your doctor is still just a phone call away.

Your hospice nurse becomes your primary source of caregiving, communicating directly with your doctor about your condition, checking about medications, and so on. If you are distressed or have increased pain, you call your hospice nurse, and, if necessary, your nurse will get in touch with your doctor. (Your hospice nurse is especially good at getting hold of your doctor; she often has access to his or her private line and beeper number.)

What Hospice Does

Hospice doesn't *make* you die. It recognizes the fact that you are near the end of your life and makes dying as easy and comfortable as possible. "We help you *live*. We don't accelerate death." Still, some people have the mistaken notion that a commitment to hospice invites a self-fulfilling prophecy, that saying anything as explicit as "six months to live" becomes a death sentence, a fact, no matter what the state of your illness or well-being. Actually, the "six months to live" estimate is prepared primarily for medical insurance purposes, qualifying you for access to all hospice benefits under most insurance plans, including Medicare.

Most patients report feeling immeasurably better once they've joined hospice and have started receiving hospice services. "We had this patient come in in terrible pain, and in just a little while she was back to working on her computer."

Visits from hospice workers are based on need: once a week or every day. "With technology what it is today, we don't have to move the patient back and forth—to draw blood, for instance." Your hospice nurse keeps in touch with your doctor, informing him or her of your status and your medications. Home care and hospice workers adjust pain medication to suit your needs, in the form of pills, patches, liquids, injections, subcutaneous pumps, or epidural catheters. If death is near, hospice care nurses may coordinate your care, with frequent evaluation of your condition, delivering pain medication and comfort care.

Hospice workers understand the anguish that you undergo at this time, and in addition to giving hands-on physical care, they are also able to help with your emotional state. Their insights and support extend to your family and children, helping them cope with the demands of this difficult time.

Your family has a crucial role to play, provided you want them involved and they are willing, able, and available; members are instructed in how to give medication and physical care. You can keep your children involved by letting them help in practical and meaningful ways; they can brush your hair, read you the newspaper, massage your neck, hands, or feet, tell you funny stories. (Don't underestimate the value of a good laugh—for you and for them.) They want to help and they need to feel they are contributing to your well-being. (See Chapter 25.)

If you have no family to step in for this role, home health aides may substitute. If you cannot take care of yourself completely at home, if you need twenty-four-hour care, or if you need continuous skilled nursing care, you may qualify for some form of additional in-home care, or if necessary you can go to a hospice center, nursing facility, or hospital.

If your family has been providing continuous care but they must go away, twenty-four-hour respite care is available for up to a week under the "Hospice Benefit," and this is covered by Medicare and most other policies. Depending on your insurance policy, where you live, and how long your family is away, the care may be provided in your home or at a hospice facility. Every hospice is different, and every insurance plan is different, so you'll have to investigate which benefits are available in the hospice you sign up with.

Most hospice care is team based: nurses, social workers, home health aides, and chaplains are the players. They meet regularly, review each patient's situation and each family's needs, determine whether to call for special help—a child psychologist, for instance—or request volunteer assistance for errands or social visits. (One volunteer took his hospice patient out every Friday to play bridge; it was a good time for both of them.) Hospice workers also need the support they get from one another to keep going, and to do the job they do well: "I don't know where I'd be if it weren't for my team."

Your Way

For some of you, euthanasia (painless death, or "merciful death") has a place in your philosophic approach to death. You may have joined the Hemlock Society, a group that believes in "death with dignity," using drugs to end life sooner, to end intolerable suffering. Women in a truly desperate situation might find themselves considering an extreme, such as working with Dr. Kevorkian or his followers, but even if you applaud what Dr. Kevorkian does, or you simply believe in keeping full control over your life and death, you may not have the energy, emotional stamina, or judgment at this point to arrange or evaluate this kind of "escape." Critics of what is called assisted suicide point out many flaws that blur what is claimed to be a rational appeal for an end to suffering. Fear of pain may cloud your judgment. Deep depression (which is not uncommon at this moment in this situation) drives some to premature death. But treatment with antidepressants can help you live longer and better. Fear of being a burden to one's family is another assailable reason frequently cited by sober appraisers of this life/death debate.

Another problem with this aggressive (or "logical") approach to dying is that most of the drugs recommended for this "final exit" require a doctor's prescription, and if you ask your physician to provide the prescription, you are asking your doctor to be an accomplice to an illegal action, subject to arrest and imprisonment. More important, most doctors are not comfortable with the idea of assisted suicide. Most doctors, however, are prepared to provide additional pain relief that includes the "dual effect of morphine" (serious pain relief accompanied by suppressed respiration and blood pressure, which can cause death) to a terminal patient in severe pain. The physician is intent on relieving extreme pain, agitation, uncontrollable coughing, and difficulty breathing, knowing that high doses of this medication carries a risk of death, especially for someone who is near death, whereas the intent of assisted suicide is to help the patient achieve relief through death.

Although those people who manage—discreetly—to procure the "final exit" medication may find peace of mind in having this "insurance" in hand—pills that will let them die when they choose—few end up using it. "It would give me peace to have something available as insurance, but my preference is to die naturally."

You have no need to get mixed up in that whole messy stew. If controlling how you die is important to you, then you should try to find a doctor and hospice nurse who will work as partners with you to support you in your search for a peaceful and painless, dignified, natural death.

Leslie had refused all treatment. We knew what lay ahead, and it was grim. Having taken care of Leslie for some time, I knew something of her attitude about cancer care, but we had never discussed end-of-life issues. It was important for me to understand her wishes. "I really very much want to be clearheaded until the moment I die— but I know the pain may keep that from being an option." Having made her wishes crystal clear, Leslie entrusted herself to my care.

Leslie's cancer was unusually virulent. Just six weeks after the diagnosis of liver metastases, she was on a morphine drip in hospice care. Following her explicit request that she be spared any symptoms of pain or distress, I increased her medication. This was something her family knew Leslie wanted, but something they were too uncomfortable to initiate themselves, even though they couldn't bear seeing her agitated, in pain, and suffering. The higher dose of morphine took away all Leslie's suffering, but it also hastened her death by lengthening and deepening her sedation. She passed away peacefully soon after.

I find it a challenge and a privilege to take care of women throughout their lifetime, and to uphold and respect their wishes to the very end. I try to do what needs to be done "their way," without violating the code of ethics I live by and the Hippocratic Oath of care I took when I became a physician. The women who are my patients have taught me many things, most especially those who have made the transition out of this life with dignity, courage, and great feeling for those they love.

25

Endings

I wanted to know the worst and I wanted to know it all. I
wonder if I will see my two boys graduate. Time is the
thing I lack most. I try to imagine taking life easy—what if
these are my last few years or months?

No one can accurately predict just how long you—or anyone—will
live, but if you have progressive metastatic breast cancer, you may be
approaching the end of your life. Despite encouraging stories of remission and amazing recovery, you inevitably think about death and
want to be prepared for whatever happens. This uncertainty, of itself,
is probably making you feel incredibly anxious. Your family is undoubtedly anxious as well. Knowing what to expect, getting honest
answers to your questions, dealing with as few surprises as possible—
and being treated with respect—gives you some way to hold onto a
measure of control.

Before you can gather your feelings and cope with helping your
children and family face what is happening, you need to find support
for yourself and assurance that you will not be abandoned or forgotten—emotionally as well as physically—by family and doctors. Jenny
was told she probably had six months to live; her doctor wanted to
give her all the help he could: "I'll be here for whatever I can do for
you at any time of the day or night." Leslie's husband never left her
side. Joan's partner was always there for her, but she also knew when
to back off and let Joan have time alone. If you are on your own, without someone close to you, or living in an unfamiliar place where you
have few friends or family, you may feel desperate and lonely and
scared. I urge you to seek support from your religious leader or
church group, cancer support group, or individual counselor, or from
professional connections, neighbors, or other people in your community or spiritual center.

All kinds of worries and concerns crowd in on you and overwhelm you, things you thought you could take years to deal with. Once you begin to handle some of these issues and recognize that you're doing all you can as well as you can, you may be able to achieve some peace of mind, a sense of serenity you might not have expected to feel. I have known women with intense religious convictions and spiritual beliefs who look toward death with a kind of hope, look forward to it as a release from suffering, dependency, and worldly cares. Religion is an enormous source of comfort and reassurance to women with this kind of faith. "I know I'm part of a plan; there's a reason for what's happening to me. God doesn't make mistakes."

Facing Your Mortality

Any discussion about your death is hard—especially if it means giving up your hope for a cure or remission. "I was with this woman on the West Coast also with end-stage disease who did every kind of medical thing you could think of—she tried to have bone marrow transplant twice. She went through the most horrible torture. It didn't help. I have come to accept what is happening to me: I had treatment for pain—and in between tortures, some marvelous times. What's the point of ruining what little time I have left?"

In fact, studies show that over 40 percent of people nearing the end of their lives are prepared to endure additional rigorous treatment for the promise of three more months of life. The desperate search for experimental or alternative treatment may represent a fierce determination to live, or it may be denial of what is so difficult to believe and accept: the end of life.

There is no generic approach to death. How my patients face their mortality is profoundly affected by their personality, life experience, and cultural values. Our culture's up-front presentation of a grim diagnosis is shocking to many other cultures; what we might call denial, other cultures view as a kinder, gentler approach to a terrible reality. In the old days, almost no one was told they were dying; the subject of death was not discussed. Doctors and families "protected" patients from the truth; everyone tried to maintain the semblance of normalcy and peace. Perhaps it spared patients anguish, but in many cases it deprived them and their loved ones of the opportunity to maintain control as life gradually slipped away. And the opportunity to find closure, to say good-bye to one another, was lost forever. "Nobody ever told me how sick my grandmother was, and I never got the chance to tell her how my life was going, how good it was going to be, and to give her that last jolt of pleasure before she died. I keep hoping that somehow she knows."

I see patients who fiercely deny the seriousness of their illness, convinced that this episode is just a bad turn that will soon right itself on its own or with some newfound cure. They just can't deal with death straight on. Denial for them is an elemental coping mechanism, the only way they can handle this terrifying situation. If it doesn't exist, then it can't hurt, and, *ipso facto,* they protect themselves and their families. Denial can be impenetrable—but it doesn't protect your family. If you are very sick, they know, and they want to be able to reach you, to talk to you about real issues. They find themselves deep in anguish, frustration, anger, and helplessness.

There are families, too, who want to avoid any direct talk about cancer and any discussion of death. A family member may pull me aside and ask that I not use the word *cancer,* or that I avoid anything that might "take all hope away" from their loved one. I find it hard to take care of a patient and her family with this approach. My normal approach is to be straightforward and honest and to tell my patient what is going on, how I can help, and how we can all work together to help her live as well as possible. But if the family doesn't want me to say anything, do I let them make decisions for my patient, or do I involve the patient anyway? I usually dodge the issue, by talking to my patient about "the problem," outlining the type of care that would be most helpful but omitting specific reference to the gravity of the situation. All the while, I'm listening very carefully to my patient and looking for signals that will let me know just what she really knows and what she wants to hear. Whatever questions she asks, I answer honestly.

Dealing with Your Fears

You may not have had experience handling the death of anyone close to you. You may never have seen a dead body or someone actually dying. Death is terrifying to think about on many levels. A lot of what's frightening is the unknown, so the more you know about what to expect, the better prepared you'll be for whatever may happen, and the less frightened you'll be.

Dr. David Spiegel, author of the book *Living Beyond Limits,* writes that it's best "to face the worst rather than simply to hope for the best. Facing death can intensify living. Rather than denying dying, we confront its inevitability and use that fact to help reorder life priorities, to focus on living better." When Dr. Spiegel spoke at one of Living Beyond Breast Cancer$_{SM}$'s conferences (May 1994), he contributed real information and a down-to-earth, fundamental message for women with metastatic disease. "Convert your anxiety to fear, and convert general fear to specific fears, to structure those fears into a series of problems that you can focus on and do something about. You do have things to do, to make your life rich and meaningful, to live more fully, to live your life right up to the end." Dr. Spiegel doesn't look or act like a guru, but for many women he is their inspiration and support, a mentor who helps them over the last boundary.

A sensitive physician can be very helpful, gathering you and your family together to talk honestly, to establish values and priorities for the future, and to ask each other the questions you must ask, to find answers for each other before it's too late. It's important for your doctor to establish "permission" to talk about what may trouble you (and your family) and to answer any questions you may have. "How long am I going to live?" "How will I die?" "How will you help me?" And for the family: "How will we know whether she's in a coma, or she has temporarily stopped breathing, or she is dead?"

Death is a process; it comes about in many steps. Sudden death—one moment you're fine, the next you're gone—is rare in breast cancer (although not uncommon in other illnesses, such as heart disease). There's no "right" way to talk about dying—except that any discussion must respect *you,* your personal way of doing things, your ability to make your own decisions, and the quality of your death, like the quality of your life. You and your family must be helped to develop a realistic understanding of what to expect each step of the way.

There is no way your doctor can answer what may be the most compelling question on your mind: "How long will I live?" No one has a crystal ball with the answer. Any specific amount of time that is mentioned feels finite and frightening—an ultimatum? a self-fulfilling prophecy?—and generally is not therapeutic. But it is important to know if you're likely to have years, months, weeks, or just days.

Not all doctors can or will be there when you need them. They may be too busy; they may have their own discomfort with death and with their perceived failure to beat the disease; they may lack interpersonal skills, or fail to take the time to reach out to you, to give you a chance to talk about what's worrying you. But a doctor who cares about you will listen and guide you through palliative care. Every doctor I know—just like any other human being—has strengths and weaknesses; we can hope that your doctor will care for you at this time of your life with affection, and that he or she will rise to your expectations.

Other professional caregivers may help you in many significant ways. Social workers smooth out all kinds of problems: "I couldn't make it without my social worker. She got my insurance to cover hospice and ambulance service, and she helped me figure out how to talk to my children." Many of my patients find great support from their religious counselor.

If you think you'd find comfort in the presence of other women in the same situation as you, a support group may be for you, if you have the energy to get involved—and get to meetings (see Chapter 2). You may find that meeting with a psychotherapist can be the most valuable support line for you. I have known women who were able to handle a grim prognosis knowing they had a dedicated therapist available when needed.

What Matters Most

What matters most to *you* at this time? "My kids. My daughter and my two sons are my life. My husband is a great dad, but he doesn't have the same intuitive knack with my daughter as he does with my boys—and I worry about the profound loss she will suffer when I die.

"My parents and my sisters have promised me that as long as they live they will be there for my children, but I don't want my kids to be motherless any longer than possible. I've made it clear to my husband that I want him to remarry—the Right Person—as soon as he can. I've even made a few suggestions—and warned him off some less-than-appealing candidates who'll likely be knocking at his door."

Jenny knew she didn't have much time. With two young children, she needed to prepare them as best she could for life without her, and she needed to provide them with memories of her love for them. "My body may go, but my spirit will always be with you." Jenny and her husband debated allowing their six-year-old to come see her—looking so weak and unnatural—in the hospital, but they finally decided to allow the child to visit. As her little girl was leaving, she told her mother, "I have to say good-bye because you may die and I'll never see you again." It was in fact the last time she saw her mother; how important and precious a memory—even though upsetting—that visit would always be for her.

The hardest departure may be that of a divorced mother who knows her children will be taken by an ex-spouse whose nurturing skills she mistrusts. What power does she have to protect them, what people can she engage to watch over them—who won't inflame a potentially unstable father? She should try to communicate her wishes in some way with her ex-spouse, just as she needs to encourage members of her family or her good friends to try to do what they can to oversee the children's welfare. And she should explore any legal protection a creative lawyer can manage, and formally document her wishes. At least she'll find some comfort doing all she can.

A younger woman wants to know that her children will be okay and safely cared for; an older woman may worry how a sick husband or elderly parent—or even a beloved pet—will survive without her. Almost every woman I've taken care of expresses one of these concerns.

You may want to record greetings, messages, and hopes, on paper, tape, or video, for your family to store for the future. "I'm recording favorite stories, from *Goodnight Moon* to *Rikki Tikki Tavi*." And Jenny wrote each of her children an inspirational letter about her love for them and her hopes for their future. When Esther's grown children were told she was dying, they flew in to be with her till the end, crowding onto her bed, holding and hugging each other. Her son David was consumed by a need to ask questions, to benefit from her quiet, earnest wisdom: What had been most important in her life? What did she hope he and his sisters would do with their lives? What did she believe to be the goals they should pursue? Esther, who had always worked in public service, was happy to talk about her life to her children. David also recorded his mother's memories of the family's history. "And I wrote down her recipes for all the great stuff she cooked."

You may have all kinds of ideas for preserving memories for your children, but find it hard to get around to doing them. It's not an easy thing to accomplish, but perhaps it will help if you think of it as a meaningful exercise for anyone—in good health or not—who wants to leave a permanent record for later generations. Whether you live another five decades, five years, five months, or five weeks, you'll be glad you assembled this material: messages, letters, notebooks, photographs. It's a commitment to the future, no expiration date at issue.

A lot of women I treat talk about wanting to be there for their child's wedding, especially if they know it's going to happen relatively soon: "My daughter became engaged just before I found out about the metastasis. All I can think about is how much I want to dance at her wedding." Yet no mother I've talked to wants to personally urge her child to move up the date. "She's always dreamed of a big wedding, and they had to reserve this place a year in advance and line up this big-shot caterer and order the gown months and months ahead of time. How can I ask her to change the date? Instead, I tell her I'll be there, I'll be there. But will I?"

It's a delicate situation, how much you can intrude on your children's lives as you think about the end of your own. In the case of a wedding, it doesn't have to be all or nothing; I've suggested that a civil service might satisfy my patient, and the large formal wedding can happen later on. Maybe someone else should raise the subject with the prospective bride and groom: a dear friend, a close sibling, your clergyperson, or your doctor (or this book). Staying out of this initial discussion will minimize the emotional load on your kids. Then your doctor can suggest a realistic prognosis of how long you have to live and what sort of time frame is possible for planning the wedding.

I have talked to both daughters and sons about this dilemma. I discuss the mother's medical status and how she feels about the wedding. Often, making it to this event becomes the driving incentive in the struggle to stay alive. I let them know how special a gift it would be to reschedule at least some part of the wedding so it takes place while their mother is still alive. And something usually gets worked out.

You should save your energy for healing and for resolving relationships that are important to you; you may decide, however, not to deal with relationships that don't work or that cause you pain and anger— even if it's a relationship with a child. Although most people see their impending death as their last chance to heal old wounds, one of my patients chose not to tell her estranged daughter that her breast cancer had become terminal. I talked to her about her decision, and I felt I had to point out how devastating it would be to her daughter—not to make my patient feel guilty but to have her consider the consequences of her decision. "If you don't say good-bye to your daughter, you'll deprive her of the final opportunity to be involved in your life and to do something meaningful for you. She'll feel terrible if she finds out you've excluded her. You may never see her again." My patient wouldn't change her mind.

Comfort and Support

Support and comfort, the feeling of being loved by your family and friends, are essential to maintaining your spirit; you can sustain much tribulation if someone is there with you, available and listening, holding your hand—or holding you—maybe not even talking, just being there.

On the other hand, you may want to keep your illness private so you're not badgered by family and friends calling and asking how you feel, how you *really* feel, and how they can help. Time is precious; save it for the ones you love most, those especially dear to you, those worth the emotional energy necessary for talking, sharing, seeking comfort.

Many people turn to religion, to a religious counselor, even if they have not been particularly observant. Rabbi Harold Kushner (author of *When Bad Things Happen to Good People*) says, "Those who have a religious outlook are blessed, believing in a power greater than one's self. Talk to each other, to your clergyman, to yourself. We may not be able to cure you, but we can heal you. We can share sorrow, help cherish and care for those you love, and help each other to enjoy this last part of your life." The end may be bearable when it is filled with the love of those who matter to you, with the vision they represent of a future beyond your own lifetime.

There are some people who turn to alternative sources: to meditation, yoga, or philosophic dialogue. Jane and her husband went to Michael Lerner's Commonweal in Bolinas, California. "At first I thought it might be too 'California' for me, but I got past that. I wasn't looking for a cure, but for help. And I found it. I came out feeling very serene, with a core sense that it didn't matter whether I lived or died—I had *lived*. I did not have to beat this illness to continue enjoying what time I had."

If your family won't talk openly with you—if it's just too hard and the strength and courage aren't there to make it work—perhaps a support group will help fill the gap, if you feel well enough to take on something new outside your home. Rita had to find some kind of comfort. When she and her husband were told she was dying, he burst out, "What's going to happen to me?" (See Chapter 2.) Support groups can be a major source of strength, relief, warmth, comfort, and love, significantly improving your quality of life. Women with advanced metastatic disease who were part of Dr. David Spiegel's support groups were less anxious and depressed, experienced less pain, and were generally in better spirits—and lived longer—than similar women who did not participate in support groups.

Don't overlook the support possible from the written word. Rabbi Kushner's book has been remarkable comfort to people of all faiths. Dr. Spiegel's book *Living Beyond Limits* has been valued by cancer survivors with a range of illnesses. Elisabeth Kübler-Ross's many books were pioneers in the study of death and dying. Bernie Siegel's books about inspirational living have been best-sellers. Laurence LeShan's book *Cancer as a Turning Point* is warm and compassionate. (See the Selected Readings section at the back of this book.)

And don't forget joke books. My friend's last weeks were lightened by the daily joke her husband shared with her from a treasury of old jokes. Humor can be a godsend to you, even laughing about dying. Rabbi Kushner tells the joke about the old man on his deathbed, sniffing the odors wafting in from the kitchen as his family prepares for the funerary repast. "How I'd love a bit of that chopped liver." "Sorry, Dad, but that's for 'after.' "

Drawing Close to One Another

How do you manage the passage of each day? There are things you must do, people you must see; you need to connect with those you care about and be as honest and direct as each of you can manage. Maybe there are things you've always wanted to say. " 'You have been such a generous friend all these years' are words I treasure, that *my* generous friend told me during our last visit together. I knew she felt that way, but now I have the words, and the picture of her as she said them as a memorial, in my memory."

Two friends in their sixties, married to older men, one telling the other, who was dying: "I always expected that someday, when we were little old ladies in tennis shoes, the two of us would travel together, on the cheap, doing what nobody but us would want to do." Friendship that had started in grade school had lasted through the births of grandchildren, but it wasn't going to last into old, old age. Instead, the one to outlive the other was asked: "Will you be grandmother to my grandchildren?" With the promise from her friend came assurance that the children she loved would be watched over, that life would go on, and that memories of a grandmother would be passed to the future.

It's often hard to find the right words. Some people can manage to say the right thing at the right time; others may say nothing when they should say something—right time or wrong time. And you can be sure that someone will say the wrong thing at the worst time, whether it's something stupid in front of your children—"Have you told them yet?"—or something clumsy when you're alone together: "If you're going to die I hope I'm not alive to see it."

Sometimes the wrong remark can set you off. "How can you say you know how I feel? You're not dying! You have no idea how I feel!" Most people are not confronting death, as you are, but there is still much of value they can share and offer you and your family. The quiet and thoughtful ways that friends and family show they love you can be so important to your spirit and resilience.

"Tell your children how much you love them. Tell them that you want them to think about you when you are no longer here. And that when they do, they may feel sad and happy and maybe even angry because you are not there—and that all those feelings will be very normal."

Doctors Can Help

Even after you have decided to stop your treatment, your doctors can continue to help you, by being available and accessible, and by showing that they care, that they're ready to step in and guide you in making the right choices. Holding hands, listening, and telling things honestly in unadorned language can be a most effective treatment. Leslie had just learned that liver metastases were the reason for three months of gnawing belly pain, and she and her husband and I were all in the room together, all terribly upset. We'd known each other a long time and had grown close. Leslie was a woman who always told it like it was. I gave her a long hug, held on to her hand and her husband's, and said "Leslie, I love you and I hate that @#$*@/f—g breast cancer!" They laughed through tension and tears, and the three of us let go of our feelings with further outrageous expletives.

Sally couldn't bear her medical oncologist (who had supervised her original chemotherapy). When she was diagnosed with terminal metastatic disease, she worried about whether she should change doctors. I insisted that she follow her feelings and helped her find a doctor she really liked, who would help her at this important point in her life. Sally was enormously gratified; as someone who always went out of her way to please others, she needed the encouragement and permission to do what *she* wanted to do.

For you to get the most help possible from your relationship with your doctor, the two of you should have similar approaches to your care, and your doctor should know how you feel about end-of-life issues, expressed verbally and also in writing as a living will or advance directive. You may be very different from one another in every other way, but that doesn't matter. What counts is your understanding and mutual respect for each other's humanity. I'm Jewish, but I take care of many Catholic nuns who are devoted to pro-life issues. They believe that both life and death have purpose and should be protected; they do not pursue aggressive treatment to the very end, nor do they believe in heroic measures. "Let God take me. I'm ready." I have also had a Jewish patient cared for by a Catholic hospice; she and her family felt totally at home, cherished by dedicated, loving caretakers.

Preparing Your Children

How do you prepare your children for what might happen to you? Young children may be comforted believing you will be up in heaven or out among the stars; older children want more reality-grounded answers. Whatever you say, talk as much as you can with your children; let them know you are able to face this tragedy as part of life. Children can appreciate what is happening to you, and they can learn very special lessons about life. Jane had hoped to join her grandchildren down at the beach during what she knew would be her last summer in Maine. Instead, she had to stay up inside the cottage, but her grandchildren brought her stones from the beach: "healing stones to make you better."

Don't assume, if your children aren't asking any questions, that they don't have questions in their heads, that there aren't things they want to know. They may be afraid to ask, afraid to upset you. They may not know how to put their concerns into words. Or maybe they sense your reluctance to talk about what's happening to you. It really is better if you can get some conversation going. Of first importance, let them know that your cancer is not their fault, that they had nothing to do with your illness. Until Brenda's doctor explained to the whole family that Brenda's cancer was in no way related to any past injury, Brenda's nine-year-old son was sure the blow he accidentally inflicted on his mother when he was swinging his baseball bat was what caused her cancer. Younger children may even believe that their bad thoughts about you caused your illness.

You want to establish a safe environment, open to continual dialogue. "If there is anything you want to know, ask me. Do you have any questions?" "No, unless there's anything you need to tell me." Ten-year-old Pete was afraid to know and afraid not to know. Give information one step at a time.

Keep talking, and answer whatever your children ask. There is little you can tell them that will be worse than what they can imagine. Tracy had nightmares that went on for years after her grandmother died. She was only five years old when it happened, her family gave her only partial answers to her questions, and she was too young to visit her grandmother in the hospital (because of hospital policy) before her grandmother passed away. Somehow, Tracy connected remarks about her grandmother's "last struggle" with a recent visit she had made to the zoo, and Tracy's nightmare featured her grandmother in a ferocious and deadly struggle with a huge, scary gorilla.

Children catch bits of conversation; they see you with heads together whispering, arms tight round each other, somebody crying. They usually figure out that something is very wrong, and they go right to the most dreaded conclusion. You want them to know the truth, and you want them to hear it from you. But in the beginning, don't answer more than they ask until you know what they want to know and what they can handle. "I was totally honest, but I held back details, and I never gave more than they asked for." Go slowly, encourage their responses and reactions. "That is an important question. Let's talk about it. I won't tell you anything that isn't true." If you can't answer every question, promise that you'll ask your doctor at your next visit. The older the child, the more you can tell. People who have studied children say even a child of three understands that death means an end, so even a child of three must be given some kind of truthful explanation.

A prominent Boston psychoanalyst whom I admire greatly says not to deprive your child of hope. You can't know *absolutely* that you're going to die—just leave it at that: "I'm very sick. I might die, but we are all hoping I'll get better."

Those who love you have to be angry that you are dying and leaving them. Anger and frustration swirl through the family, and sometimes these feelings are directed straight at the person who is dying. "I know! You're going to die! I hate you!" yelled Nancy's five-year-old daughter. Nancy let her yell and cry, and she hugged her and told her, "It's all right, it's all right. I love you." You do your best not to leave any lingering guilt generated by this anger. Children need to know it's all right for them to be angry, and that their feelings can't damage you: not now, not before, not after.

How much should children participate after their parent's death? The Boston psychoanalyst says children should be part of whatever the family does to mourn and celebrate the departed. If the family will be gathering for a funeral, the child should be included. Whatever is part of the family culture will help the child with his or her grief, help make the death real, help the child get past the very natural effort to deny what has happened.

These ceremonies are sustaining, part of the mourning process, and children need all the help they can get to do their mourning. You might say they need to learn how to do it—and the adults are there to show them the way, with the appropriate ceremonies, rituals, and memorial days, with hugging and talking and crying. Everyone who loses a loved one feels some sense of abandonment, and it helps a child to see how adults respond to this loss and then move forward. Without help learning how to mourn and to grieve, children may carry too many unresolved issues of loss into their emotional future, compromising the important relationships of their life.

How much you include a child is a very individual decision and depends very much on the age of the child. "Should the child go along to the cemetery, should she or he watch the coffin go into the ground?" Psychoanalyst: "You don't want the child to feel left out, but

I think this can be very scary for a young child, who thinks in very concrete terms of what is happening. (If the child is still trying to understand what *dead* is, he or she may imagine that burial is doing further harm to the parent.) It's spooky enough for adults. You have to be very careful about this.

"A lot depends on the kind of family, and the rituals that are generally observed. If there's a lot of singing and spiritual rejoicing, it might work. It's probably helpful to visit the grave later on, but watching the interment could be very frightening. Adults and children search for a place in the physical world for the person who has died, so going to visit the grave and talking to the departed is a good thing.

"It depends on the age above all. The intuitive thing to do may not be the best thing to do; kids and grown-ups think differently. It's important to get advice if you have questions about a particular situation, about how to explain what has happened—and to explain how a person lives on in your memory. People have very different gifts at explaining these hard things.

"As for the long view, so much depends on how well cared for the child will be in the future, on finding a good substitute for the deceased parent."

Practical Matters

With limited time, you may feel propelled to sort through your responsibilities and obligations, and then set priorities. Focus on what is fulfilling, meaningful, and pleasurable for you. You may have to make some tough decisions—where you will direct your limited energy, what you must try to finish, what you will decline to do, whom you will decline to see. Getting your affairs in order is a top priority for most women—it needn't relate to whether you're dying or not. Reexamine your will; assign or distribute personal possessions of special sentimental value.

Have you checked out pension and life insurance arrangements for your beneficiaries? (If you are hard-pressed for money, you may be able to get access to these funds early with a "viatical" [meaning money for a journey] tax-free settlement, whereby some companies pay you up to 80 percent of the value of your life insurance in advance of your death.) Have you discussed college plans for your children? Disposition of your family home? Have you spoken to your family and your physician about an advance directive or living will and end-of-life medical decisions such as life support and other heroic measures? Hospice care? Asked whether two dear friends' last weeks together were spent in tears and hand-holding, Helen said, "Of course not—we had too much to do."

Elsie had planned for years to get an appraisal for what she thought might be a valuable pottery collection, but she had always been too busy to get around to it. Assembling the collection, finding an appraiser, and arranging for the disposition of the collection was a welcome distraction for her during her last weeks, and it represented some kind of meaningful closure.

What responsibilities do you normally shoulder that must be passed on to someone else? Can you educate someone else in the family to take on the job? It may be useful to take a chunk of time to outline what has to be done—verbally and on paper or computer—such as collecting and paying the bills at various times of the month, tracking expenses for medical insurance and income tax filing, scheduling routine medical and dental checkups for the children, and checkups and license registration for the car—and the dog. Managing significant parts of your life, even as you pass on that control, gives you some measure of satisfaction, even pleasure, through this hard time.

Don't pass on all responsibilities to others. Hold on to what is most significant to you, what defines your relationship with your family and those you care most about. A well-intentioned family member may leave you feeling useless, even invisible: planning the meals, walking the kids to the school bus, putting them to bed. "Some people want to take over for you, doing things for you, but my sister doesn't do that. 'You can do this,' she says. I feel almost cheerful when I'm doing something that matters."

If you find it difficult to accept help from others, try to relax your attitude. You must allow others to come in and help you with all kinds of stuff you shouldn't be doing. There really is a middle ground of what you do yourself and what you let others do for you. Don't hesitate to call on your family and close friends for help. Those who love you are suffering in their own way, feeling helpless, unable to make you better. Anything they can do for you provides some relief, some sense that they are contributing to your well-being. Kim's friends got together and delivered dinner every day for months. Maybe you need a ride to and from the doctor, or medicine from the drugstore. Asking for help is a gift from you to others, and from others to you.

"I'm letting go of things that deplete my energy." Keep doing what pleases you—give up the dirty work. Forget dust and clutter—take that as a doctor's order, direct from me. Even if you're a cleaning fanatic, let it go. Memories last, cleanliness doesn't. Save your energy for your family and close friends. Write and phone. Long distance is cheaper than it's ever been and worth every penny. Talk, talk, talk.

Don't let a day go by without connecting to your immediate family. Sit down together as often as you can for some kind of time together.

Your Way

I hope you have lived your life your way. Dying should come about your way, too. You need to manage your life through to the end, especially at the end. Other people's ideas about illness and suffering, and about dying, may intrude, but don't let them get in your way. Too many people worry their whole lives about how others perceive them, how others talk about them, how others judge them, and about whether what they are doing is right. I tell my patients, "This is your time; you call the tune." Your loved ones—especially your children—are looking to you to see how you're coping, how you're managing, how you live and how you die. It's not that you're being judged; it's more that you're showing them how to face this *big thing*. "I want to do this right for my children, to set an example for them, an example of living."

To My Children

> *If I ever stop breathing,*
> *the flowers will inhale for me.*
> *If I ever stop writing,*
> *the grass will dot my i's.*
> *If I ever stop listening,*
> *the shells on the beach will hear you.*
> *If I ever stop talking,*
> *the rain will sing my song.*
> *If I ever stop loving,*
> *the sky will embrace you.*
> *But if I ever stop living,*
> *then you must live on for me.*

—Susan Weisgrau

SIX

Employment, Insurance, and Wills

26

Job Issues and Health Insurance

My primary physician made all the difference for me when I was sick; he was aggressive about my care, and I had no problem with health insurance coverage during my treatment. He made a convincing statement about my capacity to work and settled any of my employer's doubts. The new law lets me carry insurance with me if I change jobs, but I may not get to keep this doctor I'm so close to, and I'll probably have to pay more than I did in the past.

Job Issues

Your health may be a nonissue at work. Your boss may be sympathetic and understanding and allow for flexible scheduling of your responsibilities—and you may have missed very little time. If your co-workers are equally sympathetic and helpful, your workplace may actually be a source of support and comfort for you. But not all women are so fortunate. Part of the fallout of a breast cancer diagnosis is the effect it can have on your financial security, health care benefits, and career opportunities.

What are the issues that concern you? Getting hired. Not getting fired. Securing benefits and insurance. Getting a promotion, not getting demoted, not being transferred or forced into early retirement. These matters can be of crucial importance to you, stretching into your future, determining your quality of life, your lifestyle, and sometimes even the bottom line of your existence. The last thing you need at this moment in your life is a hassle with your job situation and a struggle with your health insurance company.

Although the majority of employers are supportive, one hard-nosed individual can turn your world upside down. Employers—and employees—may believe common myths about cancer: "Cancer: She can't possibly do the job." "It's contagious." "She's going to die." Some employers think the woman who is fighting breast cancer won't be up to the mark, and that more problems are on the way: days off, unbalanced work load, higher health insurance costs, lower profits. Some co-workers may be convinced they'll have to pick up the slack, and they may feel resentful. Contrary to what employers and employees assume, cancer survivors tend to have no higher absence rate than other employees.

Applying for a Job

How is applying for a job different for you now, as a woman who has had breast cancer? One point you may want to bear in mind: Most laws that protect your job rights and access to health insurance can protect you only if you work for a company that employs at least fifteen people. Depending on the kind of work you do, where you live, and a range of other factors, you may not have the option to choose what size company to work for. If you can, choose an employer who appreciates diversity, who has a good labor history, and who has more than fifty employees, which provides a larger employee pool that can lower the cost of insurance.

In 1990, the Americans with Disabilities Act (ADA) was passed, and jobs in companies with fifteen or more workers fell under protective regulation. Prior to that law, there was little support for someone who suffered discrimination because of cancer or other diseases. Now, anyone who has suffered serious illness is protected along with people traditionally classified as handicapped or disabled.

The ADA requires that employers treat all workers equally and fairly, and that they not single out or exclude any employee who may be or has been disabled, or who is perceived to be disabled. This includes cancer survivors. During interviews and on job applications, employers may only ask job-related questions and are not allowed to inquire into past medical history. The only factor at issue is whether you are able to perform the requirements of the job description. Unless you are thinking of applying to Victoria's Secret as a bra model, your breast cancer history is not relevant. Barbara Hoffman, a founder of the National Coalition for Cancer Survivors and a legal expert on employment issues, advises: "Don't volunteer any information about your cancer history. Keep the focus on your current ability to do the job in question."

In addition to the ADA, each state may extend federal laws to further protect against disability-based employment discrimination. (In case of conflict or differences between state and federal regulations, federal law prevails.) New Jersey leads the way as the state with the best and most innovative health care legislation, prohibiting restrictions to health insurance because of a preexisting condition long before the Kennedy-Kassebaum bill addressed the problem.

But how do any of these laws help you when you are sitting there filling out a job application that just happens to include the question Have you ever had cancer? Strictly speaking, the question is illegal, but there it is and there you are, poised with pen in hand to fill out the form. You may feel you have no choice but to go ahead and answer this potentially explosive question, illegal or not. It happens. One authority suggests you pass such a question by, leave it blank. What's the worst that can happen? You could be asked why you left the question unanswered, and you could respond, "I assumed it was an out-of-date application form because the question is illegal—so I just left it blank." That may be as nonconfrontational an approach as you can manage.

Advisers say, if you do answer the question Have you ever had cancer?, emphasize your current state of health, that you are fully capable of performing the job requirements as described, that your past medical history in no way interferes with present performance, and that for all intents and purposes you are cured. Some experts recommend including as much supportive material as you can within the confines of the application form, to lay to rest any questions about your condition and your ability to do the job. Include your doctor's name for reference and support, and if you think it will help, a letter from your doctor that affirms your ability to perform the job. (Don't let your extra notations mess up the clarity or look of the application. Keep it neat.)

Every authority on survivor rights says you must be honest. If you lie about your history and are discovered—and with information storage banks being what they are, discovery is quite possible—you may lose your job for dishonesty and your medical insurance on the basis of fraud. "I was very tempted to lie, but I knew that the facts were available somewhere and I was afraid I'd be found out. Anyhow, I got the job."

If you depend on your job for health care coverage, the National Coalition for Cancer Survivors advises looking for a job with a company that has a large pool of employees (say 300 or more), where health benefit costs will be reasonable or even completely covered by the employer, and where even a waiting period for a preexisting condition may be waived. The costs of covering a high-risk employee can be readily absorbed in a large company; the more people involved in a plan, the more the costs can be spread out among them.

Résumé Recommendations

To present yourself in the most positive light, you want to pay particular attention to your résumé: your written description of your job qualifications and history. If you have no experience putting a résumé together, seek professional assistance at a career service center (check the Yellow Pages), or ask a friend with professional experience, which will cost you less. This is your opportunity to sell yourself in the best light possible, so make the most of all your experience and accomplishments. (Be sure the résumé is neatly typed, with no spelling errors or typos; some employers will throw out a résumé with these kinds of errors.)

In your résumé, minimize any gaps in time during which you were in treatment or recovery by downplaying chronology and emphasizing your skills; be prepared to explain any blank stretches of time in an upbeat, favorable manner.

Informing Your Employer and Co-workers

You may be happily employed, but you find yourself suddenly stressed out because of your cancer diagnosis and treatment, and you're wondering, "How do I tell about my illness? Whom do I have to tell? How much do I have to tell? Do I *have* to tell? And how do I negotiate for a flexible work schedule to manage my treatment?"

Just as when you apply for a job, once you have a job you are under no legal requirement to reveal your cancer diagnosis or treatment unless it interferes with your ability to perform your job or you anticipate that you will need time off. In that case, it is best to inform your employer as soon as possible so you will have sufficient time to negotiate your work schedule and leave-time.

If you work for a company with more than fifty employees, the federal Family and Medical Leave Act of 1993 requires employers to provide up to twelve weeks of unpaid, job-protected leave for illness—either one's own or that of a child, parent, or spouse. A reduced or intermittent work schedule is protected and possible when "medically necessary," but you must have worked at least twenty-five hours a week for one year with this employer to receive this benefit. You are also entitled to all previous benefits due you during your leave. At the end of your leave, you are entitled to return to your previous position or its equivalent.

Under the Family and Medical Leave Act, you are obligated to give thirty days' notice for medical leave unless you can indicate that your leave was unexpected and inflexible. Behaving honestly and in good faith operates in your favor if there is any form of dispute. For this reason, try to document any requests for leave. Use E-mail and keep a copy; write a memo and hand it to your boss, even if you sit down and talk about the issue in person. Avoid confrontation if at all possible.

If you think it will help, ask your doctor to call your boss to resolve potential misunderstandings and to explain your treatment schedule. This information gives your employer a realistic expectation of how your treatment will affect your work obligations. Good communication can promote a positive relationship between you and your employer.

Many survivors tell inspiring stories of co-workers' empathy and support. "When I came into work wearing a cap to cover my hair loss, everyone in my office showed up the next day in caps—and they wore those caps till I finally got my hair back." Another survivor told about co-workers who started a "sick-time bank," donating hours that totaled up to six months' leave for her.

Documentation

Even if you don't anticipate any difficulty protecting your job and future promotions, keep a personal file of all verbal and written material that applies to your position, including times, locations, names, and addresses; a record of all communications between you, your boss, and co-workers; and records of everything that happens during your workday that might be relevant to your career prospects, suggests Barbara Hoffman. Keep track of all positive commendations of your work, as well as any incidents or remarks that you consider damaging to your reputation. You can't tell when you might need this documentation to support your bid to secure your position or move up the career ladder.

If you do find yourself in dispute with your employer, you'll be grateful for any piece of substantiating documentation you can produce. Do you have any kind of daily journal where you noted a conversation about a promotion? If you discussed that conversation with a fellow employee, a friend, or a family member, ask him to provide an affidavit (a written statement sworn under oath, witnessed by a notary) about what he remembers your telling him at the time. Sometimes something as casual as a scribbled memo note will help.

Redressing Wrongs

Maybe you think you have been unfairly treated by your employer: Your position may have been threatened, eliminated, or downgraded. Or you may have been working toward a promotion, a move upward. What if you don't get your job back or your promotion doesn't come through? What were you promised? Was it verbal only? Do you have any kind of written notation about keeping your job or getting the promotion? What are your options?

First, think about what it is you actually want: your job back and secured, a change of position, full-time work, part-time employment? A promotion? An apology? A legal suit with damages in the form of a cash settlement? Consider this part carefully. Weigh the potential tension and hostility against your need for employment at this particular company. Look for options such as restoration of money lost in missing wages and legal defense. Balance all that against the possibility of an unfair reputation as a troublemaker and the stress this might create as you force your cause forward.

Whenever possible, assume a positive approach to your employer or union representative. The best way to accomplish what you want is through a reasonable representation of your position and through amicable discussion and negotiation. Be well prepared for your discussion. Never talk to your boss when you are angry and not in full control of yourself. Wait till you cool off and have had time to think things over, again and again. Speak slowly and calmly, and never raise your voice.

Review your record of communication and memos so you can speak to the issue with confidence. To build your confidence, practice for this discussion with a family member or friend; consider role playing—you as employee, the other as boss, and vice versa.

The best initial approach is to avoid confrontation and maximize mediation and negotiation on your own. To support your personal attempts to resolve conflict, you can hire a private lawyer to help you understand and address the situation. Learning about the law and your rights before you meet with your employer's representative will give you the clout to work out a compromise—or better.

If all else fails, a lawyer at your side is empowering and very useful, and he or she can back you up with important legal facts and prior rulings. (Advice on your rights is also available by calling 800-ADA WORK.)

Counsel might also be a union officer, personnel representative, social worker, or legal aide. Check with the National Coalition for Cancer Survivorship in Silver Spring, Maryland, for specific job advice. (See Helpful Organizations.)

Negotiation may be fine for some, but you may have cause and determination enough to want to go to court and sue for your rights. Keep in mind that the cost in time, money, and emotional energy can be more than you or anyone else, including a government agency constituted to protect your interests, considers worthwhile. Any government agency to which you present a complaint will first try to resolve your problem through negotiation or mediation, no matter what kind of documentation you provide. Going to court typically involves a long, costly, arduous process and should be viewed as an absolutely last resort. If, in spite of all these considerations, you are determined to follow through with a court case, be sure you file your grievance within the appropriate state or federal deadlines. The Equal Employment Opportunity Commission at 800-669-4000 will provide you with guidelines.

Whatever you decide, know your rights. Speak from strength. Information is power that reinforces your position. And document, document, document.

Health Insurance Issues

"When I took on my new job and became a union employee, I was promised Personal Choice. My doctors were at Jefferson Hospital, and I wanted to keep them. Then I was told I had to take the Kennedy Hospital doctors after all. I offered to pay more to get Personal Choice, but as a union employee I was given no alternative. I wasn't allowed to stay with the doctors who had seen me through my treatment with such dedication and skill. I was very upset and I thought about looking for another job, but it hadn't been easy for me getting this job. Talk about a rock and a hard place!"

Your experience with breast cancer may be the first time you find out what your health care insurance can or cannot really do for you. You may not have worried very much about your health insurance when you were feeling well. Now your good health can be largely dependent on your access to quality health insurance.

Most health insurance is acquired as a benefit of employment, through your job or from your spouse's insurance. (In rare cases, same-sex partners can get insurance through one partner's plan.) If employer-based health insurance is threatened by illness, coverage for the whole family may be at risk.

Many of you must find your own health insurance—often to cover your family as well as yourselves. It may be that you work at home, or part-time, or for a small independent company, or you are a single parent. Or health care comes completely or in part from the federal and/or state government as Medicare or Medicaid. There are many millions of people who have no health care coverage at all.

The U.S. Department of Health and Human Services will send you information on health care and a listing of state insurance counseling offices that will answer questions about Medicare and other health insurance options.

Understanding how health care plans differ, what they cover and what they cost, and which would be best for you, can be a daunting process. You need clear, simple information to make intelligent health insurance decisions. One example of a step in the right direction is a walk-in center for Medicare and Medicaid recipients in downtown Philadelphia. Sympathetic experts are available to the elderly to help them figure out the basics of the plan and how it applies to each of them. Many people in need are turned down for Medicaid simply because "they fail to comply with procedural requirements"—they don't know exactly how to fill out the forms.

Outlined here is a general picture of the health insurance scene. Change is the byword; plans are in constant flux. Before you make any commitment, make sure you know the details and that what you know is current and applicable to your particular situation.

Cost-Driven Health Care

Health care has become a fiercely competitive, cost-driven, often profit-driven, industry. Traditional fee-for-service medicine is fast disappearing, replaced by a spectrum of managed care plans. These shifts can threaten the autonomy of the physician and the patient, as it is replaced by group care arrangements and policies, obtained individually or through organizations such as AARP (the American Association of Retired Persons), whose minimum age of membership is fifty, or as a component of job benefits.

Health maintenance organizations (HMOs) have become the vehicle of choice for many, generally offering the lowest cost for employers and employees, with an enormous range of benefits, along with limitations and restrictions. Over the years HMOs have become more hybrid—mixed models of health care delivery. Managed care as a whole is constantly evolving; benefit packages expand and contract with and without the forces of competition and cost containment.

The ideal plan for health care insurance would come from an employer with a large number of employees, who supplies you with a health plan, at no obvious cost to you, that allows you to choose your own doctors, with no waiting period or prior conditions. This ideal (and costly) plan would also allow you to go to any specialist you or your doctors think you should consult and to have any procedure your doctors want you to undergo. But given the realities of today's market and economy, most plans are far less generous—and they're shrinking. Benefits that in the past have covered family members are now under siege, as are benefits that extend into retirement. Employers are hiring more part-time workers for whom they don't have to provide any benefits.

Although no law requires an employer to provide health care insurance to employees, if insurance is provided for one, it must be fair and equal for all. But an employer can legally avoid providing health insurance for a high-risk employee if the employer can prove that the drastic increase in the company's insurance premiums, because of that one high-risk employee, would make the company unprofitable or make the insurance too expensive for everyone else. If your employer can prove this would happen, you could be forced to find and pay for your own health care plan. (This provides strong incentive to work for a large-scale employer, where the impact of one employee's health or health insurance is barely felt.) If you find you must pay for your own insurance under these circumstances, be sure you are at least given the same contribution toward your plan that your employer contributes to everyone else's. (The check should be made directly to your insurer so that it's not considered income to you by the Internal Revenue Service.)

There is always a hidden cost to health care, such as deductions taken out of your salary. Consider health insurance part of your employee compensation (i.e., a lower-paying job with great benefits may be worth much more than a higher-paying job without).

"The health care policy I had at the time of my breast cancer treatment did not adequately cover radiation therapy, and I was left with a whopper of a bill to pay off. It has made the details of health insurance policies the primary issue in job negotiation for me."

In fact, there's a price tag on everything related to health care, particularly as not-for-profit HMOs are being supplanted by for-profit corporations. Selection of an HMO is usually determined by the employer, and benefits are offered cafeteria style—you pick and choose the benefits you want, depending on personal preference and ability to pay. If you pay less, you get less.

But paying more for your health insurance doesn't always mean you get more. Sometimes you have to pay more just to keep what you've got. And sometimes your ability to obtain or to keep your health insurance may be threatened by unaffordably high premiums once you've been diagnosed or identified as having a high-risk family history of breast cancer. (If your family has an abnormal breast cancer gene, that information only belongs in a research file (not in your hospital chart or insurance application) until we know what the genetic results really mean. (At least, that's my opinion.) (See Chapter 28.)

If you aren't provided with health insurance by your employer, and you don't qualify for Medicaid or Medicare, you may have to look into high-risk pool insurance, which usually has fewer benefits and costs a lot more. As your risk diminishes over the years, you may be able to shift to less expensive coverage.

Making a Choice

Irene Card, president of Medical Insurance Claims in Kinnelon, New Jersey, and a patient advocate and adviser on medical insurance to the National Coalition for Cancer Survivorship, as well as insurance adviser to the Post-Treatment Resource Program at Memorial Sloan-Kettering Cancer Center and a participant in Living Beyond Breast Cancer$_{SM}$ conferences, says, "I want complete freedom of choice. I won't have that with an HMO. If I elect to go to a national treatment facility, it is highly possible that the treatment would not be covered by an HMO." If you are someone who expects a full range of choice, who wants time to connect with your physician, who wants the full line of studies and tests at the best possible medical center, you may have to go beyond the standard health care maintenance options available to you at work, and pay for supplemental health care insurance.

Some advisers suggest you use the doctor to pick the plan, not the plan to pick the doctor—if you have that option and can pay for it. Ask your primary care doctor for advice, ask which plan allows him or her the most freedom to do the best job possible, which has the least amount of paperwork, and which includes the hospital that will give you the best care. Then be sure that the doctor you want is indeed on the list of the plan you may choose. Ask your doctor directly—don't rely on any administrator's assurance—especially a published listing. Lists go out of date: doctors are added, leave, or are removed from the list. Make sure that you have access to your doctor, and that his or her practice is not overcrowded and you will not be kept waiting to join his or her patient enrollment. Speak with your health plan administrator, and get any assurance or statement in writing.

Health Care Insurance Options

What are your options for managed health care insurance? The most common choice is an HMO, the cheapest form of health care coverage. But as HMOs expand and multiply, it becomes more and more confusing for consumers to figure out how various health plans (not just HMOs) differ and which best suit their needs. One phrase going the rounds of health care advisers is, "You've seen one HMO—you've seen one HMO." There's no way to generalize from one to another. In trying to help you find your way in this sea of offerings, here are a few of the most common types of health plans presently on the scene.

HMOs

Overall, HMOs are expanding at a staggering rate. In essence, these organizations contract with large numbers of patients to achieve a volume discount on health care costs. They are regarded as an efficient, low-cost way to provide health care, with minimal paperwork in the process—a big plus for a lot of busy people (but the required referral forms are themselves a burden). Young people in particular are drawn to HMO coverage, which often includes routine checkups for all family members as part of the package. Older people with more complex medical problems are the ones least likely to find HMO coverage adequate or satisfactory, although many older Americans, offered a choice by Medicare of staying within the Medicare system or going into an HMO, are choosing the HMOs.

This is how an HMO might work for you: You are assigned a primary care physician who manages your care, arranges tests and hospitalization, and refers you to specialists within the plan only when clearly necessary. You pay a fixed premium, and your doctor is paid a yearly capitation fee (a flat rate of payment for each patient, sick or well) for having you on his or her list. The primary care doctor's capitation fee may be reduced by a moderate charge for the tests ordered and the in-system specialists he or she refers you to. (Payment systems are constantly changing; this is simply an example of a common model.)

As HMOs are evolving, not all of them work by capitation fees alone; some include a fee-for-service arrangement (or various other combinations). Care is designed to be delivered within the HMO system, all costs carefully monitored to provide appropriate services at the lowest price, aimed at keeping you in the network. If you are determined to go out of the system, you may have to pay for the service or your primary care doctor may pay for it (by its being subtracted from the capitation fee).

Problems can surface when the HMO you are considering is new to your location. It may need time to develop its roster of doctors, to include complex medical procedures, to establish the availability of so-called super specialists. Patients with unusual medical conditions or in advanced stages of disease who join at this point in a developing network may find they are restricted to doctors with whom they have no prior relationship and who have no experience with their particular condition. (The doctors who have been caring for them may or may not be included in the directory of the new HMO.)

Medicare

Medicare is available to all Americans sixty-five or over, and to those who are disabled or on renal dialysis. It has been a traditional fee-for-service plan with reimbursement based on fixed allowable charges for each service. Participants are responsible for a deductible portion and a co-payment (typically 20 percent of the total) for service. If you are part of a fee-for-service plan and want Medicare coverage benefits, always check with the doctor and hospital you wish to work with to be sure they will accept your Medicare payment.

Medicare premiums are deducted from Social Security benefits, if you qualify (you or your spouse must have worked or paid Social Security at least ten years). If your work history is not adequate, you may need to pay the Medicare premiums yourself.

With the growth of HMOs and their managed costs and efficiency, the government has expanded Medicare to include HMOs prepared to contract with the government and to accept its fixed payment schedule. Participants like HMOs because they eliminate co-payments and deductions, provide prescription drugs, and cut down on participants' paperwork. Critics say the HMOs pressure doctors to hold down costs to keep up HMO profits, especially when costs for older Medicare participants often run higher than the premiums paid by the individual and the capitation paid by the insurance company to the doctor.

A monthly capitation fee is paid for each Medicare participant in an HMO to cover a full range of health care services; these fees vary from state to state and from county to county. As rulings accumulate to ensure complete access to services within an HMO for Medicare recipients, as well as the right to protest denial of claims, more and more Medicare participants are joining HMOs.

Point of Service

A point of service plan allows you to choose a doctor within a plan's network of physicians, or to go out of a plan's network to providers of your choice. (Premiums are generally higher than an HMO's.) This is a fee-for-service arrangement that pays each of your doctors for each of your visits. Second opinions are available without much hassle. You may find, however, that some treatment recommendations require approval, and you may be responsible for part of your doctors' fees. Most members of a point of service plan, however, tend to stay within the plan's network of physicians to keep their costs lower.

Preferred Provider Organization

A preferred provider organization is similar to a point of service plan. You can use the network's panel of doctors for a small co-payment fee, or you can go out of the network to doctors of your choice. If you choose an out-of-network doctor, you must pay the balance between the scheduled fee and the billed amount, which corresponds to a higher co-payment and deductible. A deductible is a fixed amount taken off the top of a doctor's or hospital's charge that you are responsible for paying, before your health care insurance contributes its obligatory share. Medicare has a $100 deductible per year that you pay before Medicare starts to pick up your charges.

Indemnity Insurance

Blue Cross/Blue Shield is a traditional health insurance carrier that allows you to go to any doctor or hospital you select, anywhere in the United States, or even abroad. (Blue Cross/Blue Shield may serve you best if you find you travel a good deal or have residences in more than one region of the country.) You can choose from a broad menu of options; what you select depends on your health needs and what you can afford. Contracts vary. You may be responsible for a deductible and out-of-pocket charges, and/or co-payments for various services, such as office visits that exceed your basic coverage. There are so many permutations now within Blue Cross that providers can't keep up with all the different rules. "We find out how a plan works when we send in the bill," said the financial officer of a large clinical practice.

Variations That Make a Big Difference

Prescription coverage varies from plan to plan. Some health insurance will completely cover the cost of medications, others will require a co-payment, and still others will not offer coverage at all.

With whatever plan you join, expect to pay some kind of deductible (each year) before your insurer's contribution kicks in, and recognize that almost every policy has a maximum lifetime benefit cut-off point. To balance that negative side, there's "stop loss." This means that at a certain point, your contribution to your health costs stops, and your insurer takes over 100 percent of the expense. However, when you are getting 100 percent from your insurer, you'll be approaching your lifetime benefit cut-off point faster. Be sure you look at that lifetime figure carefully, if you're in a position to choose your insurance; for instance, for cancer treatment, $100,000 is a drop in the bucket. Your policy should have at least $1,000,000 as a maximum, or you'd better look for supplementary insurance.

If you don't have health insurance from your work, and you don't qualify for Medicaid or Medicare, you may want to look into high-risk pool insurance. It's probably expensive, but it may well be worth the cost, and it may even be a financial imperative.

"This is *insurance*," an adviser reminded a prospective enrollee. "That means you gamble on what you think your expenses might be against what you are willing to spend for protection." If you expect you'll need a lot of medical care in the future, buy insurance now. Protect yourself against the large costs that may come later.

If You Can't Afford Health Insurance

Almost a third of Americans are without health insurance and many more have real difficulty paying for health care. Many young people don't worry about health care insurance; they don't want to spend money on what they don't think they'll need.

If you have no insurance because your employer doesn't provide it or you don't work, if you don't think you qualify for government medical assistance, and if you can't afford individual health insurance, you'll need to explore other possibilities. Discuss your options with a social worker or the hospital health insurance office to find out if you qualify for medical assistance. If you are single and your gross income is below $8000 ($10,700 for a couple), you may qualify for Medicaid. Hospital funds may be available for individuals who don't qualify for Medicaid and are unable to pay for their own care; most hospitals have special funds to cover some uninsured patients.

Discuss your financial situation with your doctor. Most doctors want to help, and they may set up a payment plan or even write off part or all of your bill. Be prepared to show your doctor your income tax returns or other evidence of your financial situation to document your inability to pay. (It is unlikely that your doctor would ever ask you for this, but if you are desperate, you may feel your case can be justifiably supported by presenting documentation of your situation.)

Several of my patients who couldn't afford health care and who didn't qualify for medical assistance obtained their care at no cost through a National Cancer Institute treatment study. There may be local studies where you live that could provide care at no cost to you. (Call 800-4-CANCER.) Breast cancer organizations such as the Susan Komen Foundation and the American Cancer Society might also provide funds for your care. (See the Helpful Organizations section at the back of this book.)

Even if you are covered by Medicare, you may not be covered for annual mammograms, but legislation is pending to change federal guidelines so that annual mammograms are authorized for all women over fifty. Current policy covers mammography only every other year. (Federal guidelines that exclude women under fifty are being reevaluated now that annual mammography for women forty and older has been recommended by the National Cancer Institute, the American Cancer Society, and the American College of Radiology.) If you need help with the cost of a mammogram, call your local branch of the American Cancer Society or one of the local or national breast cancer organizations.

Investigate. Be creative. A member of the board of Living Beyond Breast Cancer$_{SM}$ raised money from a group of friends to pay for a colleague's bone marrow transplant when the woman's health insurance wouldn't cover it.

You can also call or write your congressperson and state representative and share with them your personal struggle to obtain health care coverage, in case your elected official can come up with some form of public assistance.

Know Your Plan

Familiarize yourself with your health care contract. Read it through carefully and get help interpreting those parts you don't understand. You won't get the full benefit of your plan if you don't know your benefits and your limits. Some plans, for instance, require precertification for certain services, including hospitalization, even emergency care. If you don't follow policy requirements, you may find yourself in for a fair amount of hassle, if not a huge amount of expense. For instance, if you're in a plan that requires a referral before you can see your oncologist, yet you go to see him or her without first getting the referral, someone's going to have to pay for that visit, and most likely it won't be the insurance company. Either you'll end up paying out of pocket for the consult, or the consulting doctor will not be paid.

To keep some measure of control over your health insurability, it may be useful, on a periodic basis, to obtain copies of your medical records to find out what information is made available to your employer and insurer. You have a legal right to secure access to any of your records.

Learn what your annual and lifetime maximum coverage amounts are, so you know whether you're approaching your limit. Find out and keep track of what you have already totaled in health care costs. You may decide you need to buy an additional individual health care policy. If you are on Medicare, you may want to buy a Medigap (supplemental) policy from a private insurance company, to cover further treatment, medication, and hospital charges. Be sure that any policy you buy is guaranteed renewable. The cost of this insurance can be dismaying, but it may be essential; if you are retired from a company that provided you with major medical benefits, you should purchase one of the ten Medigap policies that best suits your needs and pocketbook.

If you are considering a Medigap policy—assuming you qualify—the best time to buy in is during your open enrollment period, which is within the first six months after you enroll in Medicare Part B or after you turn sixty-five. During this time frame, you can buy the policy of your choice at the best possible premium. It may be wise to check in advance with a trusted insurance agent about what your options may be.

Read the fine print in your contract. As resistance to retirement benefits grows among employers, you want to know if your contract promises lifetime benefits, so that you can insist that those promises are kept and challenge any cutbacks. The federal government is considering legislation that would compel employers to fulfill the promises for benefits they have made to their employees.

Remember, *your health insurance is dependent on your paying your bills*. Don't ever let your insurance lapse. If you are going to be late with your payment or you are having trouble meeting the payment, contact your insurer and explain your problem, appeal for consideration, try to arrange a modified payment plan till you have straightened out your affairs, and *get any agreement you reach in writing*. Remind your children not to let their insurance lapse in case your history of breast cancer affects their options.

Learn to Protect Your Rights and Extend Your Limits

If you find yourself in an HMO or other plan that you are less than happy with, you should be aware of the rules that apply to your case and become alert to strategies that can maximize your health care benefits within that system.

Your most significant advocate in any conflict with your health insurance provider over specific health benefits is probably your primary care physician, who is considered the gatekeeper of your plan. He or she can fight for your right to get to see your oncologist after chemo is over, for instance, or allow you to obtain additional tests or second opinions. Decisions regarding approval of out-of-network care are carefully reviewed, so you want the system's gatekeeper, your physician, to be your advocate. Be aware that in some health plans, out-of-system referrals may take money out of your doctor's pocket, so your primary care physician may not be as willing to send you to as many doctors as you perhaps would like. Capitation forces each HMO doctor to be fiscally responsible for his or her costs, and to be accountable to the HMO for every procedure, test, and referral. In fairness to your doctor, if your doctor does not keep costs down, he or she runs the risk of being expelled from the plan, or at least the risk of a financial penalty.

Fighting for specialized care outside—or inside—your HMO can be a trying challenge for you, your doctor, doctor's nurse, and secretary. Countless hours may be required on the phone to justify a CAT scan, special medication, a second opinion referral, or extra days in the hospital. If you are having trouble getting access to a specialist or approval for new treatment, prepare to write letters, make phone calls, pester for your rights. As articles in major newspapers report and as consumer advocates tell us, it's the woman who demands her rights and who is prepared to do battle who is most likely to wear out the opposition and win her appeal.

Breast cancer pressure groups like the National Breast Cancer Coalition are watchdogs of survivors' rights. And don't forget that your elected legislators are there to help you; many are working hard for your health care rights, prepared to extend the limits on current restrictions. Legislators are fighting to eliminate outpatient mastectomies, for instance, seeking at least a forty-eight-hour hospital stay for the operation. They are also working to kill any gag rules for doctors that limit what your doctor can tell you about "medically necessary treatment options," and they are fighting to protect your access to emergency care. By late 1996, the Department of Health and Human Services had informed all HMOs that any contract that limits a doctor's ability to advise and counsel a Medicare or Medicaid beneficiary (and, implicitly, all enrollees) was a violation of federal law. You are entitled to your doctor's counsel on all treatment options, including, if necessary, more costly drugs, newer therapies, alternate surgeries, and referrals to more expensive specialists.

The Claim Process

If you are processing a claim with your health care insurer, be sure to get the details right. It may help to assign this process to one person in the household, who can keep track of all records and be completely familiar with the health insurance plan on which you rely—in particular, the time limit for filing. (You must submit your claims for reimbursement within the time frame allowed.)

Read the fine print in your employment and health care contracts.

It is extremely annoying to have a claim rejected. Reasons for rejection include the following:

1. Information on the claim forms is incomplete.
2. The diagnosis is missing or incomplete.
3. The date of appointment and test procedure is missing or incorrect.
4. The number or name of the patient is missing.
5. The material is illegible.
6. You failed to provide an explanation for why multiple visits to various doctors on a single day were necessary.
7. The referral to see a specialist was presented *after* evaluation and management by that specialist.
8. The charges are deemed to be unreasonable and unusual.
9. The person who processed your claim interpreted the rules too narrowly, or simply made a mistake.

You will learn that it is important to supply as much explanation and information as possible with any claim you submit and to make sure it's complete and correct. Assemble all pertinent material and make copies of every record you submit. Your patient number should be on every piece of paper in your file. Is the right date assigned to the right appointment? Is your file in order? Any extra time spent making your claim thoroughly and overwhelmingly complete and emphatic will save you an enormous amount of time, energy, and frustration—I promise you.

Irene Card, writing for the National Coalition for Cancer Survivorship, says that a denied claim may be paid by simply resubmitting it for payment. A more careful or sympathetic claims examiner may okay what a previous examiner decided to reject. If this doesn't work, make it clear that you're not satisfied with the decision and that you request and expect a review of the denied claim. If your claim is still rejected, indicate that you want a review by the peer review physicians. If you don't take no for an answer, you may win your case by sheer persistence.

Insurance providers always insist that a charge be "reasonable and customary," meaning comparable to other specialists' charges in your area. If your claim is rejected for this reason, it's up to you and your doctor to prove that the fees you were charged are appropriate. You can have your doctor write another letter to explain the costs in greater detail, and you can do research on your own to prove that your doctor's charges are "reasonable and customary." Professional advisers suggest you call half a dozen different doctors' offices throughout your geographic region, as well as in your own immediate area, to find out what they charge for the visit or procedure in question. (Medical procedures often have a standard code number assigned to them, which can speed your inquiry.) There is also a directory of costs for every medical procedure in every ZIP code in the country, available in medical libraries. (You can check with your local medical society or nearest medical school.) Then go back to your company with information that supports your case that your physician's charges are well within reasonable and customary limits. If you handle any of your business by phone, be sure to get the full name of the person you speak to and record the date, time, and content of the conversation. Keep a personal file of all this material.

Some insurers have refused to pay for breast reconstructive surgery, claiming it's cosmetic and therefore not medically necessary. Most insurers will pay for reconstruction of the removed breast but may object to paying for additional surgeries such as reducing the healthy breast to match the size and shape of the reconstructed breast. A woman in New York had all her surgery costs paid after mounting a strong case with empathetic support from her doctor (which included a threat to file a complaint with the state insurance commissioner and a state senator).

If you are trying to collect for experimental treatment, you'll need strong support from your primary physician and from the physicians directing the treatment study. They must affirm that your involvement in the treatment study is not simply to further science but will result in a direct benefit to you that is not available from any other treatment. HMOs are proving extremely resistant to study participation for their enrollees, on the basis of higher costs for treatment. But for new treatments to be developed so that more effective cancer care can be provided, managed care plans must begin to permit access to trial studies. You should also consider getting the support of your congressperson or state representative for participation in a study; you'd be surprised how useful political pressure can be. The National Breast Cancer Coalition is an advocacy organization, another important resource for you.

Recipients of Medicare coverage who are members of HMOs have recently won a class action suit that sought to guarantee Medicare patients' right to present additional evidence to their HMO for reconsideration of denied services. Many Medicare patients had said they had been turned down for necessary services such as emergency care, home health care, skilled nursing care, and physical therapy. It took three years to win the case, but the win shows the strength of organized patients and the importance of protest through the legal process and the courts. If you're having trouble getting your insurance company representatives to listen to your claim, remind them that others have sued and won on similar points.

Again and again, you will find you must be a forceful spokesperson for your rights. The more you do it, the better your communication skills become, the more your confidence grows, and the more likely you are to get positive results. Helen had a rough time after her breast cancer diagnosis; some of her health benefits ran out, but she put up a fight, and it paid off. "You've got to teach yourself about your rights. Get on the phone, ask questions, keep at it. You've got to be informed, patient, and aggressive." Jane added, "I'm lucky I have a big mouth: I insist on my rights and I get them. I'm convinced they give people like me more, and that less assertive members get less." Patient advocate Irene Card says, "Make a pest of yourself! Take your claim back, back, back. Finally, they'll pay just to get rid of you."

But expect it to be a time-consuming and exhausting process—at a point when you feel sick, time seems especially precious, and your energy and resources are limited. If it all seems too much for you, then turn to a medical claims adjuster or adviser (see Helpful Organizations, Medical Insurance Claims, Inc.). As claims have snowballed, a profession has developed to help people stand up for the benefits owed them. (But, so that there is no suggestion of conflict of interest, claims advisers should not sell insurance.) The adjusters know how "to speak the language" in what has become an incredibly confusing area of modern life. They can also help you find your way when you have to make choices in health care planning. Ask your doctor or hospital or someone you know who has used these services for the name of an adviser, or look in the Yellow Pages under Insurance Claims Processing. Ask how long the adviser has been in business, the nature of the adviser's background, and how you will be charged. Be sure to ask for references. If you pick your adjuster with care, you're bound to get your money's worth.

Portability of Insurance: COBRA

What protection do you have for health care benefits if you lose your job, if you retire, or if you work less than the obligatory amount of time to keep normal benefits flowing? Or if you depend on your husband's coverage and he loses his job? The Consolidated Omnibus Budget Reconciliation Act (COBRA) and the new Kennedy-Kassebaum bill are designed to keep you insured under these circumstances. Since 1986, COBRA has provided for a continuation of your group medical benefits for up to eighteen months after the specified job change, provided your employer qualifies with twenty or more employees. To continue your coverage under this COBRA legislation, you must notify your employer or your health care carrier within sixty days of receipt of notice of termination or retirement. Divorce does not alter this benefit. You will be charged your full premium, plus a 2 percent surcharge for costs, and it may be more than you expect because you are no longer receiving your employer's contributory share.

If you obtain coverage with another health plan or are eligible for full coverage under Medicare, you may be prepared to discontinue your COBRA coverage, but don't move too quickly. Be sure to read the fine print of any new plan. There may be a waiting period for a preexisting condition, which means that they will not cover any of your expenses related to that condition during the designated waiting period. If there is such a clause, it is advisable, in spite of the expense, to continue your COBRA coverage (which *does* cover your pre-existing condition) until the waiting period in your new plan is over. This way, you won't get caught without protection.

The Kennedy-Kassebaum bill of 1996 may eliminate the worst fears of cancer survivors about portability of health insurance coverage from one job to another, and by limiting or eliminating exclusions for preexisting conditions, but there are strict rules you must follow if you want to stay insured. As written, the law protects anyone with a condition that has existed for twelve months or more, and who has been continuously insured for that period of time. The insurance carrier at the new job must take you on, or you may have to buy private health insurance policies without punitive exclusions. But if you believe that provisions in the Kennedy-Kassebaum bill apply to you, be sure to get a full clarification and certification of your rights. It won't be easy; this is a complex law that some lawyers require a primer to understand. And as with most legislation, interpretation of details over time will define and determine how the law will affect you specifically. If you are confused (and plenty of people are), seek help from your benefits counselor, a claims adviser, or a lawyer who specializes in health care or employment issues.

Divorce and Insurance

If you are contemplating divorce and you have been receiving health insurance through your husband's job, you'll have to do some careful planning if you need to continue your coverage through his plan. It is possible to sew up health benefits into a divorce settlement. In fact, in some states, a divorced woman has a legal right to continued coverage from her former husband's health insurance. You or your lawyer should be especially attentive to this aspect of your divorce settlement.

Even if you have secured protection of your postdivorce health benefits, there are some pitfalls to watch for, particularly how money is returned to you, the payee. You may pay your bill to your doctor and then file for a refund from your insurer, only to find that the refund has been sent to the person whose employment secures the insurance: your ex-husband. Not a good arrangement. You may have to battle red tape on this issue. And it will probably take more than a quick phone call to change the address to which the checks are to be sent; you may have to go back to your lawyer for further adjustment and negotiation of your settlement.

Life and Disability Insurance

"What do they want from me? I got a clean bill of health after my pathology report and I walked out fine. I even had a child after that. This was five years ago. Then I applied for life insurance with all kinds of doctors' letters, and I was turned down. After all the other crap, I didn't expect this. I've been with this insurance company for twenty years!"

If you are looking for life insurance coverage, your first step may be to find an empathetic insurance broker. All companies have guidelines for providing life and disability insurance for "high-risk" individuals, but some are more flexible than others. Every company's rules are different. Each insurance broker has access to a variety of companies and can search around for the best possible opportunity for you.

There is no generalization for providing life insurance to someone with a preexisting condition. There is also no standard definition of a preexisting condition. One policy may define it as *ever* having had a diagnosis of breast cancer; another may say a preexisting condition is one that is symptomatic or requires ongoing therapy. Time will be figured from the last date of treatment, with a possible three- to five-year postponement for insurance. Insurance is bound to be expensive—one and a half to two times as much as normal, plus in some cases a fee of fifteen dollars per thousand dollars of coverage. Over the years, the rate may drop. It helps if your personal doctor paints a positive picture of your condition, even though insurance representatives may tell you rates are not negotiable. "We line up the negatives, then line up the positives. There can be a lot of flexibility in those numbers," one representative confessed. The message is clear: Agitate for your interests. Your articulate persistence can make a difference, but be sure you do it with a strong foundation of accurate information.

If you manage to get life or disability insurance, be sure to pay your bills on time so your insurance does not lapse. Encourage your daughters to get life and disability insurance while they are young and healthy, and warn them not to let their insurance lapse, in case your diagnosis of breast cancer affects their options.

Women who have had breast cancer may expect to be offered what is called a substandard insurance contract. It offers renewable insurance with an adjustable premium. A good contract is noncancelable. Disability insurance, which pays income when you cannot work (up to 60 percent of current income, tax free), is also very hard to get for cancer survivors.

Many insurance companies will consider insuring cancer survivors after seven years, some after nine years. Acceptance will depend on the number of years beyond treatment, stage, number of nodes, and so on, including the goodwill and standing of your insurance agent. If they do accept a cancer survivor, insurers will undoubtedly charge higher premiums than normal.

The Times They Are a'Changing

This chapter has tried to steer you through the confusion attendant with health care insurance opportunities in this country. Just be warned: The details are changing by the minute—within the organizations, within the states, within the federal laws and regulations. What's true today may not be true tomorrow. To inform yourself about what best pertains to your situation and what is most up-to-the-moment in offerings, check with the benefits officer at your place of employment, or press your health care plan's information office, or turn to a state insurance counseling service or an independent resource person, such as a claims assistance professional.

Good luck.

27

Wills for Living and End of Life

> After I had my breast cancer surgery, we immediately made a will—that's when it became important. I was a very young woman. It's twenty years down the line, but we keep putting off making a new one. I'm fine and I don't want to be bothered—or maybe I don't want to think about it.

You have had breast cancer, and financial matters inevitably weigh heavily on your mind: bills from treatment, loss of pay for time missed from work, health care premiums, money spent on indulgences necessary to carry you and your family through the stress of your diagnosis and after. You may be in debt, or working several jobs to catch up. You may be unemployed. You're probably more focused on present problems than on long-range ones, issues you might rather put off or out of mind altogether. But they won't go away, and they're often the ones that come to haunt you in the wee hours of the morning.

No one lives forever—sooner or later we all have to give some thought to how we will end our days, whether we can depart with dignity, and, after we go, how our wishes will be carried out and our earthly possessions divided. (Do you want your stuff to go to those you love, to those who are most greedy and aggressive, or to the federal government as inheritance taxes?) This means writing a will or two: "living" wills that determine quality of life during illness or the end of life, and property wills that distribute material assets. Most people who draw up wills do it when they're in good health.

Whether you decide to act on any of these matters is an intensely personal decision. But if you choose to ignore the reality of wills, you may lose important control of how you want to live and die, and control of what you may have worked for all your life—if you are no longer able to make these decisions yourself.

With the Patient Self Determination Act of 1991, anyone admitted into a hospital must be given the opportunity to sign a written statement about life support decisions, an "advance directive of medical care." Then, if you're unable to make decisions, the hospital knows how to proceed with your care.

The Advance Directive, a.k.a. a Living Will

An advance directive, commonly known as a living will, establishes what kind of care you would choose if you were no longer capable of making your own decisions. Some individuals want aggressive treatment no matter what—every treatment, every technical support available; others want a peaceful, noninterventionist end—comfort care only, no life support. It may be simply an oral discussion of what you believe and would choose, or a written declaration of your intentions. Many people talk about these issues, but few put them in writing. The best arrangement is to let your family and your doctor know your wishes, and also to put those wishes down on paper.

You may also want to appoint someone to act for you by signing a limited, health care power of attorney. Tell that someone, as well as the members of your immediate family, your philosophy on sustaining life with or without heroic measures, continuing or withdrawing life support. Choose as your agent or surrogate someone who is strong-minded enough to resist opposing family members or doctors, someone you can trust to carry out *your* wishes, come what may. Appoint a backup person, as well, rather than putting two people in charge.

Whatever your position on end-of-life issues, it is important to broadcast your feelings while you are healthy. My mother is in her sixties, in excellent health, with long-lived parents, but she has been outspoken about "no tubes, no nothing" in the event of any catastrophe, to all her family and close friends. A clear general verbal statement of your philosophy is important; putting it in writing will make your wishes known if you are unable to speak for yourself. The law respects such wishes, and it has allowed close family members who report a patient's philosophy to instruct the hospital not to attach, or to remove, high-tech means of life support (even without written instructions to that effect). When the parents of a young woman who had been in a violent car accident wanted to withdraw her from life support when she was declared brain dead, they took the case to the Supreme Court. The Court decided that a patient's wishes to be allowed to die under these circumstances had to be respected. But at the time of the initial appeal, the Court had no clear evidence of that particular patient's wishes. Then her former fellow employees gave testimony to remarks they recalled her making (while discussing another employee's accident) that she would never wish to stay alive if she were in a similar vegetative state. This confirmation of the woman's intentions led to her removal from life support.

Let your doctor and other members of your health care team know about your living will, written or oral. Many hospitals provide a living will sample that you can adapt to your particular circumstances.

Disposition of Property and Responsibilities

Everyone needs a will and a personal advocate who can and will truly represent you in a clearheaded, disinterested fashion.

It may be particularly important for lesbian couples who have no legal connection to one another to write a foolproof will, to pass on property or arrange for child custody. Not infrequently, families of a gay couple may be unaware of the true nature of this relationship; should a partner die, it is not uncommon for the family of the deceased to come in and sweep away all trace of the deceased partner's possessions and effects, excluding the remaining partner completely. If children are involved, the ramifications can be endless. Anticipating such problems, or for tax-directed advantages, the unrelated partner might adopt the children of the other partner, if such an adoption is legal in the state in which they reside. Laws on adoption vary from state to state. Some states are quite hostile to such arrangements; others are tolerant and welcoming. Gay residents of a liberal state that permits adoption will achieve an adoption that is binding in all other states. Occasionally, where possible, one gay partner will adopt the other partner to create a "legally acceptable" relationship. Illness does put pressure on closet gays to reveal the truth about their gay lifestyle to their families, but they may nonetheless choose to continue protecting their secret, to protect parents or siblings who really don't want to know.

Another sticky legal issue involves frozen embryos. If you went through *in vitro* fertilization and have stored frozen embryos, you must specify what you want to have happen to those embryos. Has the donor of the sperm retained any legal rights to the embryos? Is there likely to be any dispute or legal battle over their ownership? Try to resolve all variations of these issues with your attorney at the time that you draw up your will. (You may have attended to all these issues before you even started the process of *in vitro* fertilization.)

Many people have very definite ideas about other personal end-of-life issues, such as the kind of funeral arrangements they want: cremation versus interment, ceremony or not, pallbearers, speakers at the memorial service, or charities to receive bequests. These wishes should also be included in your will.

A vital part of anyone's personal assets is pension benefits. Generally speaking, the largest personal assets you're likely to acquire during your lifetime are your home and your pension. How any of your assets—money in the bank, stocks and bonds, mutual funds, real estate, pension—are legally titled may change over your lifetime, depending on circumstances such as children, divorce, and death. You may, in fact, alter the beneficiaries of your estate a number of times over the course of your life. As a woman who has had breast cancer and had your sense of mortality shaken, you would be advised to keep entitlement in each of your assets up to date with your interests.

Elsie had worked for thirty years and had accumulated a sizable pension, but because she was apparently in good health and her husband—who was ten years older than she—had his own adequate pension, she had elected a single life annuity. (If the annuity [pension] is based on only one person's life, that person will collect considerably more per month than if two people—joint life—are named to the pension.) When Elsie developed a sudden and virulent form of breast cancer, she had a small window of time before she officially retired to change her pension plan assignment to joint life, to include her husband, so that he at least would get the pension for which she had worked so hard.

You can specify who gets what in your will, or you can pass things along now. Women tell us, "As soon as I was diagnosed with cancer, I started giving my things away." Personal effects may be the hardest things to give up, to distribute: "A long time ago I had breast cancer, and I kept thinking about giving my jewelry away. But my son was so young. Now he's old enough to appreciate what I have, and he has a girl, and I want him to enjoy the stuff—but I haven't given it to him yet." "I remember relatives coming in after my mother-in-law died and just grabbing up her things and running off with them. I don't want that to happen to the things I love, so I'm going to start giving them away, soon."

It may be easier to give away money than possessions you're attached to, and the government offers certain incentives that encourage such giving. You are allowed to reduce your estate by giving away

$10,000 a year to each of as many individuals you choose: If you have a large estate and a large family, you can dispose of a lot of pre-estate-tax money in one fell swoop. (There is no restriction concerning legal relationship.) If you are married, each of you can give $10,000 to as many people as you like. If your estate totals more than $600,000 (or $1,200,000 for a married couple), anything over $600,000 will be subject to inheritance tax. (This limit may be increased within the next few years.) Although $600,000 may sound like an enormous sum, the value of your house and your pension might quickly put you over the top. With any sizeable assets, we expect you will check with a lawyer rather than depending on advice that is beyond the scope of this book. I am just trying to alert you to possibilities you may not have suspected might apply to your situation.

You may want to consider "joint ownership with right of survivorship" for your major assets (cars, real estate, stock funds) so that these assets can pass to the surviving owner without any legal interference. This is the way people skirt probate (which is the legal process of proving the authenticity of your will). Probate laws vary from state to state. *How to Avoid Probate* is a popular book that advises you on the ins and outs of avoiding legal hassle in the disposition of your property; its tips can save you money, energy, and time. When Rosie reached eighty, she added her daughter's name to her bank accounts and mutual funds. When she died a few years later, there was no will, no lawyer, no probate, no taxes. Everything she owned just shifted over to her daughter.

If your estate is not complicated, you can draft a will for under fifty dollars. Any library will provide you with reference books designed to help you set up an estate and write a will. Computer software is available for writing a simple will (as well as for drawing up a living will, for issuing an advance directive for medical care, and for organizing and planning your estate). The will must be witnessed, and it should be notarized. Secure two witnesses who are not related to you and are not beneficiaries of your will.

You should choose an executor, either a close relative or a friend you trust, or a bank, or a lawyer. Your friend or relative should be paid a reasonable fee for being your executor, which can consume a fair amount of time and energy; your bank or lawyer will charge your estate at the going rate.

Drawing up a will with the help of a lawyer will obviously be more expensive than doing it yourself, but a lawyer should protect you from loopholes, errors, and ambiguities in your will that you might not be able to anticipate and that might seriously delay or complicate the disposition of your estate. If you have large assets or an involved family situation, you will undoubtedly need a lawyer to prepare your will.

Creating a will is an emotional issue—it's a written acknowledgment that you're mortal—but taking control will give you peace of mind and help you clarify who and what are most important to you. It's a job worth doing well.

SEVEN

Hope on the Horizon

28

Understanding the Breast Cancer Genes

My mother has breast cancer and I have the abnormal BRCA1 gene. What do I do? I'm only twenty five—I want to get married and have a family. But now? What do I tell my fiancé? When do I tell him? *Do* I tell him? The doctor says that to protect myself from cancer I should actually think about having my breasts and ovaries removed! I can barely take it all in. Can't I wait? Till I have some kids at least? But then is it fair to have a child if I'm going to pass on this horrible gene? How do I make any sense of all this?

What Are the Breast Cancer Genes?

A major step toward understanding the biology of breast cancer, leading to better techniques for breast cancer prevention, detection, and treatment, has been the identification of the two breast cancer genes: BRCA1, which stands for breast cancer gene one, and BRCA2, or breast cancer gene two. Knowing the precise location of the BRCA1 gene on chromosome 17, and BRCA2 on chromosome 13, makes it possible to determine whether your genes are normal or not. These two large genes can contain many different abnormalities, and they may account for 5 to 10 percent of all breast cancers. There is a lot to learn about these two genes, and about other genes that must also have an effect on breast cancer development in women with and without a family history of the disease. Women diagnosed with breast cancer who have the abnormal gene usually have a significant family history of breast cancer (and in some families, ovarian cancer), but 75 percent of women with breast cancer have no family history of the disease.

What Are Genes?

Genes are long, spiraled, threadlike molecules made of DNA (deoxyribonucleic acid); the cells of the breast and the rest of your body are built on the instructions that come from DNA. Genes are packaged in chromosomes. Your body is made up of billions of cells, and each cell has a nucleus that contains the chromosomes that carry the genes.

You have two copies of every chromosome and therefore two copies of every gene, one from your mother and one from your father. Each chromosome (we humans have forty-six) has a characteristic shape and order of genes.

Abnormal genes can be recognized by a shape and order that are different from normal. Think of your genes as an instruction manual for cell growth and function, where abnormalities are like misprints or typographical errors; a given edition of the manual will have the same misprints. Examples of such a "misprint" are the four common abnormalities on the BRCA1 or BRCA2 genes that appear to have greater frequency among Ashkenazi Jewish women (whose ancestors came from Central or Eastern Europe).

Genes regulate the function and growth of each cell; normal breast cells grow, rest, and die in a defined, orderly manner; they behave as they should. Breast genes regulate the behavior of these breast cells.

How Do Abnormal Genes Cause Cancer?

In their normal form, BRCA1 and BRCA2 are suppressor genes, whose job it is to produce a protein that suppresses uncontrolled cellular growth, preventing breast cancer. There are two copies of each of these genes in all women (and men), and as long as at least one gene is working properly, breast cell growth is normal and under control. But if both copies of this breast gene are abnormal, abnormal growth cannot be suppressed. Breast cells can now escape control, multiply, invade healthy tissue, and spread to other parts of the body: breast cancer.

All breast cancers are caused by abnormal genes whose defects are either *acquired* or *inherited*. If you were born with an abnormal gene that one of your parents passed on to you, you have an *inherited* genetic abnormality; you will then have one impaired gene from that parent and one healthy gene from your other parent.

If you were not born with an abnormal gene, but one of your genes became defective as a result of wear and tear, toxic, environmental, dietary, hormonal, or unknown factors, or an error in gene replication, you have a *nonhereditary* or *acquired* abnormality. Eighty-five to 90 percent of breast cancers are due to an acquired genetic abnormality.

Whether you inherited an abnormal breast cancer gene or acquired it, as long as you have one working gene, you have enough suppressor power to prevent cancer. But if this one working gene, because of wear and tear from damaging or harmful circumstances or from some error in its process of replication, breaks down, then uncontrolled growth—cancer—occurs.

How Common Are the Abnormal Breast Cancer Genes?

Inherited abnormal breast cancer genes probably explain only 10 percent of all cases of breast cancer. Most women who get breast cancer do not have an inherited abnormal breast cancer gene.

The abnormal breast cancer genes were first discovered in studies of families in which many young women were affected by breast and/or ovarian cancer. Either one of the abnormal genes, BRCA1 or BRCA2, is expected to account for many of the breast cancers in these families.

Your likelihood of having an abnormal breast cancer gene goes up if (1) the breast cancers in your family were diagnosed in blood-related members before age fifty; (2) there is both breast and ovarian cancer in your family, particularly if there is/was both breast and ovarian cancer in a single individual; (3) there are many women in your family who have had breast and/or ovarian cancer; (4) women in your family have had breast cancer in both breasts; (5) you are of Ashkenazi Jewish descent.

If one family member has an abnormal breast cancer gene, it does not mean that all members of the family will. If your mother or father has the abnormal form of the breast cancer gene, before testing anyone else, basic statistics will predict that you have a 50 percent chance of inheriting the abnormal gene, and your children have a 25 percent chance of inheriting the abnormal gene—50 percent of your 50 percent risk since you get only one of your parent's two genes.

Breast cancer gene abnormalities are more commonly found in women diagnosed with breast cancer before age forty. As many as 25 percent of younger women with breast cancer will have an abnormal breast cancer gene—usually BRCA1.

Specific abnormalities in BRCA1 and BRCA2 are more commonly found in Ashkenazi Jewish women than in non-Jewish women. Approximately one out of fifty Ashkenazi Jewish women—with or without breast cancer—will have a genetic abnormality on BRCA1 or

BRCA2. In a recent study of over 5000 Ashkenazi Jews, male and female, 120 people had one of the three most common abnormalities of BRCA1 and BRCA2 (2.3 percent). No individual had more than one abnormality in their breast cancer genes. You may wonder if it's possible to inherit the same abnormal gene from each of your parents—and thus have two of the same abnormal breast cancer genes—but no study so far has observed this double whammy. Another one of those so-far-unresolved puzzles.

Cancer Risk and the Abnormal Breast Cancer Gene

Women who have an abnormal BRCA1 or BRCA2 gene are at very high risk for developing breast cancer, ranging from 40 to 85 percent by age seventy. In contrast, the average woman without an abnormal breast cancer gene has a 12 percent risk of developing breast cancer over her lifetime. Women with an abnormal BRCA1 gene are also at increased risk for developing ovarian cancer: a 5 to 65 percent lifetime risk. The level of risk described in published studies varies significantly, depending on which group of women is under study. Studies of women who have an extensive family history of both breast and ovarian cancer show a breast cancer risk closer to 85 percent; women with no or minimal family history are at lower risk, maybe even lower than 40 percent. Where you fall within this range of risk depends on multiple factors: the extent to which breast cancer has affected other members of your family who share the same genetic abnormality, your age, and a combination of lifestyle and environmental influences. The recent study of Ashkenazi Jews showed a breast cancer risk of 56 percent and an ovarian cancer risk of 16 percent in women with an abnormal breast cancer gene.

The fact that the genetic abnormalities resulting in cancer are inherited does not mean that these cancers are more virulent. Recent evidence suggests, in fact, that women with the abnormal gene who develop breast or ovarian cancer may have a *less* deadly version of the disease.

Men who carry the abnormal BRCA1 gene have a higher risk of colon and prostate cancer. Men who have the abnormal BRCA2 gene are at increased risk for developing breast cancer; 6 percent of men who carry this gene will eventually develop breast cancer.

Impact of Genetic Information: Possibilities and Limitations

Anyone seeking information about her—or his—genetic makeup needs to know the possibilities and limitations such information brings with it.

The potential benefits or possibilities in obtaining genetic information include the following:

1. If there is a specific breast cancer genetic abnormality in your family and your test is normal, then your genetic counselor can tell you with greater certainty that you have the same relatively low risk of developing breast cancer and ovarian cancer as women in the general population. Routine breast cancer surveillance (self-examination, mammograms, doctor visits) will still be important for you, as it is for all women. (There are no accepted ovarian cancer screening guidelines for women at average risk for the disease.)

2. If you have an abnormal breast cancer test result, you may benefit from a close and vigilant program of surveillance to monitor the health of your breasts and ovaries. The benefit comes from finding a cancer in its earliest stage, when it is most treatable and curable.

3. You may decide to participate in clinical trials to see whether drugs such as tamoxifen can prevent your getting breast cancer.

4. You may even consider options as extreme as surgical removal of your breasts and/or ovaries before cancer has an opportunity to form.

5. An abnormal gene test result may influence your treatment choices if cancer develops, giving you more information from which you may form your decisions.

6. If you obtain genetic testing in a research setting, or if you participate in other clinical studies, you will be contributing to the clinical scientific research that eventually should lead to the prevention and cure of breast cancer.

7. Finally, knowing that you carry the abnormal breast cancer gene may lead you to make significant lifestyle and family planning changes to help improve your odds.

The significant limitations and potentially adverse reactions to learning about your genetic makeup include the following:

1. We still don't know how to prevent breast cancer; the value of drugs such as tamoxifen is still uncertain.

2. Prophylactic removal of breasts and ovaries does not eliminate every single breast- and ovary-related cell, and therefore does not eliminate all risk entirely. Even after such surgery, a woman with an abnormal breast cancer gene must continue to be monitored regularly, because the risk for breast and ovarian cancer remains significant. It may be easier to find an early-stage breast cancer in or under the skin where the breast used to be, compared with finding it in the breast itself, but if reconstruction is done after the mastectomy, the physical examination of the area can be challenging. Close follow-up remains necessary.

3. For families in which there are many women with breast cancer who all test normal for the known breast cancer genes, this test result may be only partially reassuring; these families may still have an inherited form of breast cancer that just hasn't been identified as yet. A woman from such a family still must be followed very closely.

4. You cannot assume that close surveillance will always result in early detection of breast cancer in all women; some women may end up being diagnosed with later-stage disease despite the best surveillance techniques.

5. An abnormal test result can produce tremendous anxiety, depression, anger, denial, and isolation in some women; if you don't feel you can handle this heavy information, knowing that nothing you can do will guarantee the prevention of breast cancer, perhaps you should refrain from taking the test till more is known that can help beat the disease.

6. An abnormal breast cancer gene test does not mean that a woman will necessarily get breast cancer; some women manage to escape its curse. But no woman knows if she's going to be the one who is going to get it, or the one who won't. (Most women with the abnormal gene will assume they are bound to get it, and all of them will undoubtedly suffer stress and anxiety.)

7. If you find that you've passed the abnormal gene on to your children, the burden of guilt can be exceedingly difficult to handle.

8. Discrimination based on genetic information is a serious potential risk of genetic testing. Genetic results are like a crystal ball predicting your future, influencing your ability to find a partner, get a job or develop a career, obtain life and health insurance, and keep your personal affairs to yourself. In few other areas is confidentiality so vital as it is in the matter of genetic testing.

9. Testing for the breast cancer gene may not answer all your questions. Families who carry an abnormal breast cancer gene may have other factors involved in their high risk of breast cancer that

are not at present understood. So far, nearly all testing and risk calculations that have been performed on women who have the abnormal genes are based on women who also have a strong family history of breast cancer. We don't yet know how to make accurate predictions of breast cancer risk in women with an abnormal breast cancer gene who don't have a family history of breast cancer.

The Genetic Risk Assessment Process

Many women who come for genetic testing are motivated by a perception that their risk of breast cancer is much higher than it really is; they want to know if they have the abnormal breast cancer gene because a member of their family has cancer. Or sometimes, in a family with a large number of women who have breast cancer and/or ovarian cancer, everybody is most anxious to have the woman who has no evidence of disease undergo the breast cancer gene test to resolve the uncertainty.

Education is the first step in genetic risk assessment. The concerned individual or family members need basic information about breast cancer, breast cancer risk, prevention, treatment, and health issues beyond treatment. A discussion should include information about the role of genetics in breast cancer, a description of the testing process, and the value and drawbacks of the gene test, as outlined previously. Group sessions and individual conferences can be provided by a genetic counselor or other health care professional specifically trained in breast cancer genetics.

If you decide to proceed with genetic risk assessment, one of these trained professionals will help you prepare a detailed family health history. This history of the family is used to generate a family tree, also known as a pedigree, establishing the family's lineage and listing members of each generation, going back as far as you have recorded information. This tree requires at least three generations' history; most people's health information about their forebears does not extend beyond their grandparents. Cooperation among family members who share high risk for breast cancer is necessary to proceed with comprehensive genetic testing.

If you identify a potential case of inherited breast or ovarian cancer, it needs to be validated, confirmed with medical records and a pathology report whenever possible. For example, if one of your aunts died of liver cancer, you need to find out if it was breast cancer that metastasized to the liver or if it was cancer that originated in the liver. This process requires cooperation of family members, persistent research, informed consent, and signed release forms to get access to relevant information. Some family members may be resolute about maintaining privacy; this is their prerogative. No one should ever be coerced into participating. Unfortunately, the breast cancer stigma persists; it wasn't that long ago that the "big C" was referred to only in hushed whispers. As a reflection of that stigma, asking elderly relatives about deceased family members may yield minimal information, because few people years back were even told that anyone had cancer.

Whether it's a carryover of the stigma or a measure of the depth of denial, pain, and anger associated with cancer, it's not uncommon for tension and hard feelings to develop between those who want the test performed and those who wish to avoid it.

After the family history has been completed, the genetic counselor analyzes the pattern of breast cancer involvement in your family to determine its significance. Your family's pedigree is categorized in one of three ways: (1) *Sporadic* means your personal or family history of breast cancer does not follow any regular pattern of inheritance. Rather, it is scattered and isolated in its appearance, and the genetic abnormality in the woman with breast cancer who was tested is probbly of acquired origin, with no higher risk factor than appears in the general public. (2) *Familial* means there may be a significant family history present, but that history does not follow a well-defined, specific pattern of inherited breast cancer, or, if the family history is strong but incomplete, there may be insufficient information from the pedigree to make a strong enough correlation to inheritance. (3) *Hereditary* means a compelling family history is present that consists of multiple blood relatives with breast and/or ovarian cancer, strongly suggesting the presence of an inherited form of the disease.

If you fall into the third, high-risk category, you may decide to go ahead with the breast cancer gene test. In one nationally known Philadelphia cancer center, just under 20 percent of the women who participated in the family risk assessment program fell into that high-risk category. Women in the second (familial) category are at moderate risk and can get the test if they are motivated to do so, although it is not medically indicated; women in the first (sporadic) category are at low risk and are thought not to benefit from the test. Based on these category-based recommendations and the individual's particular interests, roughly 25 percent of people initially interested in the test end up being tested for the abnormal breast cancer genes.

Who Gets Tested

If your family history of breast cancer follows an inherited pattern from one parent only, then testing of generations before yours needs to be done only on that parent's blood relatives, whether they've had breast cancer or not. Any biological child of that parent would also be a candidate for testing.

If your family history is limited, say, to your mother's side, she may be the best person to go first and get the gene test. This makes sense for three reasons: (1) If she has the gene, the information learned about her specific abnormality within the gene will help direct and shorten the gene search in your test, because it is assumed that if you inherited a breast cancer gene abnormality, it will be the same abnormality as your mother's. (2) Because she is a generation older than you, she is likely to be much closer to retirement than you are, and therefore much less vulnerable to employment and insurance discrimination. (3) If your mother doesn't have the abnormal gene, then she could not pass the abnormal gene on to you, and testing can stop with her.

I have a thirty-five-year-old friend without breast cancer who is from an Ashkenazi Jewish family in which her mother's sister, her mother's father's sister, and her mother's father's mother all had breast cancer. Her own mother, who does not have breast cancer at age seventy, has decided to seek testing first, because if she is tested and doesn't have the abnormal gene, she could not have passed it to her children. In this case, if the mother's father were alive, he would be the likeliest choice for the first testing.

If your parent does have an abnormal breast cancer gene, you should seriously consider being tested. If your parent from the affected side is unwilling to be tested, or is deceased, you may decide to proceed with the testing for yourself.

If a woman with breast cancer has undergone a bone marrow transplantation with bone marrow donated from another person (an allogeneic transplant), a breast cancer gene test of her blood would not necessarily be representative of her own genetic composition. Her options for having herself tested include obtaining her blood from a pre-transplant stored sample or doing a tissue scraping or biopsy.

Most geneticists advise against testing children under eighteen. A positive test could predict a female child's likelihood to develop cancer fifty years before the fact—and, even further into the future than that, the likelihood of this child's daughters to develop cancer. But there is no advantage to having information about genetic defects before age eighteen because there are currently no effective therapies available to prevent breast cancer, and the onset of breast cancer does not usually occur before age thirty. It is also quite possible that by the time these children are beyond puberty or beyond their childbearing years, a new treatment may be discovered to correct an abnormal breast cancer gene before cancer has a chance to develop. Moreover, there are profound disadvantages to early testing. The terrible psychological burden for the child's parents, and for the child as she grows to understand what these findings mean, may be too much to bear. And of course there are major discrimination issues at risk. I've already heard of parents ready to remove the breasts and ovaries of a prepubescent daughter, a radical approach that I think is unacceptable. (It is very unlikely that any surgeon would agree to perform such a procedure.) Far better advice would be to keep prepubescent daughters lean and active, as one way to delay the onset of menarche, and possibly reduce their risk of breast cancer.

Prenatal testing using amniocentesis or CVS (chorionic villous sampling) is not yet being done, not just because of ethical issues, but for the practical reason that it currently takes too long to perform the genetic test in most facilities—maybe even longer than the pregnancy itself. (Myriad Genetic Laboratories, of Salt Lake City, has a turnaround time of one month on blood samples. Presently, they do not perform pre-natal testing.)

Consent for the Gene Test

"Before you go for that test, you want to be sure you want to know the answer," says Dr. Lisa Jablon, director of a breast cancer risk program. And you need to have a good answer to the question "What will I do with the test results?" before getting the test, suggests Dr. Gordon Schwartz, a highly respected Philadelphia breast cancer surgeon. Genetic testing for breast cancer can have a tremendous impact on the lives of the people who are tested. Before being tested, they must sign an informed consent document, which states that they have been fully informed of the benefits and possibilities, as well as the limitations and risks, of the information to be gathered from the test (this would include all issues raised in the prior section).

Many centers require your participation in more than one session of education and counseling before the actual test can proceed, to help you fully understand and digest all the information available at this time, so you can weigh the reasons for and against getting the test.

Testing of multiple family members affected by breast cancer improves the accuracy and the significance of the test for you and your family. If a woman has not had breast cancer, some centers will not do the test unless there is a significant family history or someone in your family has already been shown to have the abnormal breast cancer gene. Some centers insist that a relative with breast cancer be tested first, before testing the individual who has not had cancer. If no relatives with breast or ovarian cancer are living, it may be necessary to obtain tissue from a deceased relative with cancer to complete the puzzle of a particular family's genetic picture. (Cancerous tissue is usually stored in tissue banks for many years, accessible for research inquiries long after the donor has passed on.) Genetic testing of preserved tissue is not as accurate, however, as the testing of fresh blood.

Generally, any woman who has had breast cancer and wants to have the test will be accepted for testing, even if her family history is not significant.

Quality of Testing Facilities

Ideally, genetic counseling would be available to anyone who takes the breast cancer gene test, offering the talents of a multidisciplinary team, including a geneticist and a genetics counselor, a physician, a social worker, and a specially trained nurse. However, although blood testing will eventually become readily and widely available, genetic counseling—necessary to interpret and deliver the test results—will be available in only a few centers, usually those associated with university hospitals.

Most testing centers are in university hospitals or their affiliates, with an established integrated research program. If you are part of a breast cancer gene research study, the test is usually free, and your results are recorded with a special identification number (not your name) to protect your privacy.

Commercial laboratories operate with fewer constraints than a research center; some labs ask no more from you than a signed consent form and your check. They offer the test for various charges and need never see more of you than a tubeful of your blood. Commercial tests are almost always processed through the mail, but don't imagine these tests are anything like a home pregnancy test you can do by yourself. Blood must be drawn at a doctor's office and sent off to an independent genetics laboratory, together with a completed test form co-signed by a doctor. DNA is extracted from the blood cells, then examined for abnormal patterns and shapes.

Commercial labs offer little or no personal assistance or counseling to help you interpret what the results mean. Some commercial labs do provide a resource guide to help you and your doctor identify genetic counseling services in your area. Myriad Genetic Laboratories conducts important research with the results obtained from its testing (privacy guaranteed with coding). In fact, this lab was the first to define the precise location and sequence of the first breast cancer gene.

At most other commercial laboratories, however, it may be hard for you to be guaranteed privacy, a crucial concern. You might try to submit your sample under a code number rather than your name. Some women adopt an assumed name.

One commercial laboratory charges around $500 to search for the four most common abnormal points on the BRCA1 and BRCA2 genes. If this initial test is normal, they will sequence the remainder of the genes, for a fee of $1500, to assess the 100 or more other potential weak points in the genes that can cause breast cancer. Another commercial laboratory charges $2400 to completely map out both BRCA1 and BRCA2; if an abnormality is found in one family member, subsequent family members who want the test are charged $395 for an evaluation of the presence or absence of that specific abnormality.

I prefer that testing be done in a research setting so that you can get individual counseling, protect your privacy, save on cost, and contribute valuable information to research, so that one day we can better understand how to cure, and prevent, breast cancer. An additional advantage is that your medical insurance company is not involved in your testing and is not informed of the results, and you pay very little or nothing. Few health care plans are prepared to pay for the test anyway. Myriad Genetic has counselors who can help you if you wish to seek financial support from your insurance company.

To locate a research study center near you, call 800-4-CANCER. You may find that you live nowhere near a research center, so a mail-in test with separate genetic counseling may be your only viable option.

Test Results

Results are typically sent to your doctor or genetic counselor, who then reports them to you. Expect to wait a long time for test results. Testing for the four most common sites of genetic abnormalities may take two to three months. If those four sites are normal, and the breast cancer gene abnormality in your family was one of those four, then testing can stop there. But if your family is without a known breast cancer gene abnormality and you are the first to be tested, then testing should continue, to check out the rest of the gene(s). This can take one to two years at many of the research centers. If your family's specific gene abnormality is already known, the test can take much less time.

Commercial labs may give quicker results than research centers. Myriad Genetic Laboratories, for instance, has a turn-around time of four weeks to map out both BRCA1 and BRCA2 (not just the four most common sites of abnormalities).

Results are usually sent to the requesting physician rather than directly to you. If you were tested at a research facility, you are called into the center, where the results are presented to you by the genetic counselor and her team, which may include a cancer doctor, social worker, and psychologist. The significance of the results for you are then discussed.

An essential and critical part of the genetic risk assessment program is the responsible and sensitive disclosure of test results to you. I recommend that you bring someone along with you when you go to receive your results. Receiving good news—a normal breast cancer gene test result—is a tremendous relief; it can help you regain a positive interest in life and optimism toward the future. But if you are told you have an abnormal gene, having someone who cares about you at your side can really help support you through the immediate distress. If your tests are normal and other family members have tested positive for the abnormal gene, your relief may be overshadowed by guilt, "survivor's guilt": "My cousin just died of breast cancer and she carried the abnormal breast cancer gene BRCA1. I have breast cancer and I also have the gene. My sister is distraught and she and her husband decide, that's it—off with the breasts, fast, and she makes plans for the operation. Meanwhile, I'm in touch with our oncologist, who's the one who tested my family for the gene. She calls my sister immediately and tells her she doesn't have the gene. Cancel the operation, go home and enjoy. But does she celebrate? No. She feels so guilty: 'Why am I the only one in the family not to get the gene?' "

Although you may decide to share your results from your gene tests with your family, absolute confidentiality and privacy must be assured and secured to protect whoever has been identified as carrying an abnormal breast cancer gene. An abnormal test result essentially belongs only to the person involved. There can be no compromise on this issue until laws are in place that keep results from being available to insurers and employers, thus eliminating the possibility of discrimination if the results are disclosed. Until your privacy can be guaranteed, *test results should not be written on any chart or noted on any record*. Your name should not be attached to a result lest the information leak out or be accessed by insurers, health care providers, or employers. Privacy is most easily protected if you are tested and identified with a code number instead of a name. As mentioned earlier, some women use assumed names. Personally, I don't believe that withholding genetic test information from your medical record constitutes fraud because we don't yet understand how to interpret the results, to figure out what the results really mean to you.

"What Do I Do Now?"

Regardless of the extent of "theoretical" discussion prior to consent, if the results show an abnormal breast cancer gene, you may feel hit with unexpected and overwhelming news. You will want and need comprehensive information and practical advice to sort out how to handle this new fact in your life, and to point you in the direction of health and well-being.

The best way to prevent or treat breast cancer in women with an abnormal gene is still a mystery. The discovery of the breast cancer gene abnormalities is so new that clinical studies haven't been done to give the necessary answers. But you need the best information right now, to guide your decisions and actions. I can offer you the following recommendations, based on currently available but admittedly limited information—and common sense:

If your breast cancer gene test is normal and you have no family history or your family history is minimal, or your family has a defined breast cancer gene abnormality that you don't have, then your risk of breast cancer is equal to that of a woman in the general public: 12 percent over your lifetime.

1. You should continue to practice regular breast self-examination and obtain annual or semiannual clinical breast examinations (depending on your doctor's recommendation).
2. Frequency of screening mammography should be based on current guidelines for women of average risk: baseline mammograms between ages thirty-five and forty, annual mammograms after age forty.
3. In addition, a low-fat, well-balanced, nutritious diet, regular exercise, and avoidance of excess weight will improve your sense of well-being and general health, and possibly lower your risk of breast cancer.

If your test and your family's tests are normal but there are many young women in your family affected by breast cancer, it is still very possible there is an inherited genetic abnormality present in the affected members of the family that has not yet been identified. Under these circumstances, you need to do the following:

1. Continue close follow-up care: baseline mammogram between thirty and thirty-five (mammography for women under thirty is usually not reliable), annual mammography starting between ages thirty-five and forty (note: the suggested frequency of these studies between the ages of thirty and forty is based on the age of breast cancer onset in your family, how easy or hard it is to read your mammogram, and your physician's recommendation), clinical breast examination every six months, and monthly breast self-examination.
2. Consider participation in a cancer prevention trial, such as the tamoxifen prevention trial.
3. Pay attention to a healthy lifestyle and follow recommended nutrition and exercise guidelines.
4. Stay connected to a research center in case new genetic discoveries are established.

If your test result is abnormal, and it has been double-checked and verified, you will need to consider a series of health-enhancing guidelines: (Keep in mind that there is not a 100 percent correlation between having an abnormal breast cancer gene and getting breast cancer or ovarian cancer—unlike other diseases like Down's syndrome, where having the gene means having Down's.)

1. Guard the privacy of your test results with scrupulous attention.
2. Rigorously follow early detection practices that monitor the health of your breasts and ovaries, as described above. If high resolution or digital mammography is available, consider starting annual mammography at an earlier age. Your ovarian health can be monitored by semiannual pelvic examination by a gynecologist, annual pelvic ultrasound with an intravaginal probe, and blood tests for a special protein called CA-125. Studies are under way to better define the value of these screening tests in women with an abnormal breast cancer gene. And newer technologies are also under investigation, including MRI (magnetic resonance imaging) and PET (positron emission tomography) scanning for these women. If these screening studies are available to you, seriously consider participating in them. Close and vigilant surveillance can result in finding a cancer in its earliest stage when it is most treatable and curable.
3. Participate in clinical trials that test potential cancer-preventing agents such as tamoxifen; your role in clinical studies can be sig-

nificant, leading to results that may be of direct benefit to you and other women in your situation.

4. Adopt healthy lifestyle choices to stay well and possibly reduce the risk of cancer or its recurrence, including a low-fat, well-balanced, nutritious diet, regular exercise, and weight control, and only occasional consumption of alcohol.

5. Consider family planning choices that may help lower your risk, such as having children at an earlier age than you may have planned, (this *may* lower your risk; also, some women choose to have children at a younger age, prior to prophylactic surgery), and avoiding any (or prolonged) use of hormone replacement therapy.

6. You may want to consider options as extreme as surgical removal of your breasts and/or ovaries before cancer has an opportunity to form. A woman who has an abnormal breast cancer gene and develops breast cancer in one breast, may choose mastectomy of the breast and prophylactic removal of the other, presumably healthy, breast. Before planning anything as drastic as prophylactic surgery, however, you should first carefully consider a number of important factors that bear on your decision, given your unique history. These factors, and the relevance of your family history, will undoubtedly change as new information about these genes and breast cancer is discovered.

Prophylactic breast removal can theoretically reduce your risk of getting breast cancer by 80 to 90 percent, and prophylactic removal of the ovaries may reduce your risk of getting ovarian cancer by 50 percent. (This theoretical level of effectiveness was suggested by Schrag et al., *New England Journal of Medicine,* May 1997.)

The higher your risk, the more likely you will benefit from prophylactic surgery. If your risk of breast cancer is estimated to be 80 percent, your risk could be lowered to 8 percent; if your risk of ovarian cancer is estimated to be 40 percent, your risk could be lowered to 20 percent. Be aware, however, that if you are at 80 percent risk of breast cancer and you have prophylactic surgery, there is a 20 percent chance that your surgery was unnecessary—because twenty out of a hundred women at your level of risk will not get breast cancer in the first place. There is also an 8 percent chance that the procedure will not prevent breast cancer. (The procedure is at most 90 percent effective, 10 percent ineffective—you can still get breast cancer in spite of having had the procedure.) If you do not have the procedure and you stay as you are—intact—and if you practice early detection techniques diligently, even if you are diagnosed with and treated for breast cancer it may very well be a breast cancer that is curable; you might therefore do just as well without prophylactic surgery—and its disfigurement.

To continue: If your risk of getting breast cancer is about 40 percent, prophylactic surgery reduces it to 4 percent. That leaves a 60 percent chance that your surgery was unnecessary—if you were not destined to get breast cancer in the first place—and the 4 percent chance that the procedure won't prevent breast cancer. That adds up to a 64 percent chance that the procedure might be unproductive. On the other hand, there is a 36 percent chance that the procedure will prevent breast cancer; however, if you hadn't had the procedure and you were one of the 40 percent of women destined to get breast cancer, there is a very strong possibility that the cancer might be found early enough to be cured. So the 36 percent benefit may actually be less than you may anticipate.

The younger you are at the time of prophylactic surgery, the greater the purported benefit. Breast cancers associated with an abnormal breast cancer gene usually occur at a younger age than the much more common age-related breast cancers. In addition, as you age, there are other medical conditions that may affect your health, like diabetes, heart disease, effects from smoking, et cetera; thus, as you grow older, your risk of getting a breast-cancer-gene-related breast cancer lessens, and your chance of getting sick from other illness increases. As a consequence, the purported benefit from prophylactic surgery diminishes as you get older.

If you've already had breast cancer, you may be wondering about what role prophylactic surgery might have for you. The value of any prophylactic procedure is profoundly affected by any coexisting illness, particularly breast cancer, and particularly the stage and nature of breast cancer you have had. If you have been treated for a moderate- to late-stage breast cancer, where the risk of recurrence of the *first* breast cancer is much more significant than the chance of being diagnosed with a *new, unrelated* breast cancer, then prophylactic surgery does not offer significant benefit. But if you have been treated for an early-stage breast cancer and your risk of recurrence is very low, then prophylactic surgery may be of value to you. Obviously this is a matter to carefully discuss with your doctor and genetic counselor.

You might decide to have your ovaries removed but not your breasts. It is much easier to find an early-stage breast cancer than it is to reliably find an early-stage ovarian cancer. Besides, removal of your breasts has a greater effect on your outward self-image than removal of your ovaries. While this makes some sense, the article in the *New England Journal of Medicine* argues that prophylactic breast surgery is considered more effective at preventing breast cancer than ovary removal is at preventing ovarian cancer.

The psychological implications of having an abnormal breast cancer gene are incredibly important. Women with an abnormal gene may have witnessed the death of their mother or sister from breast cancer and experience severe anxiety over their own vulnerability; these women might well be better off emotionally if they have prophylactic surgery. Other women may find that the psychological devastation that accompanies the loss of their breasts and ovaries and the opportunity to have children is too much to endure; they are far more able and prepared to deal with close follow-up and to adhere to a disciplined, healthy lifestyle in the hope of protecting their future.

If you are agonizing over this dilemma, your family history can provide invaluable information to help guide your decision. If you have an abnormal breast cancer gene and a family history of breast and ovarian cancer, look at the pattern of your family's disease history in consultation with a genetic counselor, to try to estimate the most realistic picture of your particular risk *and* at what age you might expect to develop cancer. If every woman in your family who has carried an abnormal breast cancer gene has developed cancer by age forty, and you have the abnormal gene and you are thirty and without breast cancer so far, you may decide to have prophylactic surgery as soon as possible—or perhaps take your chance waiting for a year or two in order to have a child. If, on the other hand, every woman in your family with an abnormal breast cancer gene was diagnosed with breast cancer in her fifties and ten years later each continued to do well, and you are thirty with the same gene abnormality, you may decide against prophylactic surgery and be followed carefully over the years with mammography and breast examination and a healthy lifestyle—with an ear cocked to catch the newest medical advances that might keep you free from disease—and allow you to have a family as well.

The decision to have prophylactic surgery is not an emergency. You have time. Based on the theoretical model described in the *New England Journal of Medicine,* there is no significant loss of therapeutic advantage when these procedures are done at age forty, after childbearing, than at age thirty. Also, breast reconstruction can be done after breast removal, and for a woman who has not had breast cancer, hormone replacement therapy can be provided, at least until the time of natural menopause (say, from age thirty to age fifty), to replace the hormones that her removed ovaries would have produced. These are very individual, complex decisions that must be made in consultation with your physician.

If you intend to apply for reimbursement for prophylactic surgery from your health care provider (and forgo privacy), be sure to muster a very strong case. Assemble letters of support from your primary care physician, and your surgeon, laying out the details that have established the reasons for this drastic step. Some doctors are able to persuade the medical insurance company to cover the cost of prophylactic surgeries based on family history alone—no mention of breast cancer genetic results. In other situations, genetic information is needed to win coverage requiring additional input from your gene-testing center, your genetic counselors, and your oncologist.

There is little precedent for approval of this expensive procedure, which some health care providers may view as "elective." Each application will likely be evaluated on its individual merits. Prepare for an active defense and stick to your guns.

7. Concentrate on maintaining peace of mind and your quality of life by working on stress reduction, relaxation, and enjoyment through one or more of the following: support groups, meditation, prayer, exercise, music, visualization, and distraction. Individual counseling and antidepressant medications may be advisable if anxiety or depression makes it too difficult for you to manage on your own.

8. Finally, a woman with an abnormal breast cancer gene who is then diagnosed with breast cancer may need to approach treatment decisions differently from a woman with a similar diagnosis who is without an abnormal breast cancer gene. For example, it's not known if lumpectomy and radiation would be as effective as mastectomy in a woman with an abnormal breast cancer gene. Although there are no clinical trial results to provide the answer at this time, retrospective data show no obvious advantage of the more aggressive surgery in women with a strong family history of breast cancer. Clearly, optimal treatment recommendations for women with the abnormal breast cancer gene, diagnosed with breast cancer, need to be defined.

Better answers to these complex considerations and issues will continue to emerge and evolve as new information becomes available.

Into the Future

Future basic science and clinical research in genetics will help unravel the answers to the fundamental questions of what causes breast cancer and how breast cancer can be prevented. Information from genetic research is expected to define new genetic mutations in families with inherited breast cancer unrelated to the abnormal BRCA1 and BRCA2 genes. New research will determine how other genes, such as the gene for the estrogen receptor, interact with breast cancer genes to affect breast cancer risk.

Research will also lead to better utilization of genetic information to develop more accurate and reliable predictors of cancer risk, and to determine improved guidelines for genetic counseling. The risk of breast cancer and the nature of breast cancer that can develop may depend on the particular *combination* of genes a woman is born with, as well as the *site* of the particular abnormality on the breast cancer genes. One combination may predict a 70 percent risk of developing an aggressive breast cancer prior to menopause. Another combination may predict a 30 percent risk of having a less aggressive cancer after menopause. (This is also true of ovarian cancer.)

Better cancer prevention strategies must be developed—derived from a better understanding of the relationship of genes, diet, and the environment. We will then be able to offer more meaningful lifestyle recommendations. Studies of cancer prevention drugs, such as tamoxifen and new agents on the horizon, may be effective alone or in combination with other interventions. Further study may tell us how to prevent breast cancer by repairing or replacing defective genes (or the protein they are responsible for producing), so that cancer is never able to develop. Until a more effective method of breast cancer prevention is identified, women may continue to consider and elect prophylactic surgery. In the meantime, as more is learned about the significance of specific sites and combinations of genetic abnormalities, prophylactic surgeries may be more aptly tailored to each woman's unique risk profile. For example, if a woman has a specific breast cancer gene abnormality associated with a high risk of breast cancer and a low risk of ovarian cancer, then she need consider only prophylactic mastectomies, sparing her ovaries. If she has a low risk of breast cancer and a high risk of ovarian cancer, then she need consider only methods to reduce her risk of ovarian cancer, such as taking birth control pills or removing her ovaries—both with close follow-up.

The best way to treat women who have the abnormal gene and who develop breast or ovarian cancer needs to be further defined by clinical studies that incorporate genetic profiles of these women. These studies will tell us which current therapies are most effective. The value of new gene therapies will need to be studied to identify effective treatment that most specifically targets an individual's unique genetic abnormality to achieve greater benefits with less toxicity.

Studies with an emphasis on quality of life will help people with a genetic predisposition to cancer find effective tools to deal with premature menopause, chronic stress, damaged self-esteem, anger, fear, and depression.

As our knowledge evolves, the women and men who participate in these clinical studies—and their immediate families, as well as many others—will benefit from this research. Whatever advances genetic research yields must be interpreted and conveyed as quickly as possible to the women and their families who need this information to live well beyond breast cancer.

29

Don't Let Breast Cancer Define You

On the Air, in Your Face

There's always something new in your face about breast cancer. It seems as if you can never be free of it. As much as you would like never to hear those two words again, you do want the latest reliable information on breast cancer, from TV, radio, newspapers, magazines, and now the Web. There's something obviously compelling about the printed word and the television image, but there's a lot of skewed reporting, and when you hear stories of miracle cures, magic potions, and embattled prophets, don't believe everything you hear. The media are starved for sensational topics and positive results. When something doesn't work, it may not even be reported; there's a real bias against negative results. When studies showed there was no cancer-fighting benefit to melatonin and that sharks *do* get cancer, there were no headlines.

The news media like short bits of information that make a splash quickly. When the study on lumpectomy plus radiation showed benefits equal to mastectomy, the media reported the equal benefits of lumpectomy and mastectomy; radiation, a vital part of the equation was largely omitted. When women with negative nodes were told they could stop taking tamoxifen after five years, there were no recommendations for women with positive nodes, because they weren't included in the study. But most headlines told women they could stop taking tamoxifen after five years, period. Examine carefully what you find reported in the media. If something sounds exciting, look further for in-depth information.

Time Out from Breast Cancer

"Is it wise for me to hang out with other women who have had breast cancer, to keep up with the support group, to become a hotline volunteer? Or would it be better for me to get away from the whole thing, at least for a while, so I can separate myself from constant reminders of illness and give myself a little space from the issue?" Debby had finished treatment. She took a job at a breast cancer foundation, but after three months she gave it up because the breast cancer issue had become all-consuming. She had to get some distance to try feeling normal for a change. Debby had the sense to listen to her inner voice. You need to figure out what sustains you, what you find healing, what makes you uncomfortable, and what makes you happy.

There are many women who put the whole breast cancer thing behind them after they finish their treatment. It doesn't mean they're in denial. It's just their personal style. "Been there, done that. What next?" Other women can't handle all that's hit them at once, so they put some of it away, "for later." Once, when Living Beyond Breast Cancer_SM_ was organizing a conference, a thirteen-year breast cancer survivor picked up a brochure to one of our conferences and, for the first time in all those years, called to talk to someone about her buried-away diagnosis, her fear, and her anger. She had good reason to be angry; her family had ostracized her, scolded her. "No one else ever had breast cancer in our family—*you* had to be the one to get it!" She had reached a point at last where she could emerge from that blanket of shame. She came to our conference and was overwhelmed by the warmth and support of a thousand breast cancer survivors.

Thinking about the Future

Are you trying not to think about the future, with barely enough energy to cope with the "now"? The inertia that follows the end of treatment can be paralyzing. "If I do something that presupposes a future—plan a vacation for next year or order tickets for the coming season's theater subscription—will I jinx myself? Why am I unable to think rationally?"

How do you learn to live your life as if every day were your last *and* as if you have fifty years ahead of you? Can you return to the career plan you had been pursuing before it was derailed by breast cancer? One of my patients recently pulled me aside, a year after treatment, and nervously told me she was thinking about going to graduate school. Then she added that it was a four-year program, and did I think that she could do it? What she was asking was whether she would live long enough to finish the course.

Living in the moment doesn't cut it for long. "One day at a time" may help keep your head straight, but it won't pay your bills or build your future. You need to plan, for next year and ten years after that. Who is keeping you from doing it? Perhaps *you* are. It may be that you have to give yourself the okay to plan ahead, and it may help to have reassurance from your doctor that your outlook is strong enough to do so. You may need reassurance from your partner, children, or extended family, to pursue your dreams—or just to plan what goes beyond tomorrow.

Breast cancer may cause you to travel an entirely different path in life. Marnie Daniels used her skills as a beautician to develop a twist in her career; she now specializes in wigs and makeup for women who undergo chemotherapy. Amy Langer, executive director of the National Alliance of Breast Cancer Organizations, had had a big job on Wall Street, but when she was diagnosed with breast cancer, she decided to give it up and devote her strong talents to building NABCO, bringing it to new heights. Fran Visco gave up partnership in a well-respected Philadelphia law firm to dedicate herself to ending the curse of breast cancer. She is the president of the National Breast Cancer Coalition.

Don't Let Breast Cancer Define Who You Are

At one of our workshops, a woman introduced herself to me saying, "I'm a lumpectomy with radiation, stage two. . . ." I stopped her immediately and asked her to listen to what she had just said. "You are *not* your cancer: You are an individual!" Remember that. Breast cancer has had a major impact on your life, but you must stop it at the border.

You may need to remind others, too, that you are more than your breast cancer history. Overheard by a woman waiting for treatment: one radiation therapist to another, "There's a breast in room three." No! You are not your breast. You are a person, and *all of you* needs attention and support. All the caregivers in your life must always have that big picture in mind and treat and respect you as a whole human being.

The phrase is overused, but it still works: This is the first day of the rest of your life. One after another of my patients says, "I have a new perspective. Every day counts in a way it never did before." Breast cancer is not a logical disease, and it certainly doesn't treat people fairly. But you can say to yourself, "This was not my fault. I can't help what happened. I can't go back and undo it—the only thing to do is go forward, one step at a time."

Time alone may be the only thing that brings peace of mind. Fine—but at least acknowledge that some time has already passed. Take pleasure in it and use it as a stepping-stone to better things ahead. After a year, give yourself a pat on the back, and plan for the next step, however big or small.

30

Conclusion:
Turning "Why Me?" into
"Why Anybody?"

No one ever made me any lifetime promise, and no one comes with a guarantee. So I live with a big question over my head—but still, this is a second chance. I don't postpone what I want to do. I get pleasure in simple things—and every day is an adventure!

You Are More Than You May Imagine

You and I are not isolated individuals—each of us is connected to those around us, in the makeup of our cells and in the power of our spirit. Generation to generation, we pass on the DNA of our genes, and also our shared values, experience, and love. I believe I am in each of my children, in my husband, my sisters and brothers, and my parents. I am also spiritually intertwined with my home and my neighborhood and the schools I've attended—and my organization Living Beyond Breast Cancer_SM_. Many of you are spiritually enmeshed with your church and your God. If you believe in the enduring power of the spirit—including yours—in those you love, you know you will continue in some way as part of others.

The Bright Side of a Bad Deal

Breast cancer can bring out amazing qualities in you, ones you hadn't imagined you possessed. "My marriage had gone to hell, and very soon I was a single parent raising a four-year-old. And then I got breast cancer, at thirty-three. I was scared and worried—but I found an odd kind of courage. I wrote to my college sweetheart, whom I hadn't been in touch with for twelve years. He had never married—and we got together. He stayed by me the whole way, through treatment and hair loss (the worst), and now we're married. I would never have written to him if it hadn't been for the cancer. I figured I had nothing to lose, and life is too short. Anything I wanted to do, I suddenly felt I could do."

Or you learn what's important: "My husband and I fought each other on almost every issue, from how to raise our two children to what to eat for dinner. With the discovery of my cancer, we forgot all the craziness and began treating each other like human beings."

These are the paradoxical pluses from this disease, women saying, "I wouldn't have asked for this to happen—but my life has never been better." It's hard to imagine such a possibility unless you've lived this yourself. Of course, not everyone has this fortitude; there are plenty of women who can manage only by denying their fears and slamming the door tight against all talk of this disease. But so many of you take courage from every direction and forge on.

Again: Don't let breast cancer define the rest of your life. "I am better than ever. Deciding to fight for my life made me define myself and realize for the first time why my life was valuable."

Moving from Anger to Action

Anger drives a lot of women once they've been hit by breast cancer. "I never dreamed I could hold such anger!" Jill couldn't tell family or friends how she felt—her emotions scared even herself—so she wrote a fierce and hate-filled letter to her cancer, ending with, "I didn't choose you, and you're not going to stop me!" Then she burned it—and eased away from anger to a new sense of calm. Nancy told me "I kept a journal. I could put that anguish—my anger—on paper. I didn't have to carry it around with me."

The point is to turn "Why me?" into "Why anybody?"—and to make a difference. You've had this bad thing happen, now make something good come out of it. "I got handed lemons—so I made lemonade." So many women have used that expression when we've talked together.

Dr. David Spiegel advises, "Extract meaning from what is happening to you; use your experience to help someone else." One woman, well known in her community, went on radio and TV, telling how breast cancer touches everyone's world. "Scores of women wrote and told me they went out and had their first mammogram."

Another woman: "I talk to groups about breast health, teaching women how to detect breast cancer with what's called a breast board. I show it to the men: 'You won't touch this? You've touched your share of breasts in your life, I'm sure.' Maybe they're embarrassed, but they laugh, and do the check along with the women. A third of breast cancers are discovered this way, and I feel I'm helping."

Others drive patients to the hospital for their daily chemotherapy or radiation treatment, or join a hospice volunteer corps. But it doesn't have to be health-related volunteerism. "I just want to make tomorrow better for someone. I work as treasurer for a homeless shelter and feeding program." "I tutor children in a Camden school."

"My mother volunteered for a clinical breast cancer prevention study. It was the way she found to handle her distress, maybe her guilt, about my getting breast cancer. She told me, 'I want to be able to tell my granddaughters how to prevent breast cancer.'"

"I had never been politically active, but when I got cancer, I got busy: I joined the National Breast Cancer Coalition and the Democratic party. Do something. Make the cancer experience mean something." Fay took her own route to healing: "I was very angry, after treatment, with how little attention was paid to breast cancer politically. Anger is a huge force that can fuel positive things like starting up and developing a political breast cancer organization." The National Breast Cancer Coalition (NBCC) was formed because a lot of women were frustrated and angry with the lack of funding for breast cancer awareness, education, and research in the face of the rising statistics of the disease. Through the amazing leadership of individuals like Fran Visco, Susan Love, Amy Langer, Taddy Dickerson, Sharon Green, Pat Barr, Jane Reece-Coulbourne—and many more—the NBCC has fought hard to raise millions and millions of dollars for research to find a cure. *This could happen even sooner* if each of you joins this army to help fight for this cause. (You can write to NBCC, 1707 L Street NW, Suite 1060, Washington, DC 20036, or call 202-296-7477.)

"Helping others keeps your mind off yourself," says Helen. "If I don't use my experience to help others, then the experience was wasted on me. I don't intend to let that happen." You can really make a difference to a cause and an organization—the contribution of your time, talent, and resources is what fuels the battle. Direct your passion to what you care about—and bigger things can happen. I also encourage you to help other women diagnosed with breast cancer find the information and the support they need to deal with the difficult physical, emotional, social, and financial issues beyond breast cancer diagnosis through Living Beyond Breast Cancer$_{SM,}$ a Philadelphia-Delaware Valley organization with a national presence. Write to us at 111 Forrest Avenue, Narberth, PA 19072, or call 610-668-1320.

This Book's for You

Maybe you've read every word in this book; more likely, you've skipped about and read what matters most to you and studied a few parts in detail. I hope this book has helped you. You've been through a tough period, but now is the time for healing and restoring your health. I hope you've drawn support from the independent, courageous, and generous voices you've listened to in this text: the women who've shared secrets, opened up to feelings that had had been pushed out of view—remembering incidents that were painful or wonderful when they were going through treatment or learning to cope with living well beyond breast cancer.

Many of you have decided to live for each minute of the day, and every day at its fullest. "Grab hold of what's bothering you about your life and shake out the good stuff." With each year that goes by, more and more of you will get to live a longer life. Research is turning up more keys to that longer life, and someday—hopefully soon—someone will discover the cure for breast cancer, and then, more important, how to prevent it, so your daughters and granddaughters and their families will have nothing to fear, and we can all breathe free of the scourge of this dreadful disease.

"My husband told me, 'You can cry for a while, but then you have to figure out how to get yourself back together.'" "My friend wanted me to sit in a rocking chair and hold his hand. I want to explore the world. I've been given this second chance—and I'm going to use it!"

Appendix:

Arm and Shoulder Exercises

Start off these exercises a few at a time. Gradually work up to a series of ten each a couple of times a day, every day, for as long as they seem to be working for you or until you are symptom free for at least a month.

1. Sitting or standing, with your arms at your sides, lift your shoulders up toward your ears as you take a deep breath. Lower your shoulders while breathing out. Next, still with your arms at your sides, roll your shoulders forward, then backward.
2. Raise both arms out to the sides to shoulder height. Move your arms down to your sides and back up to shoulder height, gently flapping like a bird. Next, again raise both arms out to the sides to shoulder height, and move your arms in a circular pattern.
3. Standing, hold a rod* in a horizontal position with both hands down behind your back. With arms and back straight, slowly lift your arms out behind you as high as you can, then slowly lower them.
4. Lie on your back on a firm surface. Hold the rod with both hands, resting it on your thighs. Slowly raise the rod up over your head so your arms, your torso, and your legs form a straight line. (Keep your back flat against the floor during this exercise.) Relax and hold this position for fifteen seconds, then slowly return your arms to their original position and relax once more. Perform this exercise in a standing position as well.

* Or dowel, sawed-off broom handle, cane, stick—about 30 inches long.

5. Position yourself as above, lying on a firm surface, with your arms holding the rod over your head, again with your arms, your torso, and your legs forming a straight line. Then bend your arms so you bring the rod to rest on the top of your head (not your forehead). Next straighten your arms and bring the rod slowly back down to rest on your thighs. Practice this exercise in a standing position as well.

6. Stand in the corner of a room and face into the corner. Stretch your arms in front of you and touch each of the two walls that meet in the corner you're facing, and "walk" your fingers up the walls as high as you comfortably can. Then rest your hands and your forearms against the walls and slowly lean your body into the corner. Hold for fifteen seconds and return to a normal standing position.

Helpful Organizations

A Friend Indeed. Box 1710, Champlain, NY 12919-1710. 514-843-5730.

American Cancer Society. 1599 Clifton Rd. NE, Atlanta, GA 30329. 800-ACS-2345.

American College of Radiology. 1891 Preston White Dr., Reston, VA 20191. 800-227-5463.

American College of Surgeons. 55 E. Erie St., Chicago, IL 60611. 312-664-4050.

American Society of Clinical Oncology. 225 Reinekers Lane, Suite 650, Alexandria, VA 22314. 703-299-0150.

American Society of Plastic and Reconstructive Surgeons. 444 E. Algonquin Rd., Arlington Heights, IL 60005. 800-635-0635.

Arm in Arm. 302 Presway Rd., Timonium, MD 21093. 410-494-0083.

Cancer Care, Inc. 1180 Avenue of the Americas, New York, NY 10036. 800-813-4673.

Choice in Dying. 200 Varick St., New York, NY 10014. 800-989-9455.

Harvard Women's Health Watch. 164 Longwood Ave., Boston, MA 02115. 617-432-1485.

International Cancer Alliance. 4853 Cordell Ave., Suite 11, Bethesda, MD 20814. 800-422-7361.

Living Beyond Breast Cancer. 111 Forest Ave., Narberth, PA 19072. 610-668-1320.

Make Today Count. Mid-America Cancer Center, 1235 E. Cherokee, Springfield, MO 65804-2263. 800-432-2273.

Mautner Project for Lesbians with Cancer. 1707 L St. NW, Suite 1060, Washington, DC 20036. 202-332-5536.

Medical Insurance Claims, Inc. 170 Kinnelon Rd., Kinnelon, NJ 07405-2322. 973-492-2828. (Irene Card, President.)

National Alliance of Breast Cancer Organizations (NABCO). 9 E. 37th St., 10th floor, New York, NY 10016. 212-719-0154.

National Breast Cancer Coalition. 1707 L St. NW, Suite 1060, Washington, DC 20036. 202-296-7477.

National Cancer Institute (NCI). Cancer Information Service, 31 Center Drive MSC 2580, Building 31, Room 10A16, Bethesda, MD 20892-2580. 800-4-CANCER.

National Coalition for Cancer Survivorship. 1010 Wayne Ave., 5th floor, Silver Spring, MD 20910. 301-650-8868 (soon to have an 888 number).

National Family Caregivers Association. 9621 E. Bexhill Drive, Kensington, MD 20895. 800-896-3650.

National Hospice Organization. 1901 N. Moore St., Suite 901, Arlington, VA 22209. 800-658-8898.

National Lymphedema Network. 2211 Post St., Suite 404, San Francisco, CA 94115. 800-541-3259.

National Women's Health Network. 514 10th St. NW, Washington, DC 20004. 202-347-1147.

Susan Komen Foundation. 5005 LBJ Freeway, Suite 370, Dallas, TX 75244. 800-462-9273.

The Wellness Community. 2716 Ocean Park Blvd., Suite 1040, Santa Monica, CA 90405-5211. 310-314-2555. (Call for location nearest you.)

Y-Me Organization. 212 W. Van Buren, 4th Floor, Chicago, IL 60607. 800-221-2141.

This list is not intended to be all-inclusive. For more information contact the National Alliance of Breast Cancer Organizations for their free "Breast Cancer Resource List" ($3.00 to cover postage and mailing).

Selected Readings

Breast Cancer Diagnosis and Treatment

Breast Cancer? Let Me Check My Schedule
    Bombeck, Erma 1994
An upbeat, humorous, and realistic description of how Bombeck fit diagnosis, treatment, and beyond, into her over-busy life.

The Race Is Run One Step at a Time
    Brinker, N. 1990
Brinker is the founder of the Susan B. Komen Foundation. The book describes how and why this woman created and energized a successful national organization. General information on breast cancer.

High Dose Chemotherapy with Bone Marrow Transplant for
    ECRI (Emergency Care Research Institute) 1996
Excellent reference for women with metastatic disease who are trying to decide between standard chemotherapy and bone marrow transplantation. For a free copy call ECRI, 610-825-6000.

You Don't Have to Be Your Mother
    Feldman, G. 1994
The moving story of the author's and her mother's breast cancer experiences. Well written, intellectually stimulating, but not exactly reassuring.

The Truth About Breast Implants
    Guthrie, R. 1994
Strong views against silicone implants. Recommends saline implants. Doesn't address nonimplant alternatives for breast reconstruction.

Breast Cancer: The Complete Guide
    Hirshaut, Y. 1992
    Pressman, P.
Excellent comprehensive guide to breast cancer through the voice of two breast cancer specialists. Good appendixes.

Breast Cancer Black Woman
    Johnson, E. 1993
Discusses the unique problems that African-American women experience facing breast cancer. Basic breast health information and after-cancer issues.

What to Do If You Get Breast Cancer
    Komarnicky, L. 1995
    Rosenberg, A.
Straightfoward, comprehensive, accessible guide to breast cancer diagnosis and treatment. A quick read.

The Breast Cancer Companion
    LaTour, K. 1993
Excellent comprehensive guide to the full breast cancer experience, from diagnosis to beyond treatment. Brings in voices of other survivors and draws nicely on the author's own experience. A must buy.

The Complete Book of Breast Care
    Lauersen, N. 1996
Comprehensive and thoughtful guide to breast cancer diagnosis and treatment.

Dr. Susan Love's Breast Book
    Love, Susan 1996
The best book on basic breast health and management of breast cancer. Comprehensive, strong voice, all-inclusive; considered the bible by most women. Direct presentation of accurate and honest facts and statistics. (May be more than you want to know.) Excellent appendixes. The complete guide, not a quickie. A must buy.

A Step-by-Step Guide to Dealing with Your Breast Cancer
    Robinson, R. 1994
    Petrek, J.
Helps you take charge of treatment decisions, etc. Information
presented in a supportive, conversational style.

Every Woman's Guide to Breast Cancer
    Seltzer, L. 1987
Well-organized, comprehensive guide to breast cancer, parts a bit
outdated. Frequent use of cancer statistics may be frightening to
some.

The Breast Cancer Handbook
    Swirsky, J. 1994
    Balaban, B.
Survivors' guide to the diagnosis and treatment of breast cancer. Easy
to read and digest.

Breast Cancer? Breast Health
    Weed, S. 1996
A holistic approach to breast cancer. Strength is knowledge of plants,
but weakness is discussion of conventional medicine.

After Cancer

I Want to Grow Hair, I Want to Grow Up, I Want to Go to Boise
    Bombeck, Erma 1989
Optimistic and funny. Good to share with children.

Love, Laughter, and a High Regard for Statistics
    Buchanon, S. 1994
Individual story with an original insight and perspective that's worth
reading.

Cancer in Two Voices
    Butler, S. 1991
    Rosenblum, B.
Compelling story of a lesbian couple's particular experience dealing
with breast cancer treatment and recovery.

Not Now . . . I'm Having a No Hair Day
    Clifford, C. 1996
Great cartoons. Humorous, sensitive, and insightful. Short. Makes
you feel good. A must.

Dream Doll: The Ruth Handler Story
    Handler, Ruth 1994
Inspiring story of the career of a successful woman who also had
breast cancer. Ruth Handler invented the Barbie Doll and Nearly Me
breast prostheses. Discusses how her cancer diagnosis shook her
strong sense of self, and how she came back on course.

Getting Better: Conversations with Myself and Other Friends
    Hargrove, A. 1988
Quick read. Humorous and insightful.

No Less a Woman
    Kahane, D. 1990
Voices of ten women. Tells about how breast cancer assaulted these
women's femininity and how they learned to feel good about
themselves once more. Good appendixes.

Life after Cancer
    Kent, A. 1996
Compelling personal stories. Some insights into the politics of breast
cancer. Very opinionated.

The Cancer Journals
    Lorde, A. 1980
Describes the tortuous and self-empowering journey through breast
cancer diagnosis, treatment, and healing.

Triumph: Getting Back to Normal When You Have Cancer
    Morra, M. 1990
    Potts, E.
Good for families. Question and Answer format makes it very
accessible. A good general guide to cancer.

When Cancer Recurs
    National Cancer Institute, 1992
NIH Publication N., 93-2709, excellent, free booklet that can be
obtained by calling 800-4-CANCER.

Cancervive: The Challenge of Life after Cancer
    Nissim, S. 1991
    Ellis, J.
Superb general guide to living a full life after cancer. A must read.

To Be Alive
    Runowicz, C. 1995
    Haupt, D.
Very good general book about life after different kinds of cancer. Lacks depth on breast cancer issues.

A Tribe of Warrior Women
    Springer, M. 1996
Beautiful photograph portraits of breast cancer survivors, accompanied by their moving personal stories.

Stories of Hope and Healing
    Strong, L. 1994
Stories of six women are interesting and encouraging.

Breast Cancer Journal—A Century of Petals
    Wittman, J. 1993
Touching personal story. Good appendixes.

General Cancer

Everyone's Guide to Cancer Therapy
    Dollinger, M. 1994
    Rosenbaum, E.
Good general reference book on all cancers, with in-depth material on breast cancer treatment issues.

When Cancer Comes
    Hawkins, D. 1993
    Koppersmith, D.
    Koppersmith, G.
Good guide to cancer in general. Your family may benefit from the section that talks about their needs.

General Women's Health

Women and Fatigue
  Atkinson, H. 1985
Deals with broad issue of fatigue in women, not specific to breast cancer. Comprehensive and useful.

The New Our Bodies Ourselves
  Boston Women's Health Book Collective 1992
Superb, comprehensive, down-to-earth guide to general health issues for women. Minimal cancer information. A "good friend" perspective.

The Good Housekeeping Illustrated Guide to Women's Health
  Cox, K. 1995
Good easy-to-use reference guide to women's general health issues. (Minimal cancer information.)

Women's Bodies; Women's Wisdom
  Northrup, C. 1994
A well-integrated complementary and conventional medicine approach to women's health.

Menopause

The Pause
  Barbach, Lonnie 1993
Excellent reference. Original insights and advice. Good appendixes. (No specific information for women with breast cancer.)

The Herbal Menopause Book
  Crawford, A. 1996
One of the better herbal guides to managing menopausal symptoms, but provides no information about use of herbs in women affected by breast cancer.

The Complete Book of Menopause
  Landau, C. 1994
  Cyr, M.
  Moulton, A.

Strong on sexuality and myths of depression, weak on hot flashes. Information not readily accessible.

Dr. Susan Love's Hormone Book
  Love, Susan 1997
Excellent guide to understanding and managing menopause and growing older. For all women. Offers practical advice specifically for women diagnosed with breast cancer.

Understanding Menopause
  O'Leary-Cobb, Janine 1993
Wonderful collection of wise and practical advice. Well-balanced, responsible, and holistic.

Natural Menopause: The Complete Guide
  Perry, S. 1997
  O'Hanlan, K.
Excellent, straightforward, clear, practical, and accessible.

Menopausal Years: The Wise Woman Way
  Weed, S. 1992
Good guide to Western herbal remedies to ease menopausal symptoms, with an alternative medicine perspective.

Family

When a Parent Has Cancer: A Guide to Caring for Your Children
  Harpham, W. 1997
Written by a physician, cancer survivor, and mother. Provides excellent information and support for parents struggling with how to talk to their children about cancer.

Helping the Women You Love Recover from Breast Cancer
  Murcia, A. 1989
  Stewart, B.
Simple and straightforward advice from husbands of women with breast cancer.

When Someone You Love Has Cancer
  Pomeroy, D. 1996
Helps family members help people with cancer. Good appendixes; includes sample will and other legal forms, also lists resources.

Sex

For Yourself: The Fulfillment of Female Sexuality
   Barbach, Lonnie 1975
Gives support and information to women having difficulty reaching
orgasm, or who are uncomfortable with their sexuality. Old, but not
outdated.

Up Front: Sex and the Post-Mastectomy Woman
   Dackman, L. 1990
A must read. Personal experience loaded with important practical
advice.

Sex in America: A Definitive Survey
   Michael, R. 1994
Data and perspective on what everyone else is doing in bed. (But the
word *breast* is not in the index.)

Seven Weeks to Better Sex
   Renshaw, D. 1995
Friendly tone. Sex information is mostly about married couples.

Sexuality and Fertility after Cancer
   Schover, Leslie 1997
Superb guide to intimacy, sexuality, and fertility after breast cancer.
Full of practical information; warm and compassionate. A must buy.

Mind-Body

The Answer Is Within You
   Ayers, L. 1994
Insight into psychological experience of breast cancer treatment and
recovery.

When Life Becomes Precious
   Babcock, E. 1997
Sympathetic guide for loved ones of cancer patients. Very thorough.

Minding the Body, Mending the Mind
   Borysenko, J. 1987
Good tips for stress reduction, has a "Zen" approach. May be too
mellow for Type A personality.

The Power of the Mind to Heal
   Borysenko, M. 1994
   Borysenko, J.
Helpful alternative mind-body approach to health and emotional
healing.

Boundless Energy
   Chopra, Deepak 1995
Need to believe in this approach; must be highly motivated to adhere
to required philosphical reorientation and lifestyle changes.

Anatomy of an Illness
   Cousins, Norman 1982
Many people value the honest and insightful perspective on the
author's own illness.

At the Will of the Body
   Frank, A. 1991
Thoughts and insights on emotional recovery after a serious illness.
Very useful, although not breast cancer specific.

Wherever You Go There You Are
   Kabat-Zinn, J. 1994
Interesting existential approach to mind-body medicine, to lead you
to fuller awareness and appreciation of the world you inhabit.

Love, Medicine & Miracles
   Siegel, Bernie 1994
Has inspired countless cancer patients to get beyond their anguish
to heal their spirits. (But overemphasizes personal control over
cancer.)

Spontaneous Healing
   Weil, Andrew 1995
Fascinating book with mind-body emphasis; helps you take charge of
your care.

Nutrition

Six Weeks to Get Out the Fat
   American Heart Association 1996
Practical book that helps you understand and adhere to a low-fat diet.

A Banquet of Health
Block, Penny 1994
Excellent vegetarian cookbook with emphasis on surviving cancer.
To order call 847-328-6632.

The Cancer Recovery Eating Plan: The Right Foods to Help Fuel Your Recovery
Nixon, D. 1994
Excellent balanced and practical reference book on nutrition. Lots of great recipes.

Doctor, What Should I Eat?
Rosenfeld, I. 1995
Practical nutritional solutions for many ailments; includes management of side effects of breast cancer treatment.

Estrogen: The Natural Way
Shandler, Nina 1997
Easy, tasty recipes for cooking with soybean products and flaxseed to ease the side effects of menopause.

Fitness

Fitting in Fitness
American Heart Association 1997
A comprehensive and practical guide to physical fitness and how to incorporate exercise into a busy schedule.

Smart Exercise
Bailey, C. 1994
"User-friendly" guide to understanding the value of exercise, presenting effective and original ways to get in shape and stay there.

The Power of Meditation and Prayer
Kabat-Zinn, J. 1997
A how-to guide to effective meditation, with an alternative medicine perspective.

Cancer as a Turning Point
LeShan, Laurence 1994
Shares insights into emotional recovery after cancer, from the author's extensive experience as a psychotherapist.

Taking Charge: Overcoming the Challenges of Long-Term Illnesses
   Pollin, I. 1994
   Golant, S.
A good self-help guide to emotional recovery.

Living Beyond Limits
   Spiegel, David 1993
Excellent book for emotional recovery and self-awareness for anyone
whose life has been disrupted by serious illness.

Necessary Losses
   Viorst, J. 1986
Uplifting and helpful for dealing with loss of function, self-image,
even lives.

Alternative Medicine

Between Heaven and Earth
   Beinfield, H. 1991
Excellent layperson's guide to Chinese medicine: comprehensive,
responsible, easy to read.

How to Treat Yourself with Chinese Herbs
   Hsu, H. 1980
Basic how-to guide to Chinese herbal medicine. Very little on cancer.

Choices in Healing
   Lerner, Michael 1994
Excellent background information on alternative medicine. Not a
practical how-to reference.

Chinese Herbal Medicine
   Reid, D. 1987
General guide to Chinese medicine, but does not address cancer.

Breast Health
   Simone, C. 1985
Full range of issues. Combines conventional and alternative medicine
approaches. At times rather overzealous about some unproven
alternative therapies.

Chinese Herbal Medicine
    Tang, S. 1995
Comprehensive coverage of basic principles of Chinese medicine, with descriptions of herbs, and how they are used for all kinds of illnesses. Recipes included.

Herbs of Choice: The Therapeutic Use of Phytomedicinals
    Tyler, V. 1994
Sophisticated reference guide. Cancer section is short.

Financial, Legal, Social Issues

National Coalition for Cancer Survivorship
    Hoffman, B. 1996
Excellent practical guide to financial, legal, social issues. Good resource list.

If you are interested in staying up-to-date on issues of concern to women and families affected by breast cancer, sign up to receive Living Beyond Breast Cancer's_{SM} quarterly educational newsletter.

Name _____

Address _____

_____

phone ( ) _____ ; fax ( )_____

Please include a check for $35.00 payable to Living Beyond Breast Cancer_{SM} and mail to:

Living Beyond Breast Cancer_{SM}
111 Forrest Avenue
Narberth, Pennsylvania 19072

(610) 668-1320 (phone)
(610) 667-4789 (fax)

dvbiznet.com/lbbc

Living Beyond Breast Cancer_{SM} (LBBC) is a nonprofit education and support organization founded by Dr. Marisa Weiss to help all women affected by breast cancer become as healthy as possible for as long as possible, enjoying the best quality life possible. LBBC's programs include a quarterly educational newsletter, semi-annual large-scale conferences, community-based education programs for medically under-served women, and a Survivor's Helpline. (LBBC does not provide medical advice.) If you are interested in learning more about the work of LBBC, please contact us at the above address.

Index

About the Authors

Marisa Weiss, M.D., is a physician who specializes in taking care of women with breast cancer. She is founder and president of the nonprofit educational organization Living Beyond Breast Cancer, which promotes the health of all women affected by breast cancer with conferences, workshops, newsletters and a helpline. Dr. Weiss works and lives in the Philadelphia area with her husband and three children.

Ellen Weiss has served as editorial consultant to Living Beyond Breast Cancer since its founding. She is also the author of *The Secondhand Supershopper*. This is the first professional collaboration she has had with any of her six children. She and her husband live in the Philadelphia area.